HEALTH POLICY AND MANAGEMENT

Health Policy and Management

The health-care agenda in a British political context

Calum Paton

Professor of Health Policy at the Centre for Health Planning and Management
Keele University
Staffordshire

CHAPMAN & HALL
London · Glasgow · Weinheim · New York · Tokyo · Melbourne · Madras

Published by Chapman & Hall, 2–6 Boundary Row, London SE1 8HN, UK

Chapman & Hall, 2–6 Boundary Row, London SE1 8HN, UK

Blackie Academic & Professional, Wester Cleddens Road, Bishopbriggs, Glasgow G64 2NZ, UK

Chapman & Hall GmbH, Pappelallee 3, 69469 Weinheim, Germany

Chapman & Hall USA, 115 Fifth Avenue, New York, NY 10003, USA

Chapman & Hall Japan, ITP-Japan, Kyowa Building, 3F, 2-2-1 Hirakawacho, Chiyoda-ku, Tokyo 102, Japan

Chapman & Hall Australia, 102 Dodds Street, South Melbourne, Victoria 3205, Australia

Chapman & Hall India, R. Seshadri, 32 Second Main Road, CIT East, Madras 600 035, India

Distributed in the USA and Canada by Singular Publishing Group Inc., 4284 41st Street, San Diego, California 92105

First edition 1996

© 1996 Calum Paton

Typeset in 10/12pt Palatino by Saxon Graphics Ltd, Derby
Printed in England by Clays Ltd., St. Ives plc.

ISBN 0 412 55130 6   1 56593 285 4 (USA)

A catalogue record for this book is available from the British Library

Library of Congress Catalog Card Number: 95-78839

♾ Printed on permanent acid-free text paper, manufactured in accordance with ANSI/NISO Z39.48-1992 and ANSI/NISO Z39.48-1984 (Permanence of Paper).

CONTENTS

PREFACE

The fundamental aim of this book is to present an analysis of central policy and selected management issues in health care, especially British health care. The focus is at the strategic level, in that some of the most important challenges in strategic (and national) policy and management are analysed.

A primary objective of the book is to present the consequences of health policy-making. The audience is intended to include politicians, civil servants, students of health policy, doctors, nurses, other health professionals, and especially managers charged with implementing policy and achieving desired outputs and outcomes. (To that extent, the intended readership of the group includes a wide range of health service decision-makers, executives and managers: national, regional, district and other purchasing managers; health authority members and chairmen; hospital and community managers and chief executives, plus board members; hospital doctors, (especially clinical directors) but also GPs and fundholders; other health-care professionals with management responsibility; and the academic and policy community generally.

While national policy makers and managers (for example within the Department of Health and in particular the NHS Executive) are thus an intended audience, departmental and middle managers throughout the service will find the book a useful presentation of the environment of policy and strategic management within which they are operating. They will also find guidance in a number of applied areas – such as medical audit, clinical directorates, industrial relations and the management of human resources, and performance management. Part Two, on management issues, is intentionally selective, but the topics chosen are those considered to have long-term salience (beyond temporary managerial 'fads').

The book starts from the premise that – in a centralized NHS that is tightly controlled – policy objectives, in different areas of health care, provide the launch pad from which more specific management challenges flow, at various levels within the 'hierarchy' of the National Health Service. The aim of strategic management is to translate policy into procedures and services, through the process of implementation. Furthermore, the arena of policy and implementation is a complex one, and the two concepts ought not to be distinguished too rigidly. Often policy is only fully made when implementation begins! Barriers to implementing policy which confront managers may lie in power relationships in both the policy and management communities. A further complication lies in the huge agenda flowing from the NHS 'reforms'. So many potentially incompatible strands exist – and have been developed – that service managers often find themselves both 'squeezed' and grappling with an agenda full of internal tension.

The aim is to consider durable issues, to avoid 'flavours of the month'. Thus I consider the achievement of health outcomes and various debates in the territory of 'health gain', the effective allocation and management of resources, quality assurance and human resource management: these are all issues of lasting concern in healthcare (in the UK as elsewhere).

Inevitably 'the current agenda' following the 'NHS reforms' – and possible amendments to these reforms - informs much of the content of the book. The focus is, however, critical, and Part Three explains British 'reform', including its faults, in an international context.

The aim is less to consider what might be termed the 'micro-agenda' of the day, (as epitomized by pronouncements from the NHS Executive and various circulars), than to extract, from a complex and confusing territory of initiative and counter-initiative, the real issues confronting health-care systems today and the real motivation behind recent changes. While the author's views on such matters are therefore bound to play a large role in choice of topics, the topics chosen have wide acceptance as among the major territories of importance for years to come.

The format of the book is as follows. Part One provides an analysis of different policy issues at the national and strategic level – discussing the financing of health care; the making of priorities and hard choices (and who does what in this realm); the various structures and policies concerning the purchasing and provision of health care both nationally and throughout the National Health Service; and the origins and context of strategic management in the environment of today's NHS.

Inevitably there is not a consensus either on overall objectives or on means of achieving these objectives in any of the territories identified. For example, different views on the advantages and disadvantages of health-care financing systems are legion. Making hard choices (possibly involving rationing) leads to value differences as well as to more 'scientific' differences as to the consequences of different approaches. In discussing structures for purchasing and provision and how, for example, purchasing and provision ought to relate to each other, it is notoriously difficult to find an empirical basis for settling disputes as to different policies and approaches. Values and choices naturally inform the overall definition of which types

of health outcome, and what overall distribution of health outcome, are desirable – and such choices determine management challenges at the local level as policy permeates down the (still) hierarchical system of the National Health Service.

Part Two selects and analyses key management issues. Different perspectives abound in the management of human resources and industrial relations; different levels of ambitiousness concerning medical audit and quality assurance more generally are adopted in different quarters. To some, quality is a common-sense matter; to others it is an increasingly refined 'science'. There are disputes concerning the proper remit (and evidence) for different methodologies for allocating resources; and the merits and demerits of different types of business planning – and control and monitoring of performance – are discussed all over the world, continually. The recent trend towards tight performance management of providers is analysed here. The chapters overall raise issues of concern to both 'purchasers' and 'providers'.

Part Three situates British health policy and management in a comparative framework, which is then used to understand British needs better.

There cannot be one means of doing things, just as there cannot be one definition of what is to be done. Nevertheless this book seeks to articulate differences in values, and differences of approach, in an open and explicit manner. While opinions may be offered on the merits and demerits of different approaches, the author seeks to be clear about what is fact and what is value. While expressing his own views, it is made clear when this is being done. In this way, negotiating a difficult path between the Scylla of subjectivity and the Charybdis of uniformity and pseudo-objectivity is at least attempted. Where there is controversy – including party-political controversy – an attempt is made to 'unpick' what is at stake in the dispute in question. It is then left up to managers and decision-makers to make up their own minds as to 'what is going on'. But it is hoped that this will happen in a more informed and reflective manner.

There are various commentaries on British (and international) health policy. There are various books on management topics where viewpoints are brought together from different authors on different topics, or where a single topic is addressed in one book. There are also collections of case studies in international health-care management especially, with a growing British literature despite American domination of this scene. There are furthermore many books on applied or operational management issues, and reviews of issues in operational management.

This book is however written in the belief that a commentary concerned with strategic policy and management that is also a contribution to the elucidation of policy and management challenges in the NHS, written as a coherent whole by one author in a context of international awareness, fills a significant new niche in the marketplace which is currently unfilled for the NHS of the future.

ACKNOWLEDGEMENTS

I would like in particular to acknowledge the great help, over a long period, of Sally Hughes and Val Watts in preparing the manuscript, and of Barbara Goodenough in helping to organize this production. I would also like to thank Ellie Scrivens for reading the manuscript and making some valuable suggestions.

PART ONE

POLICY ISSUES

INTRODUCTION

It is a perennial question for health policy analysts and health managers alike as to the best means to produce improvements in health, and maintenance of health, for the population. Setting aside for now how such improvements are to be distributed and whether equity is to count as much as (or more than) the total quantum of benefit to be derived, it is obviously important to promote the public health in the widest sense of that term. Thus a wide range of social factors and environmental features, as well as individual and personal behaviour, affect the health of individuals and of the nation. The distribution of income, the level of unemployment, the state of housing, the presence or absence of environmental pollution of various sorts and a variety of both socially and individually determined lifestyles affect health status.

In consequence, seeking a strategy for health implies policy and action from a wide range of Government and non-Government agencies. National government has responsibility for key policy areas. So does local government – especially in the field of local environmental factors and, for example, housing and education. The National Health Service itself has responsibility not only for hospitals and direct services, whether in the community or elsewhere, but also for various forms of prevention and promotion programmes.

APPROPRIATE ROLES

It is obviously the responsibility of central government in the UK to raise appropriate finance for the National Health Service, as well as for other areas of social policy with a bearing on health. The first task is therefore to agree and coordinate a health strategy across the various Government departments and agencies. This is the responsibility of the Department of Health working (perhaps through cabinet committees) with other national departments. Securing adequate finance for the National Health Service is a primary responsibility of the Department of Health. The political battles which lie behind such a bland statement are of course legion. Nevertheless, a national health service is responsible for providing comprehensive care for the population as a whole. This causes difficulties in an age when a number of factors put pressure on budgets, under any government. Thus the growth in medical technologies and 'medical possibilities' generally, the change in demography of the population, the emergence of new diseases as well as new lifestyle-related morbidities and a whole host of other factors (including medical sector inflation) all put pressure on any health budget. Even if other economic and social policy (e.g. greater equality and better housing) helps to produce better health, the NHS will still be required for significant secondary and tertiary care as well as primary care. Indeed it is the NHS's function to care for, and cure, ill health, even when preventive strategies range across all Government departments and even when prevention is a major goal.

While it is the case therefore that not every health benefit imaginable can be funded, it is equally not the case that supply of and demand for health care arise so explosively that harsh rationing must occur. Priorities must be determined where necessary, within available resources. It is still possible, as we move towards the 21st century, for the National Health Service to deliver the bulk of the nation's reasonable health demands. In this context, it is unlikely that a formal rationing process will ration care either by care programme or specialty on the one hand or by socioeconomic groups and classes on the other. While ineffective procedures will increasingly come under question, it is unlikely and undesirable that large swathes of either health or social care will simply be removed from the sphere of public responsibility. Equally, it is unlikely that the National Health Service will be replaced by a means-tested service whereby the poor – or differential groups throughout society – are eligible for relatively more than their better-off fellow citizens.

The problem with the latter approach is that, if the better-off are to be expected to finance their own health care, then the costs of doing so will ensure that the budget left for the 'rump' NHS will be less, even *per capita*. This is so unless a move to privatization of finance for the better-off is accompanied by redistribution towards the poor – an unlikely phenomenon, given the fact that private health care is more expensive, not more economical, than the National Health Service. Thus the poor may end up with absolutely less health care than now funded through the public purse, although relatively more than the better-off funded through the public purse, under such a scenario.

Conversely, the problem with tight overall finance and rationing according to specialty or care programme – or rather, guaranteeing access to all citizens alike but to a restricted programme of benefits – is that, within a limited budget, the poor and relatively needier will receive less than they could otherwise receive with greater targeting upon them. Given that there is a direct correlation between poverty and ill health, this seems inequitable.

The advantage, then, with maintaining access to a well-funded National Health Service for all is that all citizens have an equal stake in it – and the political challenge is to ensure adequate budgets for adequate care for all, with an informal steering of priorities towards the neediest within universal budgets. This is easy to state and difficult to make effective in practice. It is however the most appropriate and indeed realistic challenge for the National Health Service of the future, as in the past.

PRIORITIES

At the broadest level there is often seen to be a trade-off between hospital services and either primary or community care, often with overtones of prevention and promotion. In many ways this is a false opposition. The most appropriate form of care, cure or prevention ought to be delivered in the most appropriate setting. Even if one believes in public health as an aspiration, with stress upon prevention, promotion, healthy living and equitable social relationships, then it may be a considerable amount of time – longer than a generation conceivably – before such an overarching policy bears fruit in terms of diminished need for hospital services (if it ever does). And what is more this assumes that such a strategy has enough political will to carry it through irrespective of the government of the day. In practice, the National Health Service will always have an important role of repair and rescue, despite the rhetoric that implies that acute hospitals are almost a thing of the past. Unless one throws the burden for healthy living on to individuals to a great extent and passes value judgements about what is acceptable behaviour and what is not, then there is severe danger in moving towards a health service that diminishes the salience of rescue and repair. Obviously the smoking debate features large here but it is only the tip of the iceberg and many aspects of lifestyle – some socially conditioned as well individually determined – create a greater statistical likelihood of ill health. There are political trade-offs here, of course: a society in which people 'die earlier' because of health-related behaviour may be a society that saves money on long term social care and social security budgets, as well as a society that raises revenue from, for example, the sale of cigarettes.

Furthermore, a society that successfully implements a broad public health strategy involving health promotion and health prevention, which feeds through to longer living for all, may well be a society that incurs greater 'acute' health care costs at the end of individuals' life-cycles – people have to die of something, and people dying at a greater age of more complex comorbidities may mean a society that needs greater hospitalization in aggregate as a result of more effective prevention and promotion.

This is analogous to the situation whereby more effective primary care may lead to more discoveries for the secondary sector to deal with.

Next, it is important to point out that the Government, by primary care, often means acute care in community settings. Primary care consists in dealing with health problems at an early stage – perhaps by preventing them altogether and by promoting good health and healthy living generally. Primary care can be carried out in the community or in hospital – if somebody is in hospital for condition X, that may be a very good location for them to receive advice on the prevention of condition Y. Equally, one can receive acute care in the community – if, for example, GP surgeries are encouraged to do more in the way of small operations.

All in all, a balanced strategy will look at which agency can best affect health in a manner compatible with civil liberties and allocate appropriate budgets – whether by direct formula or not, to local government, to

National Health Service purchasers and to other agencies where appropriate. In turn, these agencies will work with providers – whether hospitals, community services or others – to ensure that health programmes are translated into provision.

HEALTH FOR WHOM, DELIVERED BY WHOM?

One often hears talk of health in an investment. It may be an investment for society as a whole, or it may be an investment in human capital to ensure that the economy functions better. Allied to the latter strategy one often finds the Marxist analysis of health services, which paints them, even when they are publicly financed and provided, as state aid to private capital in providing a healthy workforce as economically as possible. In today's NHS – where QALYs (quality-adjusted life years) loom large, and health benefits are assessed in terms of contribution to production, *inter alia* – this analysis has a lot of truth in it. Devices for relating cost to outcome can be a good servant but a bad master.

Health of course may also be a 'consumption good'. People may spend their own money to purchase short-term health benefits. All in all, however, it seems best not to make a false distinction here either. Improvement of health ought not to be simply a matter of improvement in the economic performance of the country or of investment in particular individuals – or the whole nation – for instrumental purposes. If better health has this effect, then that is all to the good. An equitable health strategy, however, means investment in better health as a civil and human right. If, for example, one justifies investment in everybody's health for economic purposes, then, if it can be demonstrated by economists that only two-thirds of society contribute in effect to the economy, the case for an equitable health strategy embracing everybody is diminished by such a narrow criterion. This to some extent mirrors the case in the United States whereby health has hitherto been a matter for individuals and primarily for their employers, such that those who are not employed (and therefore 'invested in' by their employers) have worse access to health care.

If we can agree that an equitable health strategy implies access to health care as a right rather than as an instrumental route to some economic or other goal, then we can agree on the basis for financing the health service and also upon who the beneficiaries are to be. The question still arises as to who is employed, and how, to deliver these benefits. Pressure on public sector budgets – whether for economic or political reasons or both – leads to a stress upon efficiency and productivity. When these shade into exploitation of workers and economy for economy sake, however, there arise ethical and indeed economic questions as to 'how far productivity ought to go'. On a related note, it is all very well to address issues of appropriate skill mix, but simply to create a downward pressure on the employment of health professionals may have adverse side effects in terms of patient care and the long-term productivity of the National Health Service. Health workers are themselves citizens – and the lower paid health workers are vulnerable citizens. If health maintenance and health promotion benefits, among other things, from equitable employment arrangements it would seem ironical for the National Health Service itself to be a 'bad employer'. In consequence, overall financing levels of health care are important.

The UK spends less than most comparable countries on health care, both in terms of overall percentage of gross national product and also in terms of that percentage of gross national product going to public care. That is, although most of the UK's care (at least 90%, even after the 1980s) is spent publicly, we still spend less publicly – and therefore considerably less overall – both *per capita* and as a percentage of GNP, than comparable countries. When it is pointed out that we spend almost as much as other West European countries publicly, this also misses the point that such countries' private spending is mostly by **non-contributors** to their national health (insurance) schemes. If the UK 'excepted' the rich from taxation for the NHS, we would spend even less. Making the comparison of 'whole systems' is actually the correct procedure. And the UK spends very little. This is partly because of 'efficiency', at least prior to the NHS reforms and the resulting significant rise in administrative costs. It is also, however, because of our low-paid health workers. There is no automatically 'correct' level for pay. The market is one means of deciding; equitable public-sector-based comparisons are another; there are many others still. Nevertheless it is important to realize that a fair taxation and fiscal policy for the country as a whole can correlate with the chance to spend more publicly on health care. Even if one assumes that the ability to spend publicly (and in total) on health care is related to the country's wealth, then the UK still spends less than would be expected by such a criterion. What is more, if health is seen as contribution to society and the economy rather than simply a drain upon resources, investment in health – on an equitable basis – may equally be able to contribute to an increase in society's wealth, just as an increase in education and training, if appropriately targeted, can.

DECISION-MAKING IN HEALTH CARE: POLITICS AND MANAGEMENT

It is perhaps revealing that many societies do not have separate words for what we in the UK call politics and policy. Thus, in French, *la politique* refers to both. A hard and fast distinction between politics and policy is difficult. Politics is the arena within which political parties and other actors articulate ideologies and interests and translate these into policy. Policy as distinct from politics is the assemblage of goals and objectives for particular arenas such as health, education and housing. But of course policy is heavily infused with politics.

There are different perspectives as to how policy is made. Some stress the role of 'rationalism'. This implies the assemblage of coherent packages of policy that are internally consistent, which the political system is capable of passing into legislation. Furthermore, if such policy is implemented effectively, then the legislation (or output) would be translated into social outcome. To believe in 'rationalism' it is not necessarily to believe in the values behind the policy in question or to support that policy. It is merely to point to the coherence of that policy.

Another approach stresses the important role of standard operating procedures, and in particular bureaucracies, in making and implementing policy. In the British National Health Service right through to the 1980s, for example, it could be argued that the making and implementing of policy did not reflect a re-examination of goals and the creation of packages either to 'reachieve' or to achieve new goals. Instead, there was an incrementalism in adding to, or subtracting from, policy that reflected stable configurations of power, both within society (translated into politics) and within the bureaucracies responsible either for giving practical shape to policy (for example the civil service) or for implementing policy through strategic management (for example health authorities).

A third approach stresses the need for policy to accommodate the interests that have enough power in society to influence the policy process. Sometimes seen as an 'interest group' or 'bargaining' model, whereby interests trade off costs and benefits and come to coalitions through deals (vote trading or log rolling), this approach assumes a kind of pluralism in the policy process.

Thus in the UK it could be argued that different interests compete to 'add their

tuppence ha'penny worth' to the policy process at the national level – i.e., there is a kind of centralized pluralism whereby different interests jockey for influence in influencing central politicians or the bureaucracy. Pluralism may also refer to the dispersal of power throughout society – such that different levels of government, administration and management share power. In the UK one can point to Parliament, local government, the institutions of the National Health Service and – for example – hospital trusts. Thus a plural system would give or guarantee power to the different levels in a devolved or decentralized system, and each of these levels would have enough power in its own right such that, if different actors controlled the different levels, one could talk about a pluralist dispersal of power.

Merely to describe the latter situation is to point to its relative absence in the UK today. Responsibility for the making of policy and for the guidelines in which management operates within the National Health Service are highly centralized, and the recent NHS reforms have increased this trend. The creation of a market in health care is the creation of a mechanism to allocate resources, not the creation of a politically decentralized health service.

One can debate for some time which of the models of the policy process are most applicable in the UK today. It is worth pointing out that the NHS reforms can be interpreted as a 'rationalist' exercise in policy making, which nevertheless became mediated by the expression of interests during the period of implementation between 1991 and the middle 1990s. Furthermore, the fact that the NHS reforms contain so many strands (often contradictory or requiring resolution) perhaps suggests that the exercise was not so rationalist after all. In any case, in anything other than a totalitarian political culture, it is likely that any rationalist exercise in policy making will be mediated by different interests as policy is either refined or implemented.

Although the UK does not permit much specialized pluralist input into the passing of legislation, it is in the post legislative implementation of policy that difficulties are often ironed out (or not, as the case may be!).

Opposed to the pluralist view of policy is the view sometimes known as **elitism** – which is not a defence or normative approval of elitism but a descriptive, analytical or positive assertion that there is a relatively stable elite which controls the levels of power, and that power is not adequately spread or dispersed over society's social groupings to allow pluralism to be a convincing characterization of that process. There are various versions and refinements of elitism in the policy process (Paton, 1990).

Beyond conventional elitism, the special approach of modern Marxism argues that the tension between owners of capital on the one hand and workers or employees on the other hand is the most significant characterization of the economy, which also affects social services that are in the public sector. The state has a role in providing infrastructure to the economy (whether through transport policy, educational policy or health policy) and the state acts as a kind of surrogate employer on behalf of the private sector in 'providing' a healthy workforce, for example, as cheaply as possible. Thus, although one cannot talk about 'exploited workers' in the National Health Service in a simplistic sense, as it is publicly owned, if one views the economy as a whole one can see that a cheaply provided health service may in effect be transferring 'surplus value' indirectly to the owners of capital.

MARKETS AND PURCHASER/PROVIDER SPLITS: POLITICS AS WELL AS ECONOMICS

The idea of perfect competition is what social scientists call an 'ideal type': i.e., it is something that is never attained but that provides a instructive model of some of the dynamics at work in economics, which may be approximated to a greater or lesser extent in practice in different industries at different times. Perfect competition implies an unlimited number of suppliers, and competition to the extent that profits are reduced to zero or something resembling it (the idea of 'normal profits'). In consequence, if labour is infinitely flexible, it is argued, there be no unemployment either as all labour will be employed and all resources allocated according to the dictates of consumers under perfect competition. Any health market – such as the idea of the internal market within the British public sector – is obviously not going to obey the dictates of perfect competition. Far from it. Furthermore, a public-sector market will have characteristics significantly different from that of a private sector market, whether perfectly competitive or not (Chapter 4).

In a society with significant unemployment and disincentives to trade union activity (such as those promoted by individual employment contracts), the effect of employers (such as hospital trusts) competing for workers is likely to be overridden by the relative 'oversupply' of such workers. Only where professionals are scarce will this not apply. If the available resources for consumption in the 'public health market' are scarce, this effect will be accentuated. It is ironically the case that, in a service where the provider has a monopoly or a near monopoly, it may have enough capacity to make a 'profit' or surplus to allow greater rights and better conditions for workers. On the other hand, this effect will be overridden by the relative lack of bargaining power *vis-à-vis* the monolithic employer that the workers have – and again high unemployment and scarce finance for public health care will diminish the capacity of the worker to achieve a 'fair deal' in the health market. At the end of the day one can ask whether firms (for example, hospital trusts) are competing for workers or workers are competing to be employed in firms. It does not take too much imagination, in the context of today's NHS, to see that workers are at a relative disadvantage in their search for a 'fair deal', especially lower-paid workers whose skills are in plentiful supply.

One may also ask: is a market a transitional device to achieve a change in service mix for the future of the National Health Service, or is it an end in itself, such that markets are to continue to allocate resources through competitive mechanisms and therefore such that Government policy has to maintain markets where necessary (though maintaining spare capacity in providers, to allow competition by providers, while closing alleged surplus capacity!)? Contradictory signals have been received from the Government in the 1990s. In some cases, there is an encouragement to 'let the market work' to close hospitals and reorient services. On the other hand, in London, a planning mechanism has deliberately been chosen to supersede the market, to prevent unpredictable side effects and the possibly chaotic consequences of allowing the market to 'make the change' in health services. Elsewhere in the country, a variety of approaches are being used to close and 'downsize' hospitals. Equally, if one sees a market as a long-term guarantor of efficiency to competition (NHS Executive 1994), it may be that there are trends in the health service market – which mirror wider market trends in the economy generally – away from competition and towards monopoly. For example, successful market actors may drive out the competition – or prevent it from appearing in the first place – and then consolidate the opposition. Where it is difficult to 'enter' the market through high start-up costs and related phenomena, this effect is accentuated. Again it is not difficult to recognize that, in the health care market, the barriers to entry are great.

In practice many regions (later to be regional offices of the Department of Health) are using the market to cut labour costs through competition by providers, then making decisions as to closures and reorientated services according to national and regional plans, not according to who 'wins' and 'loses' in competition. There is, at worst, the worst of both worlds – a bureaucratic variant of competition and also a bureaucratic variant of planning. Add to this the need for business planning as both a competitive device and a centralist system of control, and it is no wonder health managers feel pressured.

One can say without being unfair that recent Government policy has been muddled as to whether the market should be used for transitional service shifts (for example closing hospitals, rationalizing services generally and promoting innovation in new services in the community) or not. Equally, policy is somewhat confused as to whether a market mechanism should continue in the long run, with distinct purchaser/provider splits guaranteeing continuing provider competition. However trends to monopoly on the supply side might ensure the necessity of a 'pro-competitive' policy by Government. This leads to the conundrum whereby although bed numbers are to be reduced in line with getting rid of alleged surplus capacity, there is nevertheless an attempt to maintain spare capacity within the new system to allow provider competition in a marketplace! It is in this context that the nature of purchaser/provider splits, both in the UK and with insight from abroad, should be examined. What are the consequences of existing policy, and what are the best means of ensuring effective provision of services in the future?

THE NHS PRE-REFORM

It can be argued that all health care systems, public and private, fall into at least one of three categories.

- There are private systems where services are paid for directly, for example by out-of-pocket payments.

- There are systems which reimburse the cost of care by a 'third-party payer' – which may be either
  - the insurance company in a private system;
  - the Government in a public system.
- Thirdly, there are systems where there is an overt purchasing function, where purchasers either
  - own the providers (as in health maintenance organizations); or
  - contract with providers – whether in a stable and long-term relationship or through constantly changing market relations with providers.

The UK before the NHS reforms was fundamentally a system of public third-party reimbursement, yet with an indirect and partial 'purchasing function' exercised by the Region. General practitioners had the right of free referral either to hospitals or to secondary, community services. There was then an attempt to 'send the money after the patient'. This occurred by regions allocating money to districts which by and large were 'provider districts'. In other words, the districts managed services such as hospitals and community health services.

Districts were also allocators of funds, of course. Regions allocated to districts according to a formula that recognized the residential population of the district (on the RAWP principle of weighted capitation) but which adjusted such allocations to account for the services provided in the district – in other words, the allocation was adjusted to take account of patients flowing in and flowing out of districts. Thus regions and districts both planned and provided secondary services, to which free referrals by GPs were made. As a result, there was – in the 'old system' also – a need for GPs to take into account 'what was possible'. At its best, the 'old system' nevertheless established new services and reshaped services to reflect GPs' and patients' wishes. A sensible reform, build-

ing on the old system rather than replacing it with rigid contracts, would have built in such 'need and demand' to the planning and commissioning process over all the country. Then broad but costed service agreements could have been 'purchased' from hospitals and community services by districts – a conflict between free referral and contracts would have been diminished.

In the old system, the aim was that the district's final allocation would reflect not only the need of its population (a Resource Allocation Working Party had created a formula – RAWP – in 1976) but would be in proportion to the amount of care provided in the districts, which was originally determined by general practitioner referrals and a variety of other factors (such as accident and emergency provision and secondary-to-tertiary referrals). Thus, as a gross generalization, such a system could be described as public third-party reimbursement – but with an additional and indeed conditioning attempt by the region to steer provision according to regional and district criteria of where care ought to be provided and what sort of care. The chance for such an overt, or rather 'back door', purchasing function to emerge occurred because – as is familiar – there was never enough money to fulfil every need. Waiting lists and waiting times were of course the biggest manifestation of the situation. In consequence, as well as regional allocations, via districts, mirroring general practitioner referrals, general practitioner referrals often had to take account of the reality of (limited) regional allocations via districts. Thus it was a two-way process. If one wants to talk in terms of purchasers and providers, the region was the ultimate purchaser, often acting through the district, and the district was responsible for provision. But the GP and patient (to the extent that the patient had a voice within the GP surgery) was a determinant of flows. The problem was that the old system of 'RAWP targets' based on patient flows worked slowly because of political constraints on 'robbing

Peter to pay Paul', given tight finance since the economic crisis of the 1970s, based on the oil crisis (ironically the very time that RAWP was introduced.)

We can compare such systems of public third-party reimbursement with the US system of private third-party reimbursement, in a fee-for-service system where the provider and the patient/user jointly determined care, which was then reimbursed by in most cases a private insurance company, the third party payer.

THE NHS POST-REFORM

The situation in the National Health Service after the NHS reforms is that there is an overt purchasing function exercised by districts, GP fundholders for a limited range of services and mixtures of the above – such as consortia (composed of more than one district) and commissioners (composed of districts and family health service authorities, and possibly incorporating GP fundholders into a district-wide or commissioner-wide plan. This reflects a trend in international health care to what is broadly known as 'managed care'. It is believed that not all demands can be recognized, for financial reasons, and that therefore there is a need for an overt purchasing function to do the prioritization, or rationing if it is more systematic and arguably harsher. The care is then 'managed' in that providers have to adopt protocols, specialty by specialty, in order to control costs. This is the sense in which trends in health care reform are similar in many Western countries: in the UK, the Netherlands and the United States, the trend is away from third-party reimbursement of open referral to 'managed care' with an overt purchasing function. That is the sense in which the UK, via the NHS reforms and the US, via the Clinton-type reforms, are moving in the same direction. It would be of course dangerous to assume that the UK and the United States are moving in the same direction in other respects – the United States

is increasing equity and the public planning component of its system, whereas the UK is doing the opposite.

A move to an overt purchasing function therefore raises the question of the relationship between the purchaser and the provider. It is not necessary to have a purchaser/provider split in order to have an overt purchasing function, as recent Swedish reforms suggest (prior to any adoption of the British model, under pressure from British advice to Sweden's former right-of-centre government in early 1994). The health maintenance organization in the United States, for example, receives money from the Government (for the poor) or from private subscribers, and then conducts purchasing through contracts with its own directly managed providers, or in the case of looser HMOs, with providers with whom it has a long-term and stable relationship). What a purchasing function recognizes, of course, is the functional need for needs assessment and the translation of such 'needs' into a service plan or contract for care. The role of the provider is then to manage itself to ensure that care is produced. Thus a functional purchaser/provider distinction is necessary. This is not the same, however, as an institutional purchaser/provider split, far less an institutional purchaser/provider split organized in order to run a competitive market.

It may be asked in the UK, if there is to be a purchaser/provider **split** as well as a functional purchaser/provider **distinction**, then what form should that split take? A number of options exist. Firstly, self-governing trusts can be fully competitive, autonomous and therefore quasi-private at least, if not actually private. Secondly, they can be free from responsibility to local purchasers yet responsible to central government through the National Health Service Executive (NHSME). This is broadly the situation that pertains at present, although when it suits the Government to say so, trusts are also claimed to be autonomous and free market agents. The advantage for the Government of trusts being responsible to the NHSME rather than, for example, to local democratic fora or to Parliament, is that the Government can then disclaim responsibility for their operation. This is done on the grounds that the NHSME is a quasi-executive agency and that Parliament and the Government are not responsible for the management functions of such an agency. There is thus a reversal of the old doctrine of ministerial responsibility, where – whether or not the minister was involved in every decision – the minister took ultimate responsibility for what went on in the Department of Health. Now those managing an executive agency are often held to account for decisions taken according to rules they were not responsible for. That is, instead of responsibility, there is a system almost of buck-passing nowadays.

All this has given rise to claims to a lack of democracy in the system. Regions are now to be part of the Ministry (the NHS Executive), with regional directors as civil servants and unable even to speak out without permission. Health authorities (and trusts) have appointed boards accountable only to the centre. Some have therefore called for elected local government to take over responsibility for purchasing, but the present author considers this a mistake (see Discussion, and Chapter 14). More promising would be elected **regional** government taking responsibility for broad regional planning of the NHS, coordinated with other social policies yet specific health authorities within such regions.

The third option, of course, is for the provider to be responsible to the purchaser – not for operational management, not even necessarily for hiring and firing of staff, but for delivery of services and indeed in order to ensure that the provider is not autonomous either constitutionally, politically or strategically, at the end of the day. Thus a purchaser/provider distinction is perfectly compatible with the system by which self-managing hospitals and community services are ultimately responsible to the local health authority. This obviously restricts the operation of a market in the radical sense. It does not, however, prevent the renegotiation of relationships over time. Whether in a market or non-market NHS, a pre-reform or post-reform NHS, it is necessary for health authority (purchasing) managers to take responsibility for the reconfiguration of services over time – perhaps the biggest challenge facing health services today, as they need to be increasingly flexible to adjust to changing needs.

In consequence, it is the responsibility of such purchasing managers to ensure that services are changed (closed and opened) over time, to ensure that needs are met. It is an open question in principle as to whether a system of direct responsibility of the provider to the authority or a market system is most capable of ensuring such transitions smoothly. Indeed it can be strongly argued that the transactions costs involved in a market of autonomous providers, jockeying for power, marketing themselves and indulging in short-term strategies, makes it less suitable for managing transition than the alternative of stable purchaser/provider links or even a constitutional purchaser/provider relationship that recognizes local providers in accordance with the service plan.

The last scenario involves agreement by purchasers with patients and GPs as to the most appropriate form and location of referral and therefore replicates the best of the pre-reform NHS, when money did attempt to follow the patient – unlike in the post-reform NHS, despite the rhetoric. Thus an appropriate pattern of primary care (based in GP surgeries) and an appropriate pattern of referrals within available resources agreed with the health authority can lead to fairly long-term contracts with appropriate providers. There is an assumption that the local providers will, *ceteris paribus*, be the appropriate ones, and that cross-boundary flows to other parts of the country will be reimbursed at appropriate costs through the intervention of a tier such as a region or regional office. Otherwise, 'extra-contractual referrals' (ECRs) may be as distortive of the budget as 'cross-boundary flow adjustments' were in the old system.

MARKET POWER

In an NHS in which finance is tightly constrained, purchasers will have the power of money. Even when purchasing is fragmented between districts and GP fundholders, providers will still need to 'put together a package' involving as much purchasing money as possible. There are therefore not so much competing purchasers as complementary purchasers – not complementary necessarily in terms of behaviour but in terms of the economic logic underlying their position *vis-à-vis* the provider. Obversely, the provider has the power of information and detailed knowledge about services – such that, although the purchaser may have desires as to outcome, the purchaser depends on the provider or 'state of the art' knowledge as to appropriate service mix and service definition. It is extremely wasteful in a market system for purchasers to ignore the expertise of their local providers and simply to seek advice 'from the outside'. This is bureaucratic and costly. It is also fatuous, for the most appropriate knowledge can be disseminated nationally and contracts made with providers then carried out appropriately on such a basis. Alternatively, the purchaser can have a productive relationship with the local provider in order to explore such issues. That is the way in which purchasing money and provider expertise can best be reconciled to produce desired service mixes and service definitions within specialties. Otherwise there is a danger of 'gaming', where purchasers seek to use their financial muscle and providers seek to deny information to the purchaser.

Examples of 'gaming' are rife as a consequence of the NHS reforms. Consider the case of the block contract, pure and simple. The purchaser often seeks to use the purchaser/provider split not as an opportunity for responsible purchasing, but as an opportunity for 'passing the buck' to the provider. The provider is given a limited sum of money, expected to provide a huge and unreasonable quantum of care from that budget – and then it is also expected that the public will vent its frustrations on the provider, as the public does not understand the purchaser/provider split and expects the hospital or other provider to be the locus of complaint.

Conversely a block contract with thresholds of extra payment for extra workload can lead to gaining on the part of the provider, simply by doing what it wants and then passing on the bill to the purchaser.

Cost per case contract, at the other extreme, may again lead to a situation in which the UK exercises its own variant of 'DRG creep', whereby providers seek to classify cases into higher-cost categories – and indeed to increase admissions under particular forms of contract that allow extra reimbursement.

All in all, therefore, costs per volume contracts probably allow purchasers and providers to share risk and define services more productively together. The problem is that such costs per volume contracts may not reflect patient wishes or GP wishes. In an appropriate system, service plans rather than strict cost per volume contracts (but based on cost and volume estimates) can allow patient wishes, GP referrals and criteria of cost control and cost effectiveness to be reconciled – and purchasing authorities can work with such actors in determining the appropriate location of particular services and service mixes. As a result, more effective management by quantifiable targets can occur (as was sometimes not the case in the pre-reform NHS) yet the perverse incentives of the post-reform NHS can be limited. No system is perfect, yet it is important to ensure that 'policy learning' takes place. It is also important to ensure that a coherent purchasing strategy incorporates the wishes and money of GP fundholders, preferably through reintegrating GP fundholding into a unified purchasing system. It is not simply a question of equity of the so-called two-tierism arising from GP fundholders having preferential treatment. It is also a case of ensuring that providers are able to plan for the future without the threat of short-term removal of funds or the 'holding back' of funds by GP fundholders (when times are harder) to ensure the survival of budgets to the end of the year. This is one of the primary reasons, along with the increased costs of running the market and ironically the increased efficiency that leads to money running out sooner, why hospitals are finding their budgets 'running out' faster towards the end of the financial year.

The best approach would probably involve services both planned and funded (i.e. both capital and revenue) according to populations' needs and desired referral patterns, yet scope for 'top-up' revenue funding as an incentive to undertake extra workload.

The aim ought to be to devise a system in which patients' rights and opinions as to appropriate care within the GP practice, criteria for referral, GPs ideas as to best, and most cost-effective, referral and purchasers' wishes can be combined. Then you have effective commissioning and procurement of care without 'overt purchasing' in the negative sense simply of rationing and managerial decision-making based on finance. The final chapter of this book sets out a strategy for improved health policy of the future.

EFFECTIVE AND APPROPRIATE CARE

Techniques such as the quality adjusted life year (QALY) (Chapter 3) and other related methodologies can help to define outcomes in health care, and the most sophisticated

versions such as the EUROQOL can also seek to combine the preference of different actors (such as patients, doctors and others) in defining outcome and its benefits. It still remains the case, however, that one must make difficult and value-laden comparisons between priorities, between specialties and within specialties as to technique or procedure.

Taking the last first, if there were two different techniques for a particular operation, for example, and one tended to produce on average or in total a better outcome but with greater risk in a minority of cases, and the other produced fewer aggregate or average benefits but less risk in these cases, then which technique ought to be chosen? Firstly, the patient might prefer one or the other, in line with his own preferences. Secondly, the doctor might recommend one or the other. Thirdly, the economist or manager might recommend one or the other on the grounds that one technique is cheaper than the other and there is no unequivocal value-free means of choosing one rather than the other.

Data over time may help to elucidate such questions. For example, one may over time be able to identify which patients are at most risk in the otherwise preferable procedure. Then, cost considerations apart, that procedure can be applied to the other patients, with less risky procedure applied to the newly identified at-risk patients. It still may of course be the case that the costs of the different techniques differ and that cost/outcome relationships therefore differ for different techniques for different groups of patients.

If one is ranking all health by a QALY-type methodology that seeks to maximize the use of money by ensuring the maximum utility or benefit, the question arises as to by whose criteria, it should be remembered. Given a finite amount of money, one may end up with a sophisticated ranking of overall priorities; of specialties within such areas (for example particular care regimes for care of the elderly, or particular surgical techniques within the arena of heart care); and particular procedures within specialties. Heart transplants by technique X may produce less QALY than kidney transplants by technique A, in turn providing less than heart transplants by technique Y, etc. When different age groups or client groups receive X rather than Y, rationing may have to discriminate by patient as well as by procedure if it is to be truly rational!

This is however a very 'rationalist' and possibly technocratic system. Firstly, it assumes agreement between purchasers and providers as to such criteria. Purchasers may, to a greater or lesser extent, be assembling such criteria over time. Providers are, however, composed of managers, doctors and other health care professionals. Simply treating them as a production line will be damaging to the professions of medicine Chapter 9), nursing and others. A balance must therefore be sought between flexibility and rational decision making. Furthermore, calculations on the basis of utility may bias advantage to the majority 'middle class' in society, which may derive benefit from procedures which are less beneficial in aggregate to those with more basic or different health needs, such as the poor. If a 'QALY methodology' is used for allocating health resources, we may therefore end up with a system with less of a 'bias to the poor' and indeed a bias away from the poor – unless **class-specific** cost/utility measures are adopted whereby specific benefits from specific services for specific classes or groups are identified. Otherwise such might be lost in an average-based calculation (Chapter 9).

All such issues show the difficulties of respectively consumerism, professional choice and indeed 'rational choice' by managers and economists, in the context of a cash-limited national health service. If there are no cost implications of alternative care regimes for a particular disease or problem, and if clinicians do not hold strong views on these alternatives, then both patients and managers (whether purchaser or provider managers) can take decisions on such matters. On the other hand this is an unlikely scenario. In practice, there will also be a central role – whether for regions or for central government – in promulgating, accepted procedures, accepted means of adjudicating between different procedures, different specialties and indeed different priorities (hard choices). Chapter 9 outlines some of the tensions between different perspectives on who should make the key decisions.

It will then, and only then, be the role of medical audit and – wider – quality assurance to ensure that appropriate regimes are appropriately carried out. The problem for a discipline such as medical audit in the context of scarce resources is that it is often pulled into the harder, value-laden choices rather than simply being a technical assessment as to whether appropriate clinical regimes and appropriate care were provided. The later chapter in this book on medical audit explores these issues. At the end of the day, fundamental issues of ethics may be involved: utilitarianism is the doctrine that dominates the QALY methodology, yet it is only one normative doctrine and maybe inadequate when set against other criteria for making social and individual choice.

CONCLUSION

This book is not an analysis or critique of the NHS reforms. But it does however inevitably engage key issues emerging as a result of the NHS reforms, in engaging topics such as purchaser/provider relationships, medical audit, the management of human resources and so forth. The NHS reforms provide both a political and an economic arena within which NHS management is currently carried out. As a result, it is inevitable that this book will also engage with issues such as the extent to which cost control is the overall agenda within the National Health Service; the protection of specialized services and centres of excellence in a market environment; the status of complex and expensive individual episodes of care in a market environment with public purchasing; the question of who benefits from the emerging National Health Service; and therefore the question of how best to manage the market or to manage a system that supersedes the market as we currently know it. That is the overall strategic agenda for senior NHS managers.

For now, it is worth pointing out that health reforms have both an ideological and a technological component. One can analyse the purchaser/provider split as a technical device for separating the definition of needs and the making of contracts by purchasers, on the one hand, and more autonomous management by providers on the other hand. The ideological dimension comes in when the purchaser/provider split is seen as a mechanism to create a market in health care. This in turn may create further momentum towards further quasi-privatization or privatization in provision, and the emergence of various interests both in purchasing and provision that make the assemblage of a 'common vision' for a truly national health service more difficult to sustain and enhance in the future. We are therefore returned to a distinction between experimentation and progress in health policy and management as opposed to the expression of social power by dominant classes through ideology, dressed up as technical innovation when it suits the powerful. To return to the earlier discussion of approaches to understanding the policy process, it should be remembered that health policy – although it has many special features – is an example of public policy generally in any country within which it is being studied.

In the UK, the NHS reforms have been accompanied by a very tight and centralist political agenda where a certain 'rationalism' in policy making has nevertheless reflected the ideology and power of what is broadly a right-wing and pro-market view of society. The Government has tolerated little dissent; senior NHS managers have therefore had to toe the line. Dissent is expressed, if at all, in private; and even policy analysts and academics who rely on Government contracts or NHSME contracts to augment or provide their finance are therefore limited in their ability to provide radical critiques of policy. The marketization of the education sector as well as of health and other sectors ensures that providers have greater difficulty in also being thinkers.

Overall, the Conservative government reorganized the NHS without cross-party consent; implemented ideologically partisan reforms; additionally uses more neutral or (eventually) accepted structures such as general management of partisan and 'tactical' political interventions; and, specifically, devolves 'management' responsibilities yet keeps managers on a tight political agenda. In the latter realm, even those here considered most suitable for devolution – human resource management, operations management, capital policy – are subject to the Government's political agenda.

Furthermore, the Government has been keen to disguise politics as 'scientific management' and has used euphemistic rhetoric to disguise the need for a more tolerant, pluralistic debate.

That is not to deny that technical comparison of the NHS pre-reform and post-reform is possible. For example, as a generalization, one can argue there was inadequate specificity in stipulation of services and service mix in the pre-reform NHS. In moving to great specification post-reform, however, flexibility in allocation and re-allocation of funds either by purchasers or providers may have been diminished. The challenge for strategic managers is to analyse in detail, in their localities, the specific instances in which this issue arises, and to seek – within the bounds of realism – to achieve 'the best of both worlds'. Likewise, there may have been – in the worst of the old system – too much of a bias towards hospitals as opposed to health and health care more generally. Equally it is the job of purchasing managers to ensure that contracts are placed with the most appropriate provider, or that service agreements are made with one's own local providers – whether hospital or community – to reflect the need for changes in priorities, more effective health strategies and indeed 'seamless care' for patients such that hospitals and community units cooperate without seeking to 'take each other over'. The final chapter in this book again sets out a scenario which covers such matters and suggests an improved structure for within which strategic managers can operate. Meanwhile, the rest of the book considers a variety of important policy issues and their management implications. Part One considers national strategic issues; Part Two considers applied topics such as management of human resources, medical audit and appropriate structures and functions for management in the long term; and Part Three considers an agenda for the future in the context of lessons from comparative health care.

DISCUSSION

- Health care systems are but one influence upon the health of nations, classes and individuals. Other social policies – such as housing policy and environmental policy, and especially the relief of poverty – are influential in affecting health status. Beveridge's five great evils – disease, want, squalor, ignorance and idleness – are all indeed influential.

Nevertheless this is a two-edged sword. While expenditure on matters other than hospitals or direct health services may be important in improving health, it is equally important to ensure that such expenditure is not left as the responsibility of the health care system – in the UK, the National Health Service. A number of Government (and non-Government) agencies must coordinate their strategy, but must also make their individual role. The most appropriate role for the National Health Service may indeed be to care for those who cannot be cured, to cure those whose diseases have not or could not have been prevented and to indulge in directly health-oriented prevention and promotion.

Other agencies, under the aegis of Government departments other than health, may be best suited for the wider strategy. Coordinating this with health care strategy is not the same as leaving everything to the health care strategy.

There is a danger in the UK today that a trendy-sounding rhetoric about holistic health is simply an excuse for leaving expenditure to the NHS. Progressive-sounding 'purchasing plans' that involve, for example, spending health authority money on improving roads or housing rather than providing hospital beds, may simply be an excuse for other agencies to do less.

- Within the health sector, one should distinguish between planning for need and reimbursing the services that exist as a result of planning. There is a danger that 'purchasing' – today's vogue term – is used to cover both and that thereby an important distinction in policy is blurred. The former – planning for need and for the provision of the services to meet that need – is not a new activity at all. What used to be known as health service planning (whether epidemiologically based or not) is a prerequisite for purchasing.

Simply to use the word 'commissioning' as the wider term is not adequate. For commissioning is also ambiguous, and may refer to the creation of specific services rather than the wider planning for need. In the sense of planning for need, there has always been 'purchasing' in British health care, formerly undertaken by regional health authorities acting in concert (where appropriate, or perhaps just by chance) with district health authorities. There was not however a purchaser/provider split in that the district health authorities also managed the services (now known as providers.)

- At its best therefore, the new 'purchasing' is simply a more appropriate or sensitive form of planning. A more effective means of gauging need, and reconciling need with available resources, may involve individuals, local communities, general practitioners, health authorities and regions, or regional offices as they are now styled in the UK.

This however says nothing about how providers are to be reimbursed, or whether there is to be an institutional purchaser/ provider **split** as opposed to a functional purchaser/provider **distinction.**

- The narrower type of 'purchasing' concerns the reimbursement of providers, by a variety of mechanisms (generally contractual). It is here that the NHS 'reforms' represent a distinct break with the past: instead of existing and newly planned providers being reimbursed directly through the District health authority (whether or not in line with workload), there is an attempt to limit – through overt 'purchasing' – the funds available in line with choices made either by managers of health authorities or by GP fundholders.

By 1996, district health authorities and family health services authorities will be merged into new unified authorities. GP fundholders will be accountable to these authorities, and a likely scenario is therefore that – even although fundholding is 'widened and deepened' to embrace more GPs and more services – fundholders' purchasing plans will have to be rendered compatible with those of the overall authority. Otherwise a major aim of post-reform 'purchasing' (cost control and rationalization of services, in order to achieve maximum value for money) will be thwarted.

- Despite some operational devolution to health authorities through the market mechanism of contracting, there is a centralization of political control of the health service – health authorities are now in effect directly appointed from the centre, as are hospitals and other allegedly self-governing trusts. As a result there is an alleged 'democratic deficit' in that local communities do not have a say in either electing or controlling their health authorities. Communicating strategies, formulated with an overwhelming stress upon financial control, to the public is not the same as control by the public.

As a result the idea of local government purchasing for all health services has revived.

- This, however, is ironical in many ways. Firstly, the idea was rejected with the creation of the National Health Service on a basis of central government control in 1948, as Health Minister Aneurin Bevan won over his cabinet colleagues.

Secondly, local government control of financing and purchasing could increase inequity, as poorer areas of the country – with less local tax base, confronting at the same time greater health need – might either be less able to finance needed services or would rely on complicated formulae by which central government sought to 'equalize the revenue' available to local government. The latter, however, creates major political and management problems, and local government finance generally has always been a bugbear in British politics.

Thirdly, the funding of specialized services would probably be required to be carried out on a separate basis. Thus the supposed unification of all spending under one authority (the local authority) might therefore end up in its opposite – a fragmentation into a hospital service and 'the rest'. This ironically could return us to a pre-1948 situation.

Fourthly, advocates of local government control are often advocates of a 'holistic health strategy' and are relatively hostile to 'hospitals and doctors', as opposed to wider community inputs into health care. Ironically, however, local government control of the health sector might well lead to less political will to reorient priorities (and, for example, to close hospitals.)

Fifthly, it is argued that the existence of a purchaser/provider split ends some of the objections to local government control of health services – principally those of the doctors, who in 1948 were unwilling to be controlled by local government politicians. This, however, depends on a naive reading of the purchaser/provider split (which in terms of British politics is a tactical device rather than a brave new concept.)

Furthermore, if there were a genuine split, such that hospitals and other providers were controlled wholly separately, there might ironically be greater difficulty in planning for the future (through indirect control of an autonomous sector) than by simply allowing authorities to control their own providers and manage change directly (rather than through contracts and incentives).

REFERENCES

NHS Executive (1994) *The Operation of the NHS Internal Market: Local Freedoms, National Responsibilities*, NHSE, Leeds.

Paton C R (1990) *US Health Politics: Public Policy and Political Theory*, Avebury, Aldershot.

BACKGROUND

If one wanted to define the major responsibility of strategic managers generally (and certainly in health care in particular) in one sentence, it would be responsibility for the translation of inputs into outcomes in the most effective and efficient manner. Already one has to use four key management terms, albeit in a dry and colourless form.

Starting at the national level – that is at the level of the health care system in any particular country as a whole – the all-embracing input is of course money. What finance is available for the health care system? To make a heroic leap to outcome, one is referring to health status of the population, or rather improvement in health status as a result of the sending of money, if inputs are to be related to outcomes by involving the hypothesis that the provision of inputs has helped to produce or alter outcomes. Later chapters will discuss different mixes of outcomes that can be sought: for example, is one seeking to maximize the total quantum of health outcome (however defined) or to concentrate on particular target groups, social classes or individuals? For now, let us accept that the purpose of providing inputs is to affect outcome positively.

An intermediary variable can be defined as outputs. The average clinical director in a hospital Department of Surgery does not generally say on a Friday afternoon, 'Well, the week's work has produced a health status improvement of X units'! Outputs are naturally services delivered – number of operations; number of inpatient episodes plus number of day cases; perhaps even number of successful interventions, by some measure or other. A successful intervention may be considered a bridge between output and outcome. That is, it is hypothesized that a successful intervention will produce a lasting improvement in health status for the patient. But without confusing the issue, outputs are the 'product' delivered, with an (again hypothetical) assumption that the product helps to produce the desired outcome.

There is also an intermediate variable between inputs and outputs. Finance is used to provide particular commodities. At the broadest level finance can be broken down into finance for revenue costs and finance for capital costs. In other words, there is money to run things and there is money to build new things, re-invest in inadequate plant and – for example – expand to provide new programmes. Ranging across both categories of revenue and capital, finance can be used to pay wages and salaries, to provide consumables and pay for utilities such as electricity, and to buy new equipment and materials generally. Considering finance's uses in this manner brings us to the original means of breaking down costs in the National Health Service, known in the older financial literature as 'subjective costing'. That is, there was a simple breakdown between the costs of employing people and the costs of providing things.

Were this a book on accounting with a health economics flavour into the bargain, one could discuss fully the implications of the distinction between fixed costs and variable costs and between direct and indirect costs. Fixed costs are those that do not vary across the provision of the particular service or unit in question. For example the cost of providing a building is not considered to vary, once it is provided, in connection with the services provided for a fixed period of time within that building (for example a surgical unit). Variable costs have a respectrum. Fully variable costs vary with each unit of care delivered – for example, the drugs administered to each patient in a department of medicine. At the other extreme of the spectrum of variable costs, one finds the concept of semi-variable costs. For example, the electricity bill may be standard week by week, unless extra operations are done, in which case more electricity may be consumed.

Direct costs are those directly concerned with providing a service or unit of service. For example, drugs for patients may again be considered to be direct costs whereas the cost of the overall hospital administration is an indirect cost. That is because, without such administration, the service would not function at all (despite the views of some in the medical profession!); yet such costs cannot be attributed directly to the provision of a particular unit of service. Instead their implications have to be apportioned by some methodology or other over all services carried out as the core business or 'point of existence' of the programme or service generally. Direct costs may therefore be variable or fixed (drugs or a piece of capital equipment, for example). Indirect costs may likewise be variable or fixed, but are more likely to be fixed if one is considering, for example, an unchanging management or administration budget or an unchanging catering budget.

The focus of this introductory chapter is, however, upon aggregate finance for health care. What are the different ways in which finance can be raised to provide a health care system and its component parts, within the component regions and areas of the country? What is the major means of financing health care in the UK? What are the most useful ideas for augmenting or changing such a system, and to what extent should managers worry about such questions?

MODELS OF FINANCING

Let us consider a spectrum of models of financing which ranges broadly from the private to the public.

PRIVATE PURCHASE BY INDIVIDUALS

One can be simplistic and consider health care as a commodity to be purchased like any other. When one is ill or requires a particular service, one buys it. It soon becomes clear that, unless one is extremely rich, the nature of medical care means that private purchase by individuals will not cover demand or need (terms to be discussed in greater detail later) at the time of requirement. The concept of the Oil Sheikh jetting in to use a private hospital on the outskirts of London and pay by credit card is not an image likely to satisfy the majority of the British public. Let us therefore move quickly to the next category, which can be considered as a kind of logical and psychological consequence of the inadequacy of the simplistic model of private purchase by individuals.

PRIVATE INSURANCE BY INDIVIDUALS

Individuals may seek to insure themselves against the costs and consequences of medical expense. The essence of insurance is quite simple. Risk is spread over the number of individuals insured, such that the revenue generated by the premiums paid by individuals covers the costs of all pay-outs. Let us consider a simple example, not drawn from health care. In a particular community, 100 individuals drive cars. There is a 1 in 100 chance that one of them will be involved in an accident, and the cost of that accident is likely to be £1000. The 'insurance company' therefore has to raise £1000, before considerations of administrative costs, profits and so forth are even thought of. Let us put these on one side for the moment. The consequence is that – if all individuals are considered to be equal risks – a premium of £10 will be paid (100 × £10 = £1000). This is the essence of insurance. Were the likely cost of accidents to increase, and were the number of individuals to increase or decrease, the premium would change accordingly. More significantly, if individuals are assumed to incur risk differentially (some are good drivers; some are not) then insurance premiums will vary for individuals to the extent they can be calculated. A basic principle of insurance is the correlation of premium with risk.

In health care, at the simplest level, one can consider a similar situation. If insurance is to be provided by for-profit companies, then profits and so forth will have to be added on, as well as administrative and overhead costs (how much profit of course depends on how the market-place functions). The textbook theory of perfect competition argues that profits are zero. This is of course an 'ideal type' situation, never approximated. If such a situation were realized, there would be no for-profit producers in the market-place. If the companies are not for-profit, then profit in the sense of distribution to shareholders is not a relevant concept, although it may be a grey area as to whether private non-profit companies differ greatly in practice from private for-profit companies. In the United States, for example, in both the insurance and hospital markets, there is often considered to be a convergence of behaviour between for-profit and non-profit companies.

If individuals are considered to be at differential risk for consuming medical care, then private companies (whether profit or non-profit, unless regulated by the Government) will seek to reflect the differential risk in the premium – a basic principle of insurance. Individuals at differential risk may be so because they are more likely to be sick, because they are sick already, because they are old and therefore statistically more likely to be sick or in need of chronic care, or because they are poor, the implication from research and other evidence being that poorer people are more likely to be ill.

Already we have a potential problem for private insurance in medical care. How can companies – and individuals themselves – know what the relative risks are, to an adequate extent? If they cannot, companies may through no fault of their own find that the premiums they have charged are inadequate – or surplus to requirements and therefore inequitable to the individuals and to society. If a company finds itself catering for sicker people with greater cost consequences, but cannot have this recognized in the premium, then there is a problem of 'adverse selection', whereby those making the greater claims cannot be screened out or 'catered for' through price discrimination. As an extreme example, people who are already seriously ill may seek insurance. The only option for the insurance company in such a situation is to seek – crudely, inevitably, given the lack of information – to screen out and deny insurance to certain individuals, groups or (most wrongly of all) people from particular social classes. How for example can one insure people who, to give an extreme example, are already HIV-positive?

Another problem for private insurance is what economists tend to call 'moral hazard'. This is a rather stern Victorian term nevertheless used eagerly by hedonistic 20th-century economists. Moral hazard simply points to the phenomenon whereby, if people are already insured, they will seek to consume as much health care as they can, or at least more than is optimal. Economists would define more-than-optimal consumption of health care as where the benefits from the care are less than the costs. Benefits are of course notoriously difficult to define, and values are involved in determining both types and quantums of benefit. Nevertheless, the point is clear at a theoretical level. Once costs are paid, consumers will seek medical care as long as there is any benefit at all, it is hypothesized. The cost to society generally may be greater than that to the individual.

Related to this problem for the private insurance market is 'the problem of the third-party payer'. This is the most interesting problem for both policy analysts and strategic managers because of the implications for how providers, purchasers and consumers ought to be related to each other. The problem of the third-party payer hypothesizes that, if the provider has an incentive to provide (for example through profit maximization) and the consumer has an incentive to consume (as long as there is some or any benefit to consumption) then, if the purchaser or financier or insurer is separate from the provider and consumer (in other words is a third party), then the provider and consumer will collude to maximize provision at the expense of the financier.

This cannot of course go on forever. If the financier has to raise premiums in order to stay in business as a result, this may eventually percolate back to the consumer's consciousness. It may of course be that the consumer is not footing all of the bill him- or herself but sharing it with an employer and/or the Government. In consequence, relating over-consumption to changed behaviour (by consumer or provider) may be an indirect and inefficient process. If one wanted to summarize the cost problems of US health care in one sentence, one could use the concept of the third-party payer: private providers have an incentive to over-provide; insured consumers have an incentive to over-consume; and third-party payers (insurance companies, whether profit or non-profit, employers and large corporations and the Government) have increasing difficulty in keeping a lid on the system. Naturally many

other (basically political) factors intervene in the United States to accentuate this problem, which is not purely one derived from economic theory. However the basic structure of the US system, combined with the decentralized nature of US politics, makes this a plausible diagnosis of the United States' major cost problem in health care.

Since this is not a book about insurance, it is judged at this point that enough has been said to point to the inadequacies of private insurance for a health care system that seeks to be both cost-effective and equitable. It is therefore again a logical and psychological move of some ease away from private insurance to what is sometimes known as public insurance

PUBLIC INSURANCE

If public insurance is truly insurance – in other words, if premiums are related to risk for health – then it is likely that the Government will pay, or significantly subsidize, premiums for the poorer, the older and the already sicker. (These categories are not of course either all inclusive or mutually exclusive.) That is, on this model, public insurance consists in public responsibility – through public finance – for paying people's (or certain people's) premiums in an insurance market which, if not publicly owned and managed, is publicly regulated.

It is common to describe various 'National Health Insurance' schemes as forms of public insurance. This is however misleading. What are called 'National Health Insurance' schemes (such as found in many European countries or Canada, for example) are in fact taxation by any other name. It would be more appropriate to call these schemes a form of 'health tax'. Naturally the health tax may not be generated solely by direct taxation (of individuals and corporations) going to the Government. In other words, contributions may come from individuals and employers through the payroll, as well as from the

Government from more direct revenues. Nevertheless, the sense in which it is misleading to call such schemes 'insurance' is that contributions by individuals, firms and so forth do not relate to the relative risk of those individuals to be covered. In other words the schemes are simply a means of generating revenue.

Often such health insurance schemes are part of, or linked to, general social security schemes, based on raising revenue through tripartite contributions from individuals, firms and Government.

Furthermore the fact that such schemes are 'public' does not in practice prevent an element of cost sharing. For example, individuals may have to pay 'co-insurance' or 'deductibles'. Co-insurance is a means of paying a **proportion** of the cost; deductibles are a means of the consumer paying a **fixed pound amount** as a contribution to the cost.

COMMUNITY FINANCING AND/OR LOCAL TAXATION

In developing countries, community financing takes various forms, and is generally more informal than through local taxation, whether direct (as in income tax) or indirect (as in sales tax or VAT). In the UK, at the foundation of the NHS, there was a debate as to whether the NHS ought to be a 'local' service or a 'national' service. It is important to draw a distinction between finance and provision when discussing whether a service is local or national. In other words, is finance to be local or national; is provision to be national or local (a separate question)?

AN EARMARKED HEALTH TAX

As already discussed, what is often called National Health Insurance may have elements of earmarked tax. What is meant under this category is a particular section of national taxation (or conceivably local taxation, although this is less likely in the UK)

that is identified specifically for the purposes of spending on the health service or health care generally. In other words, one can say so much of the proceeds from VAT go to the health service, or one can have a specific tax created for health care (hence the overlap with what is known as National Health Insurance). In the UK, earmarking a particular revenue of source of revenue for health would probably occur at the national level. In other words, national taxation would remain the source of funding for the NHS in the main. The alleged advantage of this system is that it clarifies the amount which is available for health and also allows individuals to 'feel happier' about paying extra tax if they note that the extra money is going to a favoured service. Naturally it is a truism that public opinion polls show people in favour of spending more on health, but generally not in favour of higher taxation generally. An earmarked tax is said to be a way around this conundrum, although the paradoxical opinion poll finding may simply reflect voter hypocrisy rather than a desire to have greater earmarking and therefore willingness to pay tax.

On the debit side, earmarking a tax has the disadvantage that, if the source of revenue identified as the source of health service spending is diminished (due to greater unemployment, for example, leading to less direct revenue, or fewer sales – also due to recession – leading to less indirect revenue), then health service spending is automatically diminished. Naturally taxation generally is reduced as a source of public expenditure if the economy is in trouble. Nevertheless, an absence of earmarking allows political decisions to be taken as to which ministries and types of public expenditure to protect. This has its disadvantages, but also advantages if, for example, protection of the NHS 'come what may' is preferred to protection of other types of public expenditure. Naturally the 'health service community' will tend to take this view.

There is therefore no easy answer in this realm. What is often called a hypothecated tax (that is, an earmarked tax) has been considered as a means of generating extra revenue rather than the whole amount of revenue for the National Health Service. This reflects the UK's position as a relatively 'underfunded' health financier. What is meant by 'underfunded' is a growing divergence between percentage of gross national produce (GNP) or gross domestic product (GDP) spent in the UK and that spent in other European or 'Western' countries. It is important, of course, to look at what one gets for the money as well as how much is spent. However by most criteria the UK's public expenditure as well as total expenditure on health care takes up a lesser percentage of what is often a lesser GNP. There is a general correlation between the wealth of a country (as measured by GNP, or GNP *per capita*) and willingness to spend on health. However, even by this criterion the UK is a low spender. It is often claimed that throughout the 1980s the UK's health expenditure kept pace with inflation. This is just about true. What is not pointed out, however is that, in order to meet new health challenges, comparable nations spent more and more in real terms as time went on, by comparison with the UK (Table 2.1).

Table 2.1 Percentage of gross domestic product spent on health care in various Western countries (1987) (Source: adapted from OECD, 1990)

Country	% spent	% spent publicly
Canada	8.6	6.5
France	8.6	6.7
Netherlands	8.5	6.6
Sweden	9.0	8.2
UK	6.1	5.3
US	11.2	4.6

PUBLIC FINANCE THROUGH GENERAL TAXATION

This is of course how the NHS is funded at the moment. General, national revenue provides most of the revenue going to the NHS. The separate 'national insurance' component is hardly separate, in that, in its current form, national insurance is merely an augmentation of general revenues. In other words it is not earmarked in any meaningful sense, nor is it really insurance. A number of reform proposals suggest merging of national insurance with the taxation system. Again, arguments can be made on both sides here.

When it comes to public financing through general taxation, a number of options exist.

The money could go from public sources to individuals in the form of vouchers. The argument here is that individuals can be 'consumers in their own interest'. However, a grave disadvantage applies. There is a need to adjust vouchers to the likely health needs of the individual, if equity is to be preserved in the sense of health finance being available according to need rather than the ability to pay. Thus a similar disadvantage to individual insurance applies: individuals with greater need will need larger vouchers. One can conceptualize a voucher as a ticket with a pound sign on it. It would be an actuarial nightmare to calculate exactly what each citizen of the country was going to need in the form of money for health care. If this could be done, then health planning would indeed be a simpler science! In reality, some people would have money left over at the end of year from their voucher and others would soon be running into deficit. Thus it makes much more sense to allocate to large pools of individuals, in order to spread risk. That is the basis of allocation to health authorities in the UK.

Equally, in the United States, Health Maintenance Organizations (to be discussed later) are most viable when they spread risk over adequate numbers. Professor Alain

Enthoven has estimated, for example, that Health Maintenance Organizations of fewer than 50 000 enrolees have difficulty in doing this equitably or efficiently.

Health authorities can of course be both purchasers and providers (as in the UK before the 'NHS reforms'), or purchasers only – charged with making contracts with providers in order to ensure that their populations (resident within the boundaries of the authorities) are given access to health care or certain categories of health care. The money can of course also go to GP fundholders or what in a more international setting might be called consortia of primary care doctors.

In other words, it seems to make sense for purchasers to be allocated money on behalf of large enough numbers of citizens to ensure that risks can be spread, to allow both financial efficiency and equity, in that – with large enough numbers – unexpectedly large demands or needs from particular individuals can be counterbalanced by less demand or need than expected elsewhere.

POSSIBLE CHANGES IN THE UK

Chapter 4 discusses the various configurations of purchasing and provision, in the context of the management agenda following the NHS reforms and developments of these. Meanwhile, the discussion focuses upon possible changes specifically to the financing, or extended financing, of the National Health Service in years to come.

If the aim of the National Health Service is to generate finance in what fiscal economists would call a 'progressive' manner (and furthermore then to distribute the money for health care to those with 'greatest need', irrespective of the ability to pay), then a progressive taxation system is probably the most efficient means of proceeding. In the UK throughout the 1980s, however, taxation was rendered less progressive. Direct (income) taxation was significantly reduced for the better-off, with the abolition of higher rates of

tax; indirect taxation (principally VAT) was significantly increased (from 8% to 17.5%) under the Conservative Government, placing a greater burden on those who consume a greater proportion of their income – the poor. As a consequence, funding the NHS from general taxation has more recently meant making the responsibility for paying for the NHS a greater relative burden upon the poor than in previous years.

It might therefore be more 'progressive', in the sense of raising proportionately more money from the better-off, to move to a 'National Health Insurance' system whereby particular contributions were paid by the individual, the employer and the state. If such a scheme were designed to reflect income, both of individuals and employers, and to levy a proportionately greater charge on those with greater income or profit, then more money might be generated for the National Health Service. In particular, the advantages of a so-called hypothecated tax (earmarked tax) might be realized – specific contributions would be made for a specific purpose: namely, funding the National Health Service. More resources might therefore be mobilized for the health care system. The caveat entered in discussing earmarked tax above should, however, be remembered. Earmarking a tax does not guarantee the maintenance of revenue.

Another option of course is that the tax system generally (from which the NHS is financed) be rendered again more progressive. This in itself would not guarantee more money for the NHS. Tax rates could be rendered more progressive yet in a context of overall lower taxes. Thus more progressive taxation, coupled with taxes which were higher in an absolute sense, might be necessary to guarantee stable, higher revenue for the National Health Service.

Naturally, the 'flatter' the tax system (in the sense of being less progressive) the more difficult it is to raise taxes. This is because ordinary citizens feel the pinch more directly.

The flatter the tax system, the more (relatively) popular tax cuts are likely to be with those who are neither extremely rich nor extremely poor (and therefore out of the tax bracket altogether). A difference can be noticed between the United Kingdom and the United States in this regard, in 1992. Fear of higher taxes seemed significant in the general election of April 1992 in the UK, leading to the return of a Conservative Government. In the United States however, President Clinton's electoral success was based on a perception that higher taxes would be directed at the significantly well-off. This was rendered possible because of the significant tax cuts for the very well-off which had occurred in the 1981 budget of President Reagan, reinforced in later years throughout the 1980s until very marginally reversed under President Bush.

The more the National Health Service is seen as a service funded by ordinary people, the more ordinary people will be cautious about increasing expenditure upon it. This does not mean that they will be hostile to the NHS as opposed to the privatization of finance, whereby the better-off are made responsible for their health care, perhaps on a sliding scale according to income (i.e. as one reaches certain thresholds, one has less entitlement to public health care). The reason that people might still subscribe to the National Health Service rather than being responsible themselves (even if allowed to 'contract out' from NHS contributions, as proposed by Secretary of State John Moore during the early stages of the Prime Minister's review of the National Health Service in 1988), is that the NHS might rightly be perceived as the most efficient and cost-effective means of providing health care. Therefore, although people have a perception of 'paying as they go', even if not particularly well-off, they would still rather 'pay as they go' in this way rather than in any other way involving privatization of financing.

A more progressive taxation system, or a more progressive means of raising revenue through 'National Health Insurance', would be most effective if the number of thresholds for paying higher tax or higher contributions were significant enough to prevent sudden leaps in tax threshold. In other words, a large number of bands of taxation or health service contributions makes sense in terms of economic incentives as well as in terms of equity, if that particular type of equity is considered to be important.

A CHANGING ROLE FOR THE NHS? – UNIVERSALISM VERSUS TARGETING

In early 1993, both major political parties were rethinking the role of the welfare state. The Conservative Government found itself with a rapidly increasing public sector deficit, owing principally to a combination of cuts in direct taxation throughout the 1980s and the continuing recession. As in the United States (although with a less severe deficit than there), the dictates of fiscal policy were forcing a rethink about both the extent and the structure of welfare. The Labour Party set up a Commission for Social Justice to consider priorities in welfare policy, among other things. The fundamental nature of the NHS has been its universalism – the service is available, broadly free at the point of use, to all citizens. Any radical or iconoclastic thinking, under the rubric of the debate about universalism versus targeting of welfare programmes, is even more controversial and – to many – unwelcome when applied to the NHS, which is an institution whose core values are subscribed to by the vast majority of the population. Nevertheless a basic question exists, at least at the level of theory: can the more disadvantaged in society best be helped through a public health care system that focuses on their needs or one that is universal? If there is an increasing need to ration health care, the argument might go, it would make more sense to give the poor all they need, and others only some of what they need, from the public purse. Otherwise, rationing by service rather than by population group (or social class) would allow the better-off to purchase, or insure themselves for, excluded services, whereas the poor would be less able to do so without financial hardship. In other words, such rationing is denial of care to the poor but not to the better-off. It is therefore a progressive argument for targeting – if demand and need outstrip supply or finance to create supply – geared to favouring the poor, whether or not on a sliding scale.

There are however severe difficulties with such an approach. Programmes which are 'for the poor' are likely to fall victim to spending cuts, especially by right-of-centre Governments representing 'the contented majority'. Such programmes become 'welfare wedges', like Medicaid in the United States, unless strong political correctives are available to prevent this. Furthermore, there would be a poverty or unemployment trap created, whereby one loses benefits (such as health care) as one raises one's income. Next, if the middle classes who 'exit' from the NHS to private financing were not willing to pay more in aggregate, there would be less for the 'rump' NHS – we would be back where we started. And if private care is more expensive and private finance is a more expensive system to boot, there would be less willingness by the middle classes to fund (through redistribution) even the pre-existing *per capita* expenditure on the poor who remain in the NHS.

It can equally be argued that, if the 'politics of the contented majority' (Galbraith, 1992) are rampant – in other words where electoral majorities are likely to be put together by the two-thirds who are comfortably off as opposed to the one third who are broadly poor – a universally provided service, available to all irrespective of means, is also subject to cheeseparing or diminution. In other words, the NHS as currently available may be able to meet (relatively) fewer of society's

expectations. In such a context, the worse off may be those least able to benefit from such a service, or to have their needs met fully from such a service, again in the absence of strong political correctives. It may be desirable to 'keep the middle classes in the NHS', to give them a stake in welfare. But this limits the NHS's ability to be a progressive service for the poor.

Specific aspects of the 'NHS reforms' may exacerbate such a trend. GP fundholders may have an incentive to 'cream-skim' (exclude the most expensive patients) if formulae reimbursing them are not meticulously devised. Both district purchases and trusts may seek to exclude the awkward – respectively through contracts and through admissions policy.

It is an empirical question – whatever one's ideology or policy preference – as to whether targeting or universalism will in practice help the poor (however their needs are defined), whether in health or in welfare policy generally. What can be asserted is that targeted programmes will be more effective if they are allied to an established set of 'health rights', whether constitutionally protected or not, to prevent such programmes being susceptible to gradual erosion or Government cuts at times of financial difficulty.

Likewise, in the context of a universal National Health Service, overt rights – to update the Health Services Act 1977, which is vague on the matter – might usefully be tailored to protecting the interests of the most needy in terms of those currently with the worst health outcomes, well known to be strongly correlated with lower socio-economic groupings.

Maintaining the universal nature of the NHS – if not, naturally, of all welfare programmes – is judged by the present author to be the best means of ensuring that the NHS is protected both politically and economically. This does not, however, prevent priorities from being established within the financing and provision of such a service that favour those least able to exit to the private sector when their needs or demands are not available (or available in a timely manner) through public health services. That is, national, regional and district purchasing priorities can reflect a 'bias to the poor' which walks a tightrope between favouring the poor on the one hand and maintaining middle-class allegiance to the NHS as a service capable of meeting most of its needs on the other hand. To say this is easier than to achieve it. In practice, it might be argued that the NHS is trying to achieve such a balance at the moment. But the development of QALYs and other devices which measure utility by **majority** preferences may be less useful for the poor and other groups – thus diminishing the NHS's salience for their wider needs.

A problem with encouraging – overtly or indirectly – middle-class 'exit' from public health services is of course, as stated above, the fact that their need to insure themselves to have their care provided in a more expensive private sector will create pressures for tax relief and tax reductions, which in turn might threaten the remaining public health services targeted, allegedly more effectively, at the poor. In consequence, maintaining universalism in a national health service whose international and national characteristic is efficiency as well as effectiveness is likely to be the most sensible policy.

In order to demonstrate value for money for all social groupings and classes from a publicly financed and publicly provided health service, a hypothecated health tax (whether or not contributions come in a tripartite manner from the individual, employer and the state, or whether it is simply financed from existing taxation sources, or even from a single tax earmarked for the health care system) may be an appropriate means of relating costs to benefits in health care. The danger of such an approach is that, like all direct and indirect taxes, allying the prospects for generous health care provision to revenue available from a particular tax may make fluctuations in health service spending greater than at present. In other words, during the downswing of the economic cycle, there is less money available – as fewer people are employed if direct taxation is used, or as less revenue is garnered from indirect taxation. If the NHS is financed from general revenues, it can perhaps be more easily protected, if it is seen as a priority, at the expense of other social programmes. Whether this is considered a good thing or not is a different question, but for defenders of the National Health Service, it is likely to be. That is, the smoke-filled room of the cabinet's Star Chamber may have its advantages, despite the often arbitrary nature of such centralized decision making.

PRIVATE FINANCE

Another significant trend is the growth in private care, or rather – to diagnose the trend at its source – the growth in private financing. As society becomes more unequal, even if the proportion of GDP going to public expenditure or the proportion within that going to health care does not diminish, what is 'left over' in private hands is to a greater extent in the hands of the better-off. In consequence, the growth in private care ought not to be a surprise. There is therefore nothing 'inevitable' about this phenomenon (as again some commentators have blandly assumed); it is in fact the (not always visible) result of a general redistribution of wealth. The consequence of such a trend for the public/private mix in health is not necessarily planned to evolve in this manner by conspiracy – but when it does so evolve, it becomes seemingly acceptable as a 'fact of life'.

CONCLUSION

This chapter has not sought to review in detail various options for financing health care. It has, however, reviewed briefly a spectrum of options ranging from the private to the public in financing health care, and has gone on to discuss the context in which such debates are likely to take place in the UK. As far as managers are concerned, an awareness of both financial trends and the broader debate about financing is important. The whole nature of the NHS, and the priorities it is able to address, is dependent upon the overall finance available; the sources of that finance (in that 'who pays' is likely to expect to call the tune to some extent); and the extent to which regional, district and other 'purchasing' managers have leeway in deciding upon priorities within the context of both overall finance and procedures for allocating resources to regions and districts. The next chapter considers some of the issues at stake in deciding upon priorities (what might crudely be called the 'rationing' debate) and asks who, at what level within the system, might be considered best placed to make various types of decisions.

DISCUSSION

- In considering options for health care financing, a variety of objectives ought to be taken into account. Firstly, the ability of a system to combine cost control and equity (both for patients and for staff) is important. This tends to argue for public finance and also public provision. Secondly, particular forms of public finance and public provision will vary from country to country, reflecting cultures and modes of organization.

- If there is no need for concern with either improving the basis for cost control or – more bluntly – with saving public money, then a **reimbursement** model may be more suitable. This simply means that services are planned on the basis of need – or even allowed to develop in a decentralized manner through access to the public purse for capital – and then providers are reimbursed in line with usage by patients, whether or not referred by a GP gatekeeper (as in the UK) or self-referred (as is

often the case in more open public systems such as Sweden). The essence of 'purchasing' is that reimbursement is considered too expensive.

- Fundamental motivation for a move from a 'reimbursement' model to a **'purchasing'** model is cost control. Subsidiary motives may include an attempt to control hospital doctors and to give more power to either general practitioners or the public or both. In practice, however, controlling providers directly through regulation (financial and otherwise) rather than institutionalizing a purchaser/provider split may be more effective and less costly. This is an area where close observation of the UK is now necessary.

- Mechanisms for ensuring that plans reflect need and public wishes, as well as value for money, are of course important. The question is, what is the best means of building such requirements into plans, and then paying providers in line with the workload generated by such plans?

  Arguing that the NHS 'reforms' represent a step forward on this agenda is now very common in the UK, but is often derived from facile assumptions or from no assumptions at all (i.e. simply from a trendy 'orthodoxy of the age'). This is because of more effective planning: one man's definition of purchasing may be by no means the same thing as creation of purchaser/provider splits and markets in provision.

- It is a truism that not all needs and wants in the field of welfare can be afforded, either by capitalist or socialist countries. Universalism **generally** in welfare policy may no longer be affordable. Health care is, however, a special case, in the laudable sense of that term.

  Firstly, it is likely that the British public are willing to spend more on health specifically than they are to pay taxes generally. As a result, a special 'health tax' may be possible without resort to general hypothecation in taxation (i.e. earmarking the money for public expenditure generally through specific spending taxes).

Next, universalism in health care financing and provision may guard against the phenomenon whereby 'a service for the poor is a poor service'.

Finally, if it is true that private provision and private financing are singly and together more expensive, a non-universal health care system will actually place more of a direct payment burden on the better-off, and will diminish the amount of money available through public financing for the less well-off, rather than increase it as the 'progressive' version of the argument for selectivity in public financing somewhat glibly argues.

REFERENCES

Galbraith, J. K. (1992) *The Culture of Contentment*, Sinclair-Stevenson, London.

PRIORITIES AND HARD CHOICES: TOWARDS OUTCOMES – HEALTH GAIN, DEMOCRACY OR BOTH?

3

INTRODUCTION

Before we even make a distinction between the terms 'rationing' and 'priorities', it is necessary to talk of the context in which hard choices have to be made. The more constrained total health budgets are, the more likely it is that some means of making hard choices will have to be considered and adopted. Naturally macroefficiency as well as microefficiency within health-care systems can influence how much can be done with the available money. However, once one has adjusted for such factors, it still remains the case that – in the UK – the relatively low percentage of the gross domestic product or gross national product (GNP) which we spend on health care means that hard choices (already being made) within the public health-care system (the NHS) have to be explored and arguably made more explicit.

Pressures on health-care systems, affecting the UK as other countries, naturally increase this effect. The ageing of the population (over different generational cycles), the availability of new medical techniques and therefore new 'needs' and demands, the fact that inflation appears to affect the medical care sector more than the economy as a whole and the development of new needs, including 'pandemics' such as AIDS, all lead to greater pressure on available resources for health care. Furthermore, in the UK, the legacy of the 1980s in terms of growing social inequality

and significant reductions in expenditure on other social programmes (such as housing and relief of poverty generally) mean that the NHS has to 'pick up the pieces' to a greater extent than in a age of full employment and greater social solidarity.

This is the overall social context, therefore, in which decisions as to priorities have to be taken. Once it has been decided how much total resource will be devoted to either health care *in toto* or to public health care provided through the National Health Service, it has to be decided what broad priorities should be met at the first claim on these resources. In practice, in the UK, this has been a matter for central government (lately acting through the NHS Management Executive within the Department of Health) and also, to a lesser extent, for health regions, which are increasingly accountable to the NHS Management Executive and to ministers. There is, however, still a role for district and other purchasers to decide which services and which categories of client within the population should 'have priority' where hard choices are necessary. It is a major question for the future as to what configurations of power between these relative levels within the system (national, regional and district) ought to be and indeed are likely to be according to different scenarios.

In this book, a distinction is drawn between priorities in the sense just described and rationing, which is defined as the procedure used, and choices made within such a procedure, to decide which clients and groups of clients should get what amount of care (if any at all) once it has been decided what service mix is to be offered. There is therefore a role for purchasers and/or planners in making decisions, in order to seek to mandate providers as to how to prioritize clients. At a lower level still, there is a significant role for decision makers within providing units – and especially, of course, doctors – in deciding which actual clients to deal with on a day-to-day basis.

It is bound to be a grey area as to whether it is the 'purchaser' or 'provider' who makes the latter type of decision (what might be termed the district and sub-district level rationing). It is unlikely that purchasers will either be able to, or wish to, stipulate exactly which patients shall be seen, under prevailing contracts made with providers. This would of course remove clinical freedom absolutely were it to be the case. A more likely – and developing – scenario is that, within the finance provided through the contracting process, providers decide who to treat and who not to treat. If purchasers are unhappy with the results of such decisions over time, tighter contracts (perhaps as a result of audit of one sort or another) may be made. We are currently, however, in uncharted water in the UK National Health Service, as far as this phenomenon is concerned.

CONTRACTING

One can distinguish between different types of contract in order to explore the point just made. Let us consider respectively block contracts, cost per volume contracts and cost per case contracts. A block contract leads to finance being provided for the provision of a particular service, with little or no quantification as to the number of patients to be treated (for example within the year, in an accident and emergency department or in a surgical department). Purchasers may express preferences as to priorities, in line with definitions and measurements of 'health gain' (to be discussed later). Nevertheless it will be up to providers as to who exactly is treated and who is not. We have already seen difficult decisions being made in 1992 and 1993, as non-urgent cases for treatment were denied attention until the new financial year as a result of unavailability of finance. The logic of the NHS reforms is that waiting lists and waiting times become a greater responsibility for the purchaser, who is in effect deciding what is done with the money, and which categories of patient the money is used for. In practice of course, especially under block contracts, providers have to decide on a day-to-day, week-to-week, and month-to-month basis within the financial year as to who is treated and who is not. And unless contracting becomes a much more purchaser-driven procedure, it will not just be which individual patients within particular specialties and even diagnosis are to be treated that is the real question for providers; it will also be which procedures, within specialties that have been funded, are to be given priority or formally rationed.

Therefore in practice waiting lists will be the joint responsibility of purchasers and providers. At the more 'macro' level they will be the responsibility of the purchaser. If a provider has a contract with a fixed amount of money attached to it, it is not his responsibility – given an ability to fulfil the contracts' assumptions about efficiency and so forth – if there are more patients waiting for treatment than can be met within available budgets. In practice, of course, such patients will be referred to providers by general practitioners (non-fundholding), and therefore will appear as a provider-based waiting list or will affect waiting times for different procedures offered by different providers.

As one moves to a cost per volume contract, one is stipulating through the contract an amount of money to do a specific quantity of work – with the implication (given cost per procedure assumptions and efficiency assumptions) that an identifiable number of patients per procedure (by and large) is to be treated. In this scenario, the purchaser takes greater responsibility for rationing. Certain 'types' of patient may have to be denied care – whether in any one financial year or as a result of a harder rationing which denies them care altogether on the National Health Service. When one moves to contracting by cost per case (generally in the realm of rarer, more complicated and more specialized procedures), then the responsibility is clearer to relate money to the individual patient. It is not therefore the responsibility of the provider – assuming the contract is fulfilled – to explain to the patient who is turned away why this is happening. At least that is the theory of the contracting/rationing philosophy underlying the NHS reforms. Nevertheless in practice, it may well be the responsibility of the provider to do such explanation. This is not least the case given the political environment within which the NHS is operating. Doctors and indeed managers and local providers may be unhappy at the greater responsibility they have in operational terms for turning people away, although the financial – and rationing responsibility – in fact lies with the purchaser. The intervention of the local press, the national press, or members of parliament and even ministers may well muddy such waters further.

CRITERIA FOR MAKING PRIORITIES AND FOR RATIONING

It has been pointed out quite legitimately that, if 'rationing' only applies to those who cannot exit into the private sector (i.e. the poorer), then it makes more sense to talk about denial of care rather than rationing. A classical system of rationing involves a distribution of scarce goods by political and administrative, rather than economic, means amongst the citizenry. This may mean in practice that all receive a little bit of everything, or that some get something and others get something else; or indeed that some get things and others get nothing (according to some criteria, one assumes, of need or desert). If, however, a 'rationed National Health Service' simply means that those who can afford to can turn to the private sector, then according to most criteria of equity (too broad a topic to discuss here), the rationing system is diluted.

It is interesting to note that the so called 'Oregon' approach to rationing, from the state of Oregon in the United States, runs into such ethical problems. It has been developed as a means of rationing care amongst citizens receiving public health care broadly on Medicaid, the programme for various categories of the poor in the United States. Others, covered by private insurance or other forms of finance for health care, may not have to have the same 'hard choices' made on their behalf. In the National Health Service, importing an Oregon-style form of rationing might meet less ethical objection if the rationing applied to everybody. Of course this will not be the case. And it is still possible that greater financing for health care to diminish the need for the 'cruel' side of rationing is an option that is rendered less evident as a result of an obsession with rationing. The finance for health care will never be limitless. That does not of course mean that the current level of financing is either inevitable or desirable, which is a separate debate.

Equally, one can improve 'productivity' to do more within available resources (Chapter 8), but there are clear dangers here which ought to obviate against glib assumptions of 'greater efficiency'. Recently, it has been argued that rationing is not (yet) necessary as there is still scope for more productivity, less hospital care, less 'follow up' for out-patients, fewer diagnostic tests – and, most centrally, less NHS spending on 'social care' (Roberts *et al.*, 1995). But this is only tenable if other agencies spend much more significantly on social care and 'after care'. Otherwise it is a ruthless and glib prescription.

Next, one can consider whether to ration by service or by citizenry. Two scenarios stand out here, in order to clarify the point. One can argue – on grounds of medical efficacy and other criteria to be discussed below – that certain services (and procedures within services) ought to be provided in a public health-care system and others ought not if funds are limited. That is rationing by service. Those who cannot get the procedure they wish publicly, of course, are likely to be able to 'go private' if they can afford to do so or if they wish to make the hard financial choices necessary to allow them to do so. Another scenario would ration, even in a public health-care system, according to ability to pay, as judged by level of income or some other criterion. It could be argued, that as long as a service is effective to some degree, it is more important that it is provided to those unlikely to be able to exit to the private sector rather than to 'ration it out' of the National Health Service. In other words one can envisage a scenario whereby – a progressive rather than conservative reasons – a form of means testing is introduced into the National Health Service. That would mean that, for the poor, virtually everything that was medically effective was available, whereas for others only certain categories of service were available, assuming resources were not able to do more than this. The political conundrum of course associated with such a scenario is that this would consist in a move to a non-universal National Health Service. This would therefore be significantly opposed by significant sectors of the left in politics, even if adopted for progressive reasons. This opposition would stem from reasons of ideology and sentiment, but also for harder-headed reasons. It could be argued that, to the extent the NHS becomes more clearly a 'service for the poor', it becomes a less politically universal as well

as less clinically universal social programme. In consequence, if politics and electoral majorities are dominated by the 'contented middle-class majority', then the finance available to a 'programme for the poor' would be whittled down significantly year by year and decade by decade. Pressures to reduce tax and also to ensure that Government expenditure was for the broad bulk of the citizenry or to involve significant benefit for the middle classes could undermine the effectiveness of such a service altogether. To this point can be added the more familiar argument that a universal service, covering all the population for most things, benefits from the articulate middle-class voice, and would suffer from a loss of that voice as a result of middle-class exit.

In practice if any form of hard choices, whether involving formal rationing or not, has to be made, it may be that a compromise is made between covering categories of citizens and categories of service as just described above. In other words, it may be possible to have a 'bias to the poor' without this being formalized or without the NHS formally becoming a non-universal health service. It is likely that covert rather than overt means of making such decision will be adopted by politicians. This is because seemingly socially desirable choices may ironically be more capable of being adopted if they are concealed somewhat from the public view. Another example makes this point clear: it may be thought desirable to shift priority to some extent from acute care to chronic care for socially disadvantaged groups. Although at the level of general aspiration this may be a popular policy, when it comes down to hard choices offered 'democratically' to the citizens, they may simply not choose to make such a shift a priority; it may be fiercely and vigorously opposed by sectional or even wider public interest. In consequence, if such a policy is to be achieved, it may have to be covertly!

METHODOLOGIES FOR RATIONING OR MAKING HARD CHOICES

THE QUALITY ADJUSTED LIFE YEAR (QALY)

The idea of the QALY was developed in the United States in the late 1970s. In the absence of a publicly financed, centrally directed health service in the United States, however, it has remained more of a research tool than a significant input into planning priority within the health-care system. This is to be expected, as formal rationing can only take place if there is a central body (central in this sense meaning national or district-based) which is capable of taking decisions over a significant amount of health service expenditure. The idea has been developed in the UK into a research programme, mostly at York University, which seeks to elucidate what the idea of a QALY might tell us about decision-making in the National Health Service under conditions of scarce resources.

The QALY is but one example of what might be called an outcome indicator. In other words, the argument runs, it is important to consider what outcome is obtainable from any particular health intervention or programme or interventions. Is a hip replacement worthwhile, or how worthwhile? Is a coronary artery bypass graft too expensive to be worth the candle, and how would one judge the answer to such a question? Is an anti-smoking campaign effective, let alone cost-effective?

Already it can be seen therefore that the QALY is an attempt to relate inputs to outcomes, and therefore brings us back to the basic definition of management terms at the beginning of Chapter 1. The most vehement defenders of the QALY argue that it can be a significant means for influencing the allocation of resources in the National Health Service. They argue that, since it considers outcomes and relates outcomes to costs, it is a more sensitive and effective means of allocating resources than broader measures of need which simply look at an absence of health

status, without considering the capacity of the health-care system as a whole to deal with such an absence of health status, on the one hand, or the ability of a specific indicator of an absence of health status (such as death rate) to shed any light on whether medical interventions to address that absence are effective or not, on the other hand.

It can therefore be seen that, because of current managerial preoccupation with 'health gain', the QALY is likely to figure prominently in any significant debate. What therefore in essence is the Quality Adjusted Life Year. We can consider each of the four words in the term QALY. The QALY seeks to measure how many years of life can be 'added' as a result of a medical intervention – hence the 'life' and 'year' in the title. However simply adding to life is hardly a comprehensive definition of the remit of a health-care system. It is necessary also to look at how medical intervention, even where it does not add to life or save life (and therefore prolong and add to life), can improve the quality of life – hence the 'quality adjustment' in the title.

One of the many important questions surrounding the concept of the QALY is how one trades off mortality against morbidity or, to put it another way, how one compares the importance of saving and adding to life with adding to the quality of life. This can take us into deep waters at the very beginning. For a start, what definition of health is one using – the absence of morbidity, or a more holistic and indeed social or political definition of health, such as that adopted by the World Health Organization? The latter definition crosses the boundary from the absence of any disease or morbidity to the capacity for fulfilment of all one's human faculties. It is a grey area, both philosophically and in practice, as to whether creating the conditions for humans to fulfil all their human aspirations, as a result of being healthy is any different from actually fulfilling these aspirations on their behalf. In other words, creating the capacity for freedom – to use an analogy – may involving creating the structures and 'political economy' of a particular definition of freedom. Is capitalism bad for your health? If so, should the WHO advocate its abolition?

But to return to the thorny question of how to define health outcomes and health gain in a more limited sense, value judgement will be necessary to decide the relative salience of life adding and quality adding. Many effective health procedures of course do both. The problem is that, notoriously, medical care interventions are not undertaken as a result of proper evaluation, using for example the Randomized Controlled Trial (RCT), a longitudinal survey of groups of patients or citizens, or a cross-sectional survey, which seeks to measure the effect of interventions on one population against the absence of such an effect on others. Many years after Archie Cochrane wrote *Effectiveness and Efficiency*, many medical interventions remain inexact or untested. This point can of course be overdone, as it frequently is by obsessed opponents of the medical profession. Medical science, like any science, develops by experiment, adjustment and improvement. In consequence, most doctors are capable of improving their practice by evaluating their work over time and seeking to change where necessary – a significant remit of medical audit, to be discussed in Part Two of this book.

Nevertheless the very development of outcome indicators may require both medical research (defined as the elucidation of clinically based hypotheses as to possible and actual outcomes) and also what might be termed 'audit research' (in other words the systematic use of audit in a scientific manner to evaluate the degree of attainment of outcomes). That said, what are some of the more specific issues in seeking to use the QALY (which again, it should be stressed, is but one measure of outcome)?

Firstly, there should be a traceable effect between a medical intervention and an outcome. In other words, if it is not possible to 'map back' a change in health status to a medical intervention as opposed to – hypothetically – any other cause or 'independent variable', then one cannot evaluate the salience or utility of the medical intervention. Statistical techniques may be able to help in this. One may be able to take large populations, and the data associated with them, in order to seek to trace the effect of different medical interventions and other changes upon health status, using multiple regression analysis, which seeks to disentangle the effects of different variables in producing the effect upon the 'dependent variable', i.e. the change in health status. Nevertheless, as a general warning the point stands.

Secondly, one can contrast the (relative) simplicity of saving or adding to life years with the question of quality. Quality by whose definition? There are a number of answers here, which may or may not all produce contradictory results. The Government might define the desiderata for a policy of health gain, according to its own criteria and 'scientific advice'. The scientific and medical community might – with great difficulty – come to a consensus on such matters. The population as a whole might be consulted through generalized opinion polling. The patient suffering from the morbidities in question might be consulted. Their relatives' views might be sought, not least when caring for the effects of ill health is the responsibility of these relatives. Economic decision makers might be consulted as to what type of health gain is most useful for increasing productivity in the economy.

Simply by listing these options, one can see that many thorny ethical and political, as well as technical, questions are raised. Patients are bound to emphasize the importance of improving quality in specialties with which they are most concerned, or dealing with diseases from which they suffer. Relatives will also have a 'biased' or 'partial' view. If one polls the whole citizenry, one may derive superficial answers – or if not superficial, answers that are not consistent in that (for example) procedure A may be preferred to procedure B, which may in turn be preferred to procedure C; yet procedure C may be preferred to procedure A. Polling healthy people about health priorities produces answers that may be as 'unreliable' as polling the sick people concerned. The agenda of politicians and Government decision-makers is bound to vary from the purely epidemiological! Finally, consulting industry about the health needs of the economy may make sense if one subscribes to a theory of human capital, which sees the human as a producer or nothing, but otherwise may be ethically very suspect.

To list these objections, or rather methodological problems, is not to be wholly pessimistic about the use of outcome indicators. After all, making hard choices necessitates considering who is to make them, and using which structures in what forum. Nonetheless it is important to realize that a lot of work has to be done in achieving social consensus as to how to use the QALY before it can be glibly incorporated into any informal decision-making procedure, let alone a more formal resource allocation formula.

Currently, even after the NHS reforms, resources for purchasing health care are allocated from the Department of Health to regions and down to district and GP fundholder purchasers on the criterion of morbidity, which is difficult to measure in itself. Since 1976, the NHS has used standardized mortality ratios (death rates, having controlled for the effect of the age structure of the population) as a means of finding a surrogate for morbidity – in that the two are thought, and justified by research to some extent, to be correlated. Other attempts to measure morbidity seek to measure it directly through interviews and access to medical and social data. Still other attempts seek to look at the effect of social factors upon creating hospital admissions and health-care use

generally, once one has controlled for differing availability (supply) of health care in different parts of the country in order to prevent such an exercise simply measuring what supply of health care currently exists rather that what might be 'legitimately demanded'.

Despite all the problems of these approaches, they have one advantage. By comparison with a specific outcome measure such as the QALY, they do not judge one need against another on the basis of a contentious criterion. They simply attempt to find a measure of need, and then allocate resources, which planners or purchasers can then use to address problems in their locality. It may be that a medical intervention to 'deal with' a high death rate in a particular specialty is not available or not refined. This does not, however, obviate the need to care for the morbidity, or early mortality with associated morbidity, caused by such problems. In other words, the remit of the National Health Service has traditionally been to care as well as to cure.

One can also mention the potential choice between prevention and cure (whether to deal with the same morbidity or to trade off prevention in one area against cure in another). Here the QALY may of course be of some help. One can look at the costs and outcomes of cure as opposed to the costs and outcomes of prevention, as for example with an anti-smoking campaign versus the costs and outcomes of dealing with smoking-related disease at the stage of cure, whether partial or non-existent.

What are sometimes called composite health indicators seek to measure the effect on total health status of populations of particular policies at the broad level or interventions at the more specific level. One can therefore begin to ask, through surveys or otherwise, what type of health gain is of most interest to the public. Here, however, there may be a clash between what the public wishes and what the experts define as the 'greatest' health gain.

Thirdly, QALYs have often been attacked for being 'ageist', for discriminating between the sexes (more contentiously) and for discriminating against the poor. If one is looking to maximize the number of life years saved, it is going to be less 'productive' to seek to cure old people, to put it bluntly. If one is seeking to maximize the gain to the economy, one is unlikely to give priority to the poorest or, especially, to the unemployed. It can with some degree of fairness be pointed out that this is a problem not with the QALY but with social structure and social policy. To put it somewhat whimsically, QALYs may be OK in Cuba! The point being made here is of course that, if society seeks to run its economy on the basis of a division of labour creating a particular income distribution and class of 'poor', then QALYs are reflecting rather than determining social choice.

Nevertheless, if the ethical remit of the National Health Service is considered to be to treat equally and humanely, the QALY operating in such a context may be ethically unacceptable to many people.

Fourthly, social views may colour seemingly objective 'opinion polling' on such matter. What if society is broadly homophobic, for example? It is unlikely, given both prejudices and genuine information about the causes of HIV and AIDS, that such diseases would receive priority in such a situation. It may be of course that questions are capable of being structured to prevent what has been termed 'health fascism' in the United States. For example, different stages of intervening to help HIV-positive or AIDS patients may be identified, with differing clinical and social utility. In other words, choice within a value system may be possible. Nevertheless this is likely to be a grey area, as has been discovered with the Oregon approach in the United States, to be discussed immediately below.

Fifthly, should one use the QALY to allocate resource generally or to make more informal decisions once resources have been allocated, either by the purchaser – or indeed by the provider – when deciding which groups of patient, or by the individual clinician when 'discriminating' between patients. It is here that the QALY may provide useful information, especially in the last category. Informal 'rationing' has been said to have been rampant in the NHS for many years now. Stories abound of the GP who fails to refer the 70-year-old lady with kidney malfunction on the grounds that 'I'm afraid there is not really very much we can do for you'.

Using QALYs to allocate resources formally, from the centre to regions and from regions to districts and GP fundholder purchasers, is not, in the present author's view, a viable policy. For a start, current inability to produce health gain or desired outcomes in terms of health status, may be simply a static snapshot. Such an approach would threaten the ability of new techniques and new specialties to develop that are capable – after significant research programmes and investment – of producing significant outcomes but currently seem 'ineffective' or expensive. Furthermore, if the remit of the National Health Service is to care as well as to cure, then a broad measure of need – rather than need capable of being effectively met in some technical manner – is likely to be most effective in allocating to aggregate populations on behalf of their health service requirements.

It is when one draws up league tables of health status which can be gained, and at what cost, that one may be able to provide useful information to individual clinicians and to providers – or even to purchasers who have a little bit of extra money to spend. For example if a district health authority has £500 000 extra to spend, how can it find out what health gain it might be able to achieve from different investment strategies? How many lives would an anti-smoking campaign costing

£200 000 be likely to save? How many coronary artery bypass grafts could be performed for the same amount of money? It is here that QALY research – while not eradicating the need to use value judgements – can be of particular interest and utility.

Sixthly, there are different techniques for gauging opinions as to the relative degree of 'worthwhileness' of different investment strategies. If one asks the public generally 'is enough spent on care for old people?', the answer is likely to be no. If one asks 'is it a scandal that acute units for neonatal care in Birmingham are being closed down as a result of the Governments cuts?', the answer is indeed likely to be yes! In other words one cannot gauge relative priorities, not least for the reason that the public, in most cases, do not have a scale of clear priorities in mind. When one refines the approach to consider, for example, visual analogue scales, one can seek to develop a capacity to think through relative priorities and then make taking such health-care decisions more democratic. Finally, there may be a significant trade-off, as already stated, between what the experts seek to achieve and what the public wants – in other words, if the public wants to choose medical priorities that do not, in the minds of the experts, create much health gain, is that the public's right? This is a classic science-versus-democracy issue. The answer may be that it is best to consult the public about choices between options that generate roughly the same degree of health gain as measured by research, by the least contentious assumptions possible (for example clear demonstration of life years saved, or clear demonstrations of what is meant by quality improvement). In other words, the experts can do the structuring of the question, and the scale of choice 'allowable', and the public can then make its choices. This seems a good point to move to consideration of the Oregon approach in the United States, which has been held to attempt such a procedure.

'THE OREGON FORMULA' – MODEL OR MUDDLE?

The innovation in US health care that has attracted most international attention is the 'Oregon Plan'. The Oregon Basic Health Services Plan was devised to address rising health-care costs (with an implication that there is a need for rationing) and a possible expansion of health care for the uninsured. The state of Oregon sought to expand Medicaid and life insurance to people without coverage (45 000 Oregon residents had no health coverage). The sting in the tail was the explicit decision not to cover some medical procedures – and to consult the public on what these should be. The plan sought to do five basic things:

- to extend medical eligibility from those people earning 50% of the income defined as the Federal Poverty Level to all those below the Federal Poverty Level;
- to set a public policy process for defining a basic health-care package for Medicaid clients;
- to mandate that all employers should provide universal health-care coverage for employees and their dependants at least equal to the coverage provided under the Medicaid programme;
- to establish an insurance pool for 'medically uninsurables';
- to protect providers against prosecution or civil liability for not providing services that the Oregon legislature had chosen not to fund.

As stated above, the idea was to cover more people for less. As in all public rationing procedures, there was a potential clash between expert technical judgements about which procedures best produce 'health gain' and consumer opinion – the two may not produce the same judgements. The first list of priorities produced under the 'Oregon formula' aroused criticism and was eventually rejected in the legislature. The Oregon

Health Service Commission had therefore redesigned the formula by February 1991.

It can be argued validly that rationing for the poor alone is inequitable, as it means denying care to the poor that is available through conventional medical insurance to the better-off. Furthermore, social choice as to health-care priorities may produce dubious ethical judgements, if not overtly reactionary judgements. 'Rationing' has become a buzz-word in international health care, and it is argued that where expectations outstrip resources it is inevitable. On the other hand, given the huge expenditure nationally on health care in the US, it is an open question as to whether the kind of rationing for public health care proposed by Oregon is necessary. Rationing may furthermore divert attention away from the need for redistribution and a genuine national health insurance policy.

The Oregon approach makes three assumptions:

- It is better to give everyone a basic package of benefits rather than to give fewer numbers a larger package of benefits.
- Explicit public rationing is better than implicit rationing (in the United States, of course, within the Medicaid programme as opposed to throughout society as a whole, where rationing occurs according to ability to pay).
- There should be a combination of 'experts'' opinions with democratic values making choices.

The Oregon Health Service Commission produced its first list of priorities in 1990. The commission comprised five doctors, four consumer representatives, a medical social worker and a public health nurse. The methodology used to develop the priorities was essentially one in the realm of cost-effectiveness. A total of 1600 treatments were evaluated as to both cost and 'outcome', drawing on both avoidance of death and extension of life and also quality of life, as in the QALY approach. Inevitably, such data is not wholly objective or scientific, and involve opinion and value.

The aim is to combine 'technocracy' with 'democracy' in that citizens who are not professionals are only expected to make 'hard choices' between conditions (or within groups of conditions) of roughly equivalent 'expert-defined' benefit.

The public protest following the production of the list of priorities was huge. A second list appeared in 1991. The second list was compiled after a series of community meetings and public hearings, as well as a telephone survey of randomly selected citizens. The list is interesting to note in this context that those consulted therefore were not those to be the 'objects' of the rationing experiment. It was to apply broadly to Medicaid patients who could not necessarily afford to get private health care, for procedures not available on Medicaid or in the new expanded Oregon basic health services plan for all citizens. In other words, those who could not augment what such a plan would offer from their own private income or through private insurance would be the ones to suffer. However the consultation of citizens generally led to the dubious ethical and political phenomenon whereby people were making choices for others that would not necessarily affect themselves. As in discussion around the QALY, using public meetings to allow opinions to be registered on broad priorities such as prevention versus definitions of quality versus ability to function may not produce coherent or stable results. Nevertheless, a lot of innovative work was done and 17 categories of care were ranked (Table 3.1).

When the broad categories of care had been ranked, 709 conditions were then ranked as to their cost and treatment effectiveness. As a result, it was eventually possible to list the top 10 and bottom 10 priorities in Oregon (Table 3.2)

How many of the procedures can be made available under the Oregon health services plan depends on the resources available:

Table 3.1 Health Services Commission priorities by categories (Source: adapted from Oregon Health Services Commission, Prioritization of Health Services, appendix G, pp. 11–12)

Disease-oriented	Rank	Health-oriented
Fatal conditions		
Treatment prevents death with		
Full recovery	1	
	2	Maternity and newborn care
Residual problems	3	
	4	Preventive care for children
Treatment extends life and improves quality of life	5	
	6	Reproductive services
Treatment gives comfort care	7	
	8	Preventive dental care
	9	Adult preventive care (I)
Non-fatal conditions		
Acute condition		
Treatment provides full cure	10	
Chronic condition		
Single treatment improves quality of life	11	
Acute condition		
Treatment achieves partial recovery	12	
Chronic condition		
Repeated treatments improve quality of life	13	
Acute, self-limiting condition		
Treatment speeds recovery	14	
	15	Infertility treatments
	16	Adult preventive care (II)
Fatal or neonatal conditions		
Treatments provide minimal or no improvement in length or quality of life	17	

Table 3.2 Health priorities in Oregon

Top 10	Bottom 10
• Pneumococcal pneumonia, other bacterial pneumonia, bronchopneumonia, influenza with pneumonia • Tuberculosis • Peritonitis • Foreign body in pharynx, larynx, trachea, bronchus, oesophagus • Appendix • Ruptured intestine • Hernia with obstruction or gangrene or both • The croup syndrome, acute laryngotracheitis • Acute orbital cellulitis • Ectopic pregnancy	• Gynaecomastia • Kidney cyst • Terminal HIV disease with less than 10% survival rate at 5 years (Note: treatment for earlier stages of HIV disease and comfort care for terminal stage are listed much higher in the list) • Chronic pancreatitis • Superficial wounds without infection and contusions • Constitutional aplastic anaemia • Prolapsed urethral mucosa • Extremely low birthweight babies (1–3 pounds) and under 23 weeks' gestation • Anencephaly and similar conditions in which a child is born without a brain

procedures above the line can be funded, when the line has been drawn according to the availability of resources, and procedures below the line cannot.

This is not the place to give a general 'policy' or political critique and discussion around the Oregon Plan. It can, however, be noted here that assigning priorities to medical interventions may not take into account individual circumstances. For example, to argue that 'kidney transplants are worthwhile' may not take into account different prognoses for different patients – again with the sting in the tail that social class may affect prospects.

ASSESSMENT

Both the QALY approach and the Oregon approach are attempts to rank outcomes according to effectiveness and cost, in the light of limited resources. To that extent, they may have much to contribute when considering – for example – how to deal with 'outliers'. That is, where a lot of money is being spend to produce virtually no health gain, as revealed by outcome/QALY research, it may be important to discontinue that expenditure in the light of more pressing priorities by broad social consensus. Likewise, something which could be extremely productive but which is not being funded and therefore does not raise huge ethical questions or which does not seem politically contentious, may be able to be funded at the expense of the former type of case. The fact remains, however, that the QALY and Oregon approaches, as examples of 'costed outcome' approaches, require significant refinement before any systematic as opposed to illustrative use can be made of them, let alone incorporating them into resource allocation procedures. The research is important. Data on outcomes, related data on cost, are instructive. It would however be naive to assume that the vast problems of public consultation, and public opinion revealed generally in the political and social arena, are somehow

avoided easily in the realm of hard choices in health care.

RATIONING – SOME POLICY AND MANAGEMENT CONSIDERATIONS

The word 'rationing' is currently much in vogue, not least because of the debate about the QALY in both the United States and the UK and the debate about the 'Oregon formula' (Strosberg *et al.*, 1992). Used in its pure sense, rationing would imply central decision-making as to priorities and their allocation through a public process to the whole citizenry. If 'rationing' is simply the making of choices within constrained public budgets while coexisting with the public health-care sector there is a flourishing private health-care sector, then 'rationing' may mean denial of care to the poor.

Whether we talk of rationing or simply the making of priorities, however, the key questions seem to be:

- determination of the health-care budget;
- priorities within that budget;
- specific modes of provision within those priorities;
- which categories of patients to receive such services;
- mechanisms for denying care where this is necessary, in a manner which is possible within the prevailing political system and political culture and also within the planning and management framework of the health service in question.

These various levels of rationing have to be taken at correspondingly various levels of planning and or management within any public health-care system. Some of the key questions arising must therefore be the following.

- How centralist should rationing decisions be?
- Is rationing to be done according to criteria of need as defined by experts (for example taking into account experts defin-

itions of 'health gain' defined as quantified improvements in health status for individuals classes or the nation as a whole)?

- Should such decisions be taken centrally or locally?
- Are citizens' or consumers' preferences to be taken into account, and if so what about any incompatibilities between such preferences and experts' definitions of health gain?
- Are consumers' preferences coherent in any case?
- How is formal rationing (for example by purchasers) to be reconciled with informal rationing by providers and indeed mechanisms for ensuring that those denied care are 'squeezed in ' through extracontractual referrals (in the new UK system) or simply by joining informal waiting lists decided by doctors who are not necessarily prepared to go along with purchasers' or indeed providers' managers' decisions?
- What if local variation in services provided (due to different decisions taken by different purchasers in different localities) occurs to such an extent that the concept of a 'national' health service breaks down? Will this be acceptable to the citizenry? Will citizens in one locality accept that they are denied service X (while admittedly, perhaps, having access to service Y unavailable elsewhere?). In other words, is it possible to ration by service as opposed to by person? Again, is local variation as opposed to centralism possible?
- If there is to be a significant rationing role for local purchasers, how acceptable is the current undemocratic constitution of purchasing health authorities?

It can quickly be seen that reconciling rationing (conceivably defined broadly as priority setting within available resources, as well as determination of the level of resource) with different options for giving the public a say in rationing decisions is an important challenge. There are different means by which the public can be given power in this realm, and these range from democratic representation through more informal consultation through local audit of desired priorities to formal mechanisms for consulting the public such as that undertaken in the Oregon formula. Furthermore detailed mechanisms for what are almost iterative forms of negotiating with the public can be devised, drawing on insights from service agreements developed by a number of local authorities. Another approach is to seek to establish a set of specific 'rights' to health care. The Patients' Charter in the UK allegedly does this, but in a somewhat vacuous form. The rights established are not enforceable. Furthermore the Patients' Charter deals by and large with rights to specific forms of quality in support service rather than establishing rights to specific forms of clinical care.

RATIONING – POLITICAL CONTROVERSY FOLLOWING THE NHS REFORMS

The whole issue of rationing has received much attention following the NHS reforms and the institution of a so-called 'internal market' involving a purchaser/provider split. At the time of writing this chapter, a number of significant claims have been made about refusal of treatment on the NHS, allegedly as a result of the incentives and behaviour created by the institution of an NHS market.

One particular case received significant prominence on 4 March 1993, when the *Guardian* devoted much of its front page to an allegation that 'patients were dying' through NHS market delays. This lead story was based on the discussion in a letter on page 21 of the same issue of the *Guardian* by a consultant cardiologist from St Bartholomew's Hospital in London. Thus issues raised in the claims and counterclaims around this episode provide a very useful peg upon which to hang a discussion of rationing pre- and post-

NHS-reform.

It is argued by some that, following the NHS reforms and the institution of a purchaser/provider split, providers (in particular hospitals) slow or stop treatment towards the financial year end because they have already exhausted the money made available by purchasers though contracts. In other words, only urgent cases, met from other budgets and for obvious political necessity, can be treated. Providers claim to have fulfilled their contracts, and have operated efficiently to do as much as they can. A consequence is that patients who are not technically 'emergencies' but who require relatively urgent – what might be termed semi-urgent – treatment, may be turned away. Some doctors and others therefore make the claim that patients are dying because their treatment has been delayed by the working of the NHS market.

Around this time, the Secretary of State for Health, Virginia Bottomley, confirmed that urgent cases must not be delayed, but instructed hospitals 'to pace their work to ensure an even pattern through the financial year'.

In the pre-reform NHS (before 1991, when the recommendations of the White Paper *Working for Patients* were implemented), there was not, of course, enough money to cover every referral without at least a delay, as represented by waiting lists and waiting times. Whether this is called rationing or not depends on one's definition. In the 'old system' health authorities were responsible for receiving allocation from central government via regions and then for providing services themselves. These services consisted in those offered by hospitals and other providers to their catchment populations, comprising both residents of the districts in question and those who came for treatment in the districts.

Shortages of finance meant that, towards the end of the financial year, providers in the old system might well be in financial diffi-

culty. The operation of the system, however, meant that they would do whatever they could to keep going, seeking extra cash where necessary. It was not the overt responsibility of the health authority as a purchaser to negotiate with a separate provider within its boundaries (or outwith its boundaries, for that matter) in order formally to deny treatment except to urgent cases owing to the absence of cash to provide further contracts.

In other words, the resource allocation formula used in the old system sought – albeit slowly and somewhat bureaucratically – to ensure that money followed flows of patients, as referred by general practitioners and others, without overt rationing by purchasers.

A basic argument for the NHS reforms was that providers would have an incentive to market themselves to purchasers, in order to do as much business as possible and therefore to benefit financially. The incentive for any efficient and entrepreneurial provider would therefore naturally be to do as much business as quickly and efficiently as possible. If the local purchasers were unable to provide extra contracts to do more business once the money from the initial contracts had been exhausted, providers would have an incentive to find other purchasers in order to 'keep going' through the financial year. In practice, given the ceiling on total amounts of money available for purchasing, hospitals and other providers have had in many cases to 'shut down', other than for emergencies in certain specialties, toward the end of the financial year. This is ironically analogous to the type of financial problem created in the old system, when extra workload by providers was allegedly not reimbursed. At the time of the NHS reforms, the Government claimed that this was because money was not allowed to follow the patient.

In the post-reform NHS, if the purchasing money is not adequate to fund all referrals or desired referrals, cases will have to be refused. In the old system, the responsibility lay with the provider. There was no formal rationing procedure; it was expected that the provider would cope. If the provider did not cope, waiting lists and waiting times grew, which was possible for semi-urgent cases. The logic of the new system is that the purchaser stipulates what can be done under existing contracts, or rather agrees such matters with the provider. Rationing is therefore a more overt responsibility in the new system, a responsibility held primarily by the purchaser. This does not of course obviate the fact that, in practice, it is the provider who will have to 'do the dirty work' of turning away patients. Naturally it is the front-line staff, the doctors in particular, who will have to decide which individual patients, as well as which categories of patients, will have to be turned away. The logic of this situation is therefore as described earlier in this chapter.

It is to be expected that doctors – as long as money is available in the financial year – will seek to treat all deserving cases, whether urgent semi-urgent or not. The incentives of the market are such that provider managers will seek to do whatever business they can as quickly as possible. Post-reform, therefore, the NHS appears more overtly to be suffering financial problems as a result of inadequate purchasing money – in other words the money does not follow the patient, post-referral, so much as the patient having to be referred where there is money.

The Secretary of State's instruction, in 1993, to hospitals to pace their work to ensure an even pattern through the financial year was therefore, ironically, an attempt to restore the behaviour of the pre-reform NHS, and an implicit instruction to ignore the allegedly desirable incentives of the internal market and post-reform NHS.

From a planning perspective, pacing work through the financial year makes sense. It is important to ensure that some money and resources generally are available to treat semi-urgent cases later in the year. In other words, the money should not have already been spent on less urgent cases earlier in the year. The problem with this approach, of course, is that the information cannot be available, without a 'crystal ball', that would allow doctors to identify patients whose conditions are stable, yet who may be at risk, and who – furthermore – have not yet presented but will be presenting later in the financial year!

The pre-reform NHS also suffered from this problem. If the provider had already spent the money on what retrospectively came to be seen as less urgent cases, the money still might not be available. What was different then was that there was a 'bias to treat'. In the new system, the purchaser/ provider split ensures that purchasers are adamant that no more money/contracts can be added. Providers therefore have to implement the purchaser's managerial/rationing decisions by turning away patients.

What the purchaser/provider split does achieve, in such a situation, is to highlight the gap between supply on the one hand and demand/need on the other hand. The more information becomes available as to how efficiently providers are operating and – for example – how many patients they are treating in given specialties under given types of contracting systems, the more such a gap can be identified.

Inevitably what are known as block contracts will dominate in certain large specialties. The block contract provides money for an unknown quantity of patients. To that extent, it is simply the cash limiting system of the pre-reform NHS under a new guise.

It seems likely at the time of writing that the reaction to such dilemmas will be to develop national guidelines, as the Secretary of State comes under pressure from such issues, to regulate how hospitals ought to behave in such situations. The formalities of the contracting process and the purchaser/provider split will constitute the language through which decisions are discussed. The reality, however, will be that a mix of local decision-making (through the 'market') and national political reaction will determine what happens. In other words, the rationing process inherent in the logic of the NHS reforms will be a partial process in practice.

A further consideration, drawing on the financial incentives created by the NHS reforms, is that both purchasers and providers – given financial constraints – will seek to minimize expensive work that prevents providers operating within the financial limits imposed by contracts. The ironical situation, therefore, is that, early in the financial year, providers will have an incentive to treat patients who provide 'performance indicators' suggesting high throughput and large numbers treated, but who do not lead to budget limits being broken. There is therefore a conceivable incentive to 'make' the money run out early. It is the more expensive semi-urgent cases later in the financial year which will therefore be difficult to afford within existing contracts.

PRIORITIES AND RATIONING – AN ASSESSMENT

At the broadest – and inevitably national – level, the main potential clash of priorities comes if a choice has to be made between expanding the 'high technology' and 'general acute/factory' medicine available, broadly in hospital, on the NHS, and so-called social priorities, such addressing the needs of the elderly and other groups requiring chronic care, mostly in the community. To the latter category one may wish to add the priorities of prevention and promotion rather than curative medicine. This is however a complicated area, and one may not wish to conflate the two non-acute 'priorities'. It has been argued that the institution of a purchaser/provider split enables new priorities to be forged by stronger purchasers. The evidence is, however, equivocal to say the least. It may be that purchasers come under pressure, from

GPs, patients and the marketing strategies of providers, to fund more acute medicine. In other words, the debate about who has greater power when a purchaser/provider split has been instituted – the purchaser or provider – is a complex one, which can be elucidated by drawing on economic and political theory as well as by observing trends in the post-reform NHS.

Chapter 4 considers these matters in further detail. For present purposes, it can be concluded that it is an open question as to what the longer-term priority of the NHS will be. Some commentators have argued that the NHS ought now to move away (relatively speaking) from acute medicine and address long neglected priorities in the 'community' and in 'prevention and promotion', identified since the 1960s in Government documents but never adequately quantified to receive attention.

Other commentators on the other hand argue that the 'core business' of the NHS is clinical medicine, and that 'social concerns' ought to be the responsibility of other agencies, if of anyone. This latter claim may not seem in tune with the rhetoric of 'healthy alliances' arguing that different agencies and purchasers (NHS districts, GP fundholders, local authority social services departments and others) ought to cooperate to identify global social need. This dichotomy reflects the different strands of policy that fall within what are known broadly as the 'NHS reforms'. Some of these strands stress the meeting of consumer demand/patient demand by efficient providers, which may lead to a greater acute bias. Other trends stress global needs assessment on behalf of resident populations.

In the absence of political consensus on the key priorities which should be addressed, such decisions will be difficult. Citizens are not clear in their own minds as to which priorities are to be chosen, as they themselves generally still feel that the NHS ought to be 'doing everything' within reason. This leads to an important distinction – between the citizen and the consumer. The priorities of the citizen as a reflecting member of society, not necessarily requiring health care at the present point in time, but seeking an intelligent viewpoint on future needs (not necessarily purely self-interested), may diverge sharply from the priorities of the consumer requiring a particular form of health or social care and unwilling or unable to accept that the NHS has somehow 'decided' that his/her need or demand is not a priority.

This is the sense in which general, national priorities feed down into more specific hard choices – what might be termed the realm of rationing. Can the public be consulted in this realm? Health authorities are increasingly seeking to consult their local publics – whether through sophisticated opinion surveys or through 'public meetings' – in order to determine local priorities. In the District Health Authority of City and Hackney, respondents to a questionnaire that asked respondents to list 16 health services on a scale ranging from essential to less essential ranked as the first priority what was in effect high-technology surgery. The problem was that what these people prioritized cannot necessarily be demonstrated to produce 'quality of life' or 'health gain'. The same people, however, – in a different part of the same questionnaire – emphasized quality of life rather than length of life. Unfortunately, public opinion is not 'transitive' (i.e. internally consistent).

The challenge therefore remains to develop more sophisticated testing of public opinion – both national and local – which will establish both broad priorities and consistent, more specific decisions within these priorities. But the dilemmas, both philosophical and practical, are huge. How can one prevent special interests dominating such debates? If they do not, how can one prevent 'superficial' decisions being registered by members of the public who are not thinking of the 'voice' that they would be exhibiting should more

specific needs hit them personally? There are a number of approaches to incorporating the public's views into decision-making, not all of which are compatible. The following list elucidates some of these:

- **More direct 'democratic' representation on purchasing health authorities**. This would seem to be appropriate if local purchasers are to have a greater voice in forming priorities. The NHS is now alleged to suffer from a 'democratic deficit', in which health authorities are 'business boards' yet have greater responsibility in making decisions with local implications.

- **General consultation** – it has already been noted that questionnaires and public meetings may raise as well as solve problems. More innovative schemes for using public opinion to 'agree' a set of core services to be funded by the NHS run into the fundamental problem that opinions vary; and that decision-making schemes will be arbitrary and/or majoritarian rather than consensual. Asking the public to make hypothetical choices is to pass the buck – or rather, to rephrase the question. Only individuals with purchasing power can decide – for example – to pay for, or insure for, cancer care based on a history of smoking. And individual insurance raises more problems than it solves.

- **Specific, direct decision-making by the public**. The problem with such 'referenda' is that they are likely to oversimplify complicated issues, or present simple 'either/or' choices which may be neither a full representation of the public's view nor consistent in the long term. It could be argued that rationing requires precision, but that the referendum is a blunt instrument. A 'rights' approach relating to specific types of health care could be identified and established, to ensure at least that rationing decisions were in line with such overall rights. The question still remains, of course, as to who would establish these rights. The Patients' Charter has failed to do so, in that it establishes, for example, that every citizen has the right to receive health care on the basis of clinical need regardless of ability to pay. This is not, however, an enforceable, empirical right. Currently, involvement of the courts in denial of care on the grounds of absence of resources rather than medical negligence or inefficiency is producing at the very best equivocal results. This is because there is no framework of rights, statutorily established, within which the courts are operating.

- **Service agreements** – following examples from local government, detailed local consultation, on an iterative and continuing basis, may establish priorities in a more sophisticated yet pragmatic manner than simple referenda or highly technical rationing schemes. On the other hand, the willingness of the public to invest the time to ensure that such an approach is representative of the whole community is only likely to be forthcoming if one is an optimist about participative democracy.

  Ironically, 'pragmatic' schemes to institutionalize rationing end up being utopian or inequitable, or both.

- **Market choice** – here the consumer decides: 'the consumer is always right'. In other words, neither experts nor purchasing health authorities decide what priorities are. To create such a market, one would, however, have to give vouchers to individuals – and in the absence of unlimited resources, the rationing decisions would therefore have to be made in order to allocate these vouchers! Furthermore, individuals would insure themselves, and the problems of private insurance would arise (inequity, the inefficiency of 'third party reimbursements' to private providers and the high cost of insurance against expensive or what the Americans

call 'catastrophic' health care. Markets generally operate by allowing those who have the purchasing resources to register their demands. The rationing occurs by price and ability to pay, rather than by regulation or waiting lists and times as in the NHS as currently understood. If (inevitably) direct consumer decisions are to be eschewed for decisions by purchasing authorities or by Government, consumers can only change priorities or increase the amount of money available from the health service by electing a new government, on the assumption that there is a correlation between a new government's policy at election time and what it does in practice. A further assumption is necessary: health is the salient situation that 'swings' the election – a very unlikely assumption in normal political circumstances.

Finally, both informal and formal systems of rationing are capable of subversion. Informally, local decision-makers such as doctors and both provider and purchaser managers do not necessarily take decisions according to 'scientific' or 'democratic' criteria. It is perhaps unreasonable to expect them to, acting under pressure to meet demand, within limited resources in the face of conflicting demands 'at their door'.

Formal rationing procedures can of course be subverted in a different manner. If some procedures are available on a National Health Service and others are not, treatment can simply be reclassified to allow (for example) doctors' priorities to continue to be chosen.

In conclusion, one may distinguish between ideal forms of rationing (whether formal or informal) and the emerging practice following the NHS reforms, which may or may not be ideal. The next chapter considers the main institutions and incentives created by the NHS reforms, and their likely effect upon health service decision-making.

DISCUSSION

- The need for rationing is another 'orthodoxy of the age'. There is obviously a need for the making of priorities in the public financing of health care. It may not, however, be the case that tackling of significant ill health is unaffordable from the public purse. There are questions of political will (and of course efficiency in provision) here, as well as 'inevitable economics'.

  Of course if societies and economies generally are getting absolutely or relatively poorer (as a result of increasingly internationally mobile capital, in an international capitalist economy), then hard choices may be necessary.

  Nevertheless the UK spends a relatively low percentage of its gross domestic product on health care and therefore an even lower percentage of its gross national product (i.e. the wealth produced in the UK's name throughout the world).

  Even taking into account the UK's relatively low GNP *per capita* by comparison with our west European neighbours, the UK still 'underspends'. Some of this is due to the efficiency of the National Health Service. Some of this is due to the low wages of British health workers. But some is simply a political choice, conscious or unconscious.

- It is sometimes argued that the UK is more 'in line' with such west European countries when one compares the amount spent publicly. However countries such as the Netherlands, which have a public–private mix stressing more private expenditure than in the UK, have a regulated system of financing that helps to determine the total percentage of GNP spent on health care. That is, private contributions are regulated according to income, to a greater or lesser extent. If the UK simply resorted to greater private finance without such a regulatory framework, increasing reliance on the private purse would be likely to diminish public spending – and the UK's total would not therefore rise. This gives the lie to those who advocate increasing the UK's health expenditure by relying on private finance. What is more, some countries spend much more, directly from the public purse. Although countries such as Sweden and other Nordic countries are facing financial problems in the 1990s, they start from much higher levels of public spending than the UK's.

- Methodologies for 'rationing' and prioritization vary. In the UK, arguments around the 'quality adjusted life year' tend to dominate. In the United States, the 'Oregon formula' has attracted attention. Both these methodologies stress individual health gain.

  Alternative methodologies developed in the Netherlands, and increasingly in the Nordic countries, are stressing wider definitions of health and social 'gain' – based, for example, upon one's ability to function as a member of the local community (i.e. a definition of health gain based on the European notion of solidarity as well as individualism).

  With this awareness, methodologies for allowing social participation in prioritization should be carefully considered. This is especially true in the UK where often dubious distinctions – for example, between health and social care – are being used in a tacit and hurried manner simply to cut public expenditure, without public consultation and in the context of a large degree of fatalism on the part of the British population.

- There is a real problem, of course, in financing comprehensive health care and adequate social care. Means testing of some of the latter may be inevitable, as for example recommended recently by the Commission for Social Justice.

  One of the practical problems stems

from the fact that NHS providers are not allowed to charge purchasers (whether public or private) and that therefore there is incentive to 'block beds' in hospitals when elderly people cannot be discharged to social care.

The recent obligations placed on local authorities (social services departments) by the NHS and Community Care Act, to ensure an appropriate placement of such individuals, compound the problem, especially when charters give rights to the individual not to be discharged until a chosen form of care is arranged (through a care plan). As a result, perverse incentives are set up.

It might be more sensible to ensure that an appropriate and adequate budget for social care is given to a purchaser who would then be able to reimburse **any** provider, such that a person in hospital no longer requiring medical care would have charges paid by the public purchaser (for example local government). The current problem with such a scenario is of course the inadequate funding for community care. This would need to be rectified if such a system were to work smoothly and not be discredited at the outset (as with aspects of the internal market and health care generally).

It is interesting to note that, in Sweden, municipalities (the lower tier of local government) in certain counties reimburse hospitals for social care (for example, for the elderly) and therefore have an incentive to transfer such individuals to more appropriate placements – whether in alternative forms of institutional care or in the community.

REFERENCES

Roberts, C. *et al.* (1995) Rationing is a desperate measure. *Health Service Journal*, **12 Jan**, 15.

Strosberg, M *et al.*, eds (1992) *Rationing America's Medical Care: The Oregon Plan and Beyond*, Brookings Institution, Washington DC.

THE PURCHASER/PROVIDER SPLIT AND PLANNING: FRAGMENTATION OR COHERENCE?

INTRODUCTION

This chapter considers the status of planning on the one hand and markets on the other, in health services, drawing briefly on both theory and examples from other countries in order to illustrate the current position in the National Health Service. The reasons for the 'NHS reforms' are by now quite well known (Paton, 1992; Butler, 1992). These are briefly summarized and the various trends associated with reform as it develops are outlined and explained where possible. Some future scenarios are sketched, which are basically concerned with different ways of reconciling global planning with appropriate incentives for provision in the National Health Service.

THEORETICAL PERSPECTIVES

It is important to analyse developments within the NHS from the perspective of policy analysis. From the present author's viewpoint, policy analysis draws primarily upon political science and microeconomics in order to understand both the rationale for quasi-markets and possible limitations upon the effective operation of quasi-markets within an NHS where an agenda which is both centralist and 'political' remains strong.

Microeconomics allows us to spell out the necessary conditions for a successful market. Some of these have been recently documented as a theoretical underpinning to the SAUS work on markets and quasi-markets (Le Grand and Bartlett, 1993) and comprise: appropriate market structures, such as competing providers and possibly competing purchasers; adequate information whereby providers can be monitored as to desired outcomes; appropriate motivation on the part of providers (on the principle that, through the invisible hand, 'private vice produces public good'); a situation whereby the costs of running markets ('transactions costs') rather than directly managing providers are under control and less in aggregate than the benefits of running markets; and – possibly – attention to equity (in a public sector market) such that patients/users/consumers are not disadvantaged as a result of inadequate finance or excessive need for health care by comparison with population averages.

The four fundamental characteristics of the NHS 'managed'-market can also be enumerated. They are as follows (again, a selective but salient list):

- the nature of regulation of providers;
- the fact the purchaser and user are distinct (respectively the agent and principal);
- the fact the service is globally cash limited;
- the fact that publicly defined rights must be incorporated into agreements between purchasers and providers.

Taking these in turn, the first characteristic implies that, if the regulation of providers prevents them from operating as 'profit-maximizing' or quasi-profit-maximizing institutions, then the benefits of market behaviour may ironically be lost. That is, the more 'altruistic' hospital and other self-governing trusts are, the less they may fulfil the criteria of the market's 'invisible hand'. (For example: teaching hospitals may have to eschew the benefits of marketing themselves obsessively to GP fundholders, but may suffer as a result). In essence, one may be left with neither the advantages of the market nor the advantages of coherent planning. A rationalized system may be impossible – and a comparison with the duplication and yet omission inherent in the US 'private by non-profit' hospital sector may well be an instructive one.

Furthermore, the nature of regulation of providers in the NHS – primarily of self-governing trusts in the near future – may affect the composition and nature of those trusts. It may be efficient for trusts to comprise both hospital and community units together – that is, to be comprehensive, all-embracing trusts, perhaps even embracing all the services of what was previously a health district. This would be 'efficient' if the total packages of patient care (for example, enabling 'seamless care' for particular clients who require both hospital and community services) can best be organized by a provider unit that maximizes its cost-effectiveness ratio by taking responsibility for all services.

Furthermore, a comprehensive trust will tend to avoid the problems of 'cost-shifting' between autonomous hospital trusts and autonomous community trusts. Otherwise these might seek to maximize contract income and minimize expenditure – possibly with the adverse effect that hospitals seek to 'dump' patients on to the community and *vice versa*.

On the other hand, in the pre-reform NHS, it often became a truism that hospital services swallowed-up the budgets of community services whenever hospital resources were stretched. Separate hospital community trusts

may be the best means of avoiding this. Ironically, directly accountable hospital and community services – but self-managed in an operational sense as separate provider units – may be the best means of ensuring the benefits of separation without the costs of separation.

From the present perspective it should be noted that the American health maintenance organization (HMO) operates through direct control of providers and integration of both hospital and non-hospital services into one organization. That is, the purchaser/provider split is diminished rather than increased by the operation of the health maintenance organization (although admittedly choice of purchaser – of HMO – financed either by individuals, their employers or by Government finance for the poor in the United States, exists as a counterweight to directly managed provision within the HMO).

The moot point for the purpose of the present argument is that the regulation of provision, according to political as well as economic criteria in the NHS, may mitigate the ability of trusts to be 'red in tooth and claw' and therefore to provide 'the public good from private vice'.

Regarding the second characteristic of the quasi-market, the fact that the purchaser and user are distinct may have a number of consequences. Firstly, providers may market themselves directly to users/consumers and to general practitioners (non-fundholding as well as fundholding) such that a 'political head of steam' is built up to mandate the provision of certain types of services. Purchasers may be then constrained in their choices, in the real world of a political NHS where local pressures may still be strong (although mediated now through national politicians and members of Parliament rather than through quasi-representative local health authorities). At the level of detail, the combination of this factor and the Government's defensiveness about the NHS reforms makes political interference – even in individual cases (for example, on waiting lists) – more rather than less frequent, in the post-reform NHS.

If the politics of the UK – as in so much of the 'advanced West' – is now governed by what John Kenneth Galbraith (1992) has called the values of the 'contented majority' and the 'culture of contentment', then such purchasing priorities, if so determined, may be those of the contented majority rather than the truly needy in society. That is, the discontented minority may have a raw deal if this dynamic operates in the reformed NHS. Another way of putting this is to say that the traditional argument that the NHS 'benefits the middle classes rather than the poor' maybe enhanced by a dynamic of provider power rather than purchaser power – ironically as a result of both the purchaser/provider split and the purchaser/user split in the new NHS.

Secondly, where this does not apply, purchasers may not reflect users' wishes unless a particular incentive is created for them to reflect local wishes rather than either central criteria or their own autonomous criteria. Again, the nature of regulation rather than the dictates of micro-economic theory may determine outcomes in this area.

Regarding the third characteristic, a cash-limited NHS may mean that competition by providers is competition 'to do more for the same money' – or indeed to do the same for less money, if public expenditure reviews and cuts bite in the future. That is, provider competition is a zero sum game. One provider's gain is another's loss. While this may still enable competition, it is difficult to see much of an incentive for maximizing income as a result of provision of innovative services as a result. In practice, 'squeezing providers' in this way may simply lead to greater technical productivity or efficiency at the expense of either more appropriate services or what economists would call allocative efficiency. At the very least, allocative efficiency will only be achieved in the context of greater exploitation of the NHS's workers.

It might be argued that this is an argument opposite in direction to that of my previous argument, concerning the 'autonomous provider', ironically empowered more in the post-reform NHS than in the pre-reform NHS, when providers allegedly 'did their own thing'. It is, however, possible to reconcile the two arguments. Providers can call the tune as regards priorities yet be forced to offer these priorities in a marketplace through greater productivity, due to limited finance. A further way of making the point is to say that money cannot follow the patient, but the patient must follow the contract and the money in order to ensure that referrals are kept within the NHS's available expenditure.

Regarding the fourth characteristic, one can distinguish between process rights and substantive rights. The Patients' Charter is an example of fairly minor 'process' rights whereby citizens are guaranteed certain types of treatment and providers. Purchasers therefore must be quite interventionist in dealing with providers – normally at the behest of central Government's priorities. The purchaser/provider split may be something of a myth in such circumstances. More importantly, substantive rights involve rights to specific forms of health care in specific locations. In order to guarantee these, again central regulation in alliance with local purchaser wishes (or rather a rendering compatible of the two by whatever means) may ensure that a social or political agenda prevents provider competition according to market principles. If certain services, for example, must be available and must be available in a certain locale, then the scope for provider competition is reduced to something considerably more marginal. A series of local monopolies – which would have to be heavily controlled by purchasers to prevent excessive provider power – might be the result of such regulation.

A number of specific consequences are likely to flow from such theoretical considerations, comprising the necessary conditions for markets and the specific characteristics of the NHS quasi-market. The rest of this chapter discusses some of these consequences.

BACKGROUND

The Prime Minister's review of the National Health Service was instituted in January 1988, by the then Prime Minister, Mrs Margaret Thatcher, during a television interview on *Panorama*. The motivation was to take issue with the persistent claim that the NHS was underfunded, and attempt to turn attention instead to efficiency in the provision of health services (Paton, 1992). An additional interpretation has stressed the role of the medical profession in challenging the overall amount of money going to the National Health Service. It has been argued that, as long as leading representative bodies of the medical profession were willing to work within whatever allocation was provided, the Government was willing to leave them largely to determine the cutting up of the cake in a role which was fairly autonomous of management. Nevertheless, this *quid pro quo* broke down, it is argued, as doctors began to challenge NHS financing at a political level and Mrs Thatcher in particular decided that if the informal bargain had been broken, then 'leaving the medical profession alone' would no longer apply either.

The story of how the Prime Minister's review reported in the form of the White Paper *Working for Patients*, which was then translated into the NHS (and Community Care) Act of 1990, is now a familiar one. The main planks of policy – at the political and strategic levels – flowing from the 1990 Act have included: the purchaser/provider split; the creation of self-governing trusts (opted-out units); the encouragement to a certain level (still undetermined) of fundholding by general practices; the agreeing of formal contracts (although not legal ones) between purchasers and providers; and a raft of less 'political' initiatives concerning areas such as medical audit, consultants' contracts, and so forth (Department of Health, 1989).

A question worth asking is, to what extent did the recommendations of the Prime Minister's review represent 'policy learning' from other countries or indeed from theories in the social sciences about either public management or the organization and provision of health services? The most obvious answer is that Professor Alain Enthoven from Stanford University had some considerable influence on the idea known as the 'internal market '. Enthoven had, in 1985, published a short book entitled *Reflections on the Management of the National Health Service*, in which he identified a number of barriers to efficiency in provision, which he termed 'gridlock' (Enthoven, 1985). The answer was to institute a system of direct charging between health authorities to ensure that, when patients were exported or imported, money followed the patient. At a more grandiose level, Enthoven considered that such a scheme might involve importing the idea of the health maintenance organization (HMO) to the UK. Therefore, both in the theory of the internal market (internal because it did not necessarily involve privatization, and was internal to the public sector) and in the practice of the health maintenance organization, there was 'policy learning' both from simple economic theory and from US practice.

This is in truth the extent of the influence of significant ideas or institutions from outside prevailing British practice. Earlier reviews (in 1981/82) had looked at the health-care systems of France and other west European countries in an attempt to ask whether a form of national health insurance would be either more efficient or more effective, and it had been unequivocally decided that it would not be. At the time of the Prime Minister's review in 1988/89, systematic reconnaissance of other health-care systems was not undertaken. This was quite deliberate, in that the Prime Minister's review was intended to be a cryptic exercise reporting by summer 1988 (it did in fact report at the beginning of February 1989). In line with Government practice of the day, it was less an exercise in widespread consultation than a mobilization of a quasi-practical agenda to conform with the prevailing ideology of the Government of the day. Those consulted were therefore people who were sympathetic to the Thatcher administration and made up the 'right-wing think tanks' such as the Adam Smith Institute, the Institute of Economic Affairs (Health Unit) and the Centre for Policy Studies. More formally, the Prime Minister's review committee included some advisers from business and the private insurance industry, as well as civil servants and ministers (Paton, 1992).

In terms of the new health authority and management relationships established following the NHS Act of 1990, the main trends were a move to more direct business-style health authorities rather than loosely quasi-representative health authorities, on the one hand, and a strengthening of general management – as had been instituted after the Griffiths inquiry of 1983 – on the other hand. In this regard, some 'policy learning' took place from, interestingly, New Zealand, where more radical ideas concerning 'the private management of the public service' had been under consideration and had subsequently been instituted. Indeed, in New Zealand's health-care system generally, more thoroughgoing privatization has subsequently occurred than in the UK.

Overall then the changes instituted in the British National Health Service followed a certain amount of market theory, although the extent to which this has survived the implementation of the reforms and the succession of the Thatcher administration by the Major administration is very much a question for debate (Paton, 1991). In essence, providers (whether hospitals or otherwise) were to 'market' themselves to purchasers, including health authorities, GP fundholders and (possibly) private purchasers as well.

It was understood at the time that an end to the 'localism' of the NHS, whereby most populations received their service 'on the doorstep', would be replaced by a system whereby travel to the most efficient (and possibly effective) form of care would occur. In practice, however, more localism has probably been stimulated by the NHS reforms, rather than less. Referrals now have to be sanctioned by managers from a purchasing budget, and providing services locally is generally considered more attractive. In the old system, referrals were made by general practitioners (without their own budgets) and a complicated formula reimbursed the care – although often there was not enough money to allow money to follow the patient quickly or adequately. In the new system, such referrals have to be sanctioned, and the consequence has been that, for example, purchasing health authorities from the shire counties around London will contract with local providers rather than sanctioning referrals to central London.

Part of the financial crisis confronting London's health services flows from this, although the movement of monies out of London due to the resource allocation formula is also significant.

THE PURCHASER/PROVIDER SPLIT: INSIGHTS FROM ABROAD?

The essence of a purchaser/provider split is to institute a system whereby the financing of health-care is separated from the provision. Obviously at one level this is an unavoidable truism. All health-care systems (whether public or private) consist of money to pay for services on the one hand and providers of services on the other hand. In the UK, due to both financing and provision being broadly public, the conflation of the two under the responsibility of the old-style health authority was a practical feature. In the early days of the implementation of the NHS reforms, it was believed that purchasers would be divorced from providers, and of course – to the extent that self-governing trusts are autonomous providers – this may be true. It is, however, interesting to note, on the theme of 'policy learning' from abroad, that the essence of the US health maintenance organization is to end the split between the financier and the provider, not accentuate it. The health maintenance organization in the United States has been a response to what economists would call 'the problem of the third-party payer'. This is the so-called problem that results from agreements being made between a provider and a consumer with a third party being left to pick up the bill. In the United States the third party is of course the insurance company or in some cases the employer, acting as 'in-house' insurer. The essence of the health maintenance organization is that a special type of insurance company is created whereby the financier directly employs or tightly contracts with the provider. In consequence, it is argued, both managerial and financial control can take place, and both providers and significant professionals (primarily doctors) can be given financial incentives to stay within the budget of the health maintenance organization or to help create a surplus (or a profit if the HMO is for-profit).

Thus in the UK a health maintenance organization would in theory consist in a health authority directly employing its providers – the antithesis of what has happened under the NHS reforms; and arguably this was a feature of the pre-reform NHS! What of course is true is that, in the United States, health maintenance organizations compete with traditional fee-for-service providers – where there is competition – in order to attract consumers. Thus, although there is not much competition by providers within (or contracting with) the HMO to compete for finance, there is competition to choose the

purchaser/financier. In the UK this is not the case.

In the Netherlands, health service reforms have been proposed – and partly implemented – which involve the creation both of provider markets and of purchaser markets (Dekker, 1987). In other words, providers are allegedly to compete for income from purchasers – insurance companies, merging with the non-profit) sick funds – on the basis of contracts similar to those in the UK. Additionally, however, purchasers are to compete for enrolment from the population, which is financed mostly through the Government national health insurance system (or more accurately the health tax system, organized through the payroll).

In the UK, if the consumer/patient does not like the decisions made by his purchasing health authority, there is nothing much to be done about it. In other words, any provider competition is to suit the desires of purchasing managers at purchasing health authority level, and the extent to which this is the result of democratic consultation with local population is a matter for the future. Some interesting experiments have already taken place. In the Netherlands, on the other hand, consumers can arguably move to a different purchaser if they are unhappy with their purchasers' practices or contracts. In practice this is still limited, and the reforms have not been implemented fully as proposed, on the grounds that an all-party coalition government has been developing – and reflecting the need for – political consensus. In the UK, on the other hand, the NHS reforms were the partisan creature of the Conservative government. Nevertheless, a pointer to the future in the Netherlands would argue that consumer choice of purchaser as well as purchaser choice of provider will be important.

In the UK, to the extent that GP fundholders develop as the linchpin of the new system rather than an optional extra wild card, it could be argued that choice by consumer/patient of GP fundholding practice is an exercise of consumer choice of purchaser. However, the development of GP fundholding has gone hand in hand with the development of large consortia of GP fund-holders, and local choice among rival purchasers – even were this model to become the linchpin of the system – would be unusual; the exception rather than the rule.

Furthermore, it can be argued that, in a tightly funded National Health Service as opposed to a more generously funded Dutch (public) health insurance system, choice of purchaser by consumer might in practice become choice of consumer by purchaser – whether at the margin or more generally. In other words, purchasers would seek to enrol those consumers less likely to make untenable financial demands on the system. Health maintenance organizations in the United States – as well as conventional insurers – have indulged in practices such as excluding medically or financially 'unviable' enrolees, subject to State law (which varies throughout the United States) as well as Federal law – which has in fact been loosened throughout the 1980s to allow such discrimination to a greater extent than envisaged in the 1970s when the HMO was less common but more widely discussed as a reforming element of the system.

THE NHS REFORMS IN THE FUTURE

The main problems and challenges which have emerged from the implementation of the NHS reforms may be summarized as follows:

1. To what extent should a rigid or significant purchaser/provider split be institutionalized, with minimal contact between purchasers and providers? This would be the rationale of creating an internal market whereby providers were free to market themselves without being regulated by either purchasers or 'the centre'. The other extreme position, somewhat against the original ideology behind the NHS reforms, is that

purchasers and providers 'live very closely together'. A phrase that has evolved in semi-official documents is that the relationship between purchaser and provider ought to be 'cosy'. Here, the conflict is between market logic on the one hand and the logic of a regulated public service on the other hand. The question is not just one at the level of theory or even of ideology. Taking a specific example: when it comes to quality assurance, or its subcomponent medical audit, should the purchaser be responsible for detailed regulation of the provider? It might be argued that only outcomes are of interest to the purchaser, and that it is the provider's business how quality assurance is done. On the other hand, one can look at private sector examples such as that of Marks and Spencer, which is very interventionist in terms of quality criteria relating to process as well as outcome for its suppliers. It can be argued that Marks and Spencer is a provider in the market place and the relationship with its subcontractors or subproviders is different to the relationship between a **purchaser** and provider. However the provider/subprovider link may have the same logic as the purchaser/provider link – especially in the National Health Service, where the purchaser is in a sense a 'provider' to the public. Admittedly the purchaser is using public money to buy on behalf of the public and is therefore a purchaser fair and square. The point, however, stands.

In practice, both district health authority purchasers and GP fundholders are being encouraged to set up stable relationships with providers. Otherwise the 'transactions costs' of permanent re-negotiation of contracts would be very high indeed, This is one of the areas that was relatively ignored in devising the logic of the NHS reforms. As a result, given the general nature of the prescriptions underlying the NHS reforms, the implementation process is in fact a policy-making process as well.

2. At a higher tier also, the degree of

purchaser/provider split to be allowed or encouraged is a moot point. Regions, which in many cases have been strengthened strategically while slimmed down functionally and numerically (and more recently, replaced by 'regional offices' of the Department of Health's NHS Executive), are responsible for the overall coordination of purchasing and resource allocation to purchasers – districts, consortia and GP fundholders. (After April 1996, allocations are from the centre to new 'health authorities'.) Institutions known as 'zonal outposts' were developed after 1991 to regulate self-governing trusts on the provider side, and the question therefore arises, how self-governing are trusts? The purchaser/provider split may be closed somewhat at the strategic level, just below the national level.

In consequence, purchasing decisions may be taken closely in coordination with provision decisions, and the purchaser/provider split may be an operational policy for encouraging efficient management by providers and tough commissioning by local purchasers, rather than a significant strategic plank of the NHS reforms. This is of course a grey area, and the final answer is not yet available. It is increasingly being realized that, in a supposedly 'anti-bureaucratic' reform, to strengthen the regional tier (while pretending to abolish it) and to create new bureaucracies may in fact make a nonsense of the original pretensions of the White Paper *Working for Patients*. Many regional offices, from 1994 onwards, have been promoting 'market meetings' between groups of purchasers, to ensure that one purchaser's plans do not adversely affect another's (or indeed adversely affect overall strategy). For example, one purchaser may seek to transfer services from hospital A to hospital B, to get the advantage of marginal cost pricing. Yet if another purchaser transfers **to** A – or **depends on** A – B's prices will go up, as a result of less activity and the same fixed costs. GP fundholders can equally upset the 'overall logic' of planned closures! Only

closures can lead to **overall** extra productivity. Otherwise, local purchasing may well produce a 'beggar my neighbour' situation.

3. Rationing decisions – or in some cases, decisions to deny care – have to be taken to some extent at a central level. Otherwise a series of mini 'national health services' emerges, and this is unacceptable in a political culture where a publicly funded health service is responsible to ministers, who in turn are responsible to Parliament – and in particular to the Public Accounts Committee, which has often been the most interventionist of the Commons committees supervising, and in particular planning new developments in the NHS. Niceties about purchaser/provider splits and devolution to 'agencies', as the NHS Management Executive is often seen as being (in part), often do not interest members of Parliament, as the theology to which they have to subscribe is rather different from the theology of devolved and discrete management in a public sector reorganized in the light of insights from the private sector.

Naturally there is scope for 'rationing' decisions to be taken at the local level, as districts and other commissioners undertake needs assessment and seek to form local priorities. Again, this is an area where resolution of the key issues will have to be made, but it seems at the moment that the national role will continue to be important.

4. The coordination of different purchasers – in particular GP fundholders with district health authority and consortia purchasers – poses a major challenge. The original ethos behind the purchaser/provider split was that the district health authority would undertake global 'needs assessment' on behalf of its resident population and commission services accordingly. GP fundholders have developed as a wild card – and a wilder and larger card than originally envisaged – and in many cases are making decisions as to priorities which are not in line with the decisions of district health authorities. This can have serious knock-on effects for providers, who may be

denied their marginal source of income, which makes all the difference between financial viability and financial failure, at an extreme. In other words, one may be talking 'marginally' in the language of economics, but the margin may be very wide indeed in the real world. This is especially the case if GP fundholding becomes more salient. One option is for GP fundholding to become the linchpin of the system, and recently fundholding has been both extended and differentiated into categories (from 'total fundholding' to small-scale funding) (NHS Executive, 1994). This, however, is likely to mean that, eventually, GP fundholders would become large consortia, and would in effect then become the agents of the new regulatory health authority under another name. In other words the poacher would have become the gamekeeper. The advantage of GP fundholding – promoting 'micro' innovation based on their 'nuisance value' to providers – would then be removed. On purely economic (as opposed to political or ideological) grounds, there seems little logic in such a move.

More likely – under any political party – is the increasing coordination of purchasing involving district health authorities, GP fundholders and family health service authorities (FHSAs) – and indeed DHAs and FHSAs are now being merged formally, with fundholders accountable to new, larger health authorities. Informal working relationships – also including local authorities' social services departments, for the purposes of community care – will also develop.

5. Concerning the constitutional and managerial relationships created under the aegis of the NHS reforms, 'policy learning' has primarily been from the private sector. 'Private-style' boards now run health authorities (and trusts). The management structures of health providers – and indeed purchasing health authorities – often mirror (in name at the very least) the structures of either private companies or public enterprises traditionally considered distinct from public services.

The latter change is one which is likely to be fairly long-lasting. Operational efficiency is the main goal. While adjustments may be made to the particular structures developed over time, there will be no return to the pre-general-management 'public administration' ethos, it seems. What does require to be done, however, is to incorporate a greater democracy into the management of commissioning, and arguably into the management of provision as well. Currently the NHS is widely believed to suffer from a 'democratic deficit'. Health authorities are no longer quasi-representative bodies, and the paradox for any government is that a removal of a democratic safety valve at the local level is likely to lead to greater centralization – as public unrest is focused at the centre in that local democratic institutions do not exist to handle or channel such issues.

REINVENTING PLANNING?

There is a view frequently expressed in some health service circles to the effect that 'planning is dead' and that those who advocate it are somehow embracing or retaining a philosophy or approach which has been rejected worldwide, not least in the former Eastern Europe. To the present author, simple assertion of such a view is naive. It fails to differentiate between many different types of planning. Furthermore it would be ironical if the National Health Service were to adopt the orthodoxy of the 1980s just as it is falling into disrepute elsewhere in the economy. It would, however, be familiar for the NHS to be 'one step behind', enthusiastically embracing yesterday's answer whether in the realm of political economy or managerial doctrine.

Let us distinguish between the following types of planning:

- **comprehensive planning,** including central determination of capital programmes and both mode and location of provision of health-care;

- **indicative planning**, which seeks to identify needs, identify trends in demand and supply and then seek to regulate or intervene to ensure that objectives are met (analogous to economy-wide indicative planning);
- **'Social Market' planning**, which seems to the present author to mean (given that it is a very loose and ambiguous phrase) one of the following three (not mutually exclusive) phenomena:
  - use of market mechanisms in provision yet public purchasing;
  - combination of market mechanisms and either regulation or planning;
  - the coexistence of a market economy generally with a relatively high-tax, high-welfare social sector, possibly including comprehensive planning in the health sector;
- **the planning of new developments** (such that, for example, central and regional responsibility for new hospitals coexists with the so-called 'internal market');
- **incremental planning**, whereby planning exists but is limited in its pretensions;
- **the planning of resource allocation**, whereby purchasers in the National Health Service are given specific allocations for a range of purposes, some of which are stipulated by 'planners';
- **relatively close coordination between purchasers and providers in the post-reform NHS**, for example, such that performance of providers is regulated or policed by both purchasers and possible government (through, for example, the House of Commons Public Accounts Committee as well as the Department of Health) to ensure that objectives are met.

This list is by no means exhaustive and is indeed illustrative rather than comprehensive. The aim is to point to the complexity of any debate about planning. To say that planning is dead is pretty meaningless, as well as potentially dangerous.

Some of the main challenges for 'the planning system' (in whatever institutional form) include the following:

- Mechanisms for deciding priorities generally. For example, some see the purchaser/provider split as a means for moving away from both 'provider capture' and an alleged bias to acute clinical care. Others, however, see the purchaser/provider split as a means of ensuring that the NHS concentrates on its alleged 'core business', which is defined as acute clinical care rather than social care. **It cannot be a means of doing both**, and in a public National Health Service it is reasonable to expect 'the planners' (whomsoever they may be) to make such strategic decisions prior to the placing of specific contracts by local purchasers.
- **A decision as to which tier of the National Health Service ought to be regulating purchasing, and with what degree of specificity**. For example, regions (albeit fewer) have been preserved in all but name and have indeed been strengthened to undertake this role. Providers' 'business plans' have to be created in the context of purchasing decisions. A rigid purchaser/provider split in this arena is not likely to be very helpful, at the level of efficiency, let alone ideology.
- **The coordination of purchasing, to ensure that priorities for health are tackled coherently within already tight budgets**, is a major planning challenge. Currently, district health authorities (or consortia formed from merged authorities), GP fundholders and FHSAs all have a purchasing role. Various proposals for coordinating these purchasers exist, both for formal mergers and for informal 'joint planning' (also including local authority purchasers in the case of community care).
- **Ensuring compatibility between GP fundholders' priorities and overall global health needs** (again, defined by

whomever) is a major priority for the UK.

- **The planning, or at least regulation, of the care mix to be offered by self-governing trusts** is an important challenge, as is the need to ensure that hospital trusts do not 'cost-shift' in order to unload a burden of care on to community trusts, and indeed *vice versa*. In this connection, the creation of unified hospital and community trusts has recently been discouraged, if not forbidden wholly; and this task is therefore rendered all the more necessary.

A CRITICAL VIEW OF MARKETS

Chapter 10 of this book considers resource allocation. Here it should be pointed out that the reconciliation of resource allocation on the one hand and planning on the other hand was considered a central challenge prior to the NHS reforms. There were good reasons for this. If resource allocation was the process by which allocations were made on behalf of populations to ensure equitable opportunity for access to health services on the basis of need, then planning was the means of translating that money into specific services to meet that need. This gave rise to debate about whether resource allocation ought to be formally related to plans for services (i.e. comprehensive planning) or whether comprehensive planning ought to be undertaken as a means of feeding into the resource allocation process itself.

Either way, ensuring that the criteria used in allocating resources (broadly the mobility of populations and various measures of 'need' – whether measured by standard figures such as death rates or by statistical calculations to trace the legitimate usage of health services in different parts of the country) were compatible with the criteria for actually planning the services to meet that need is self-evidently important. There is a danger that when resource allocation procedures are simplified for purely political reasons (as with the Government's response

to the RAWP review of 1988) or watered down altogether to suit other aspects of the political agenda – such as *ad hoc* allocations to GP fundholders – the result will be not only less appropriate allocations to 'purchasers' but also inadequate use of appropriate planning models. This is not least because appropriate planning models often require a supra-purchaser (i.e. regional) input. For example, prior to the Prime Minister's review of the NHS in 1988/89, some of the more innovative regions were undertaking exercises in 'regional strategic management', whereby some of the difficulties in simply using formulae to allocate resources to districts, and then expecting the districts to get on with it, were being addressed.

A significant irony here is that some of the problems with what became known as 'sub-regional RAWP' originated in the fact that district populations (at 250 000 on average) were too small to allow appropriate internal planning. The irony of course lies in the fact that now it is considered acceptable to allocate for purely political reasons to GP fundholders with only a few thousand patients.

Often the need for appropriate planning was not only the meeting of specific needs identified in the resource allocation formula and requiring transfer through to actual service provision but also the financing of flows from one district or region to another. The market is one answer to this problem, and to that extent the non-political (as opposed to the ideological) case for 'provider markets' and the internal market derives from the problems in using formulae to reimburse geographical districts but also from cross-boundary flows from one district to another, often at different implied costs for different patients. However the alternative planning models (of which 'regional strategic management' was merely one, practised briefly and embryonically in, for example, North West Thames and North Western Regions) sought a more integrated means of reconciling resource allocation and planning rather than simply saying 'let's allocate resources and then leave it up to local districts to get on with it' – albeit with a heavy dose of centralism in ordering districts what to purchase, for example, in order to meet the targets of *The Health of the Nation*! Instead, the alternative 'planning' approach was to model desired flows of patients (either by direct consultation of the public or through consultation of GPs), appropriate resource and cost assumptions and then appropriate locations and nature of services. This allowed direct control of provision by health authorities, yet not simply 'provider capture' whereby existing services and existing 'privileges' in hospitals were preserved. In other words it was 'purchasing and commissioning' at its most ambitious, although it is fair to say that the process was only beginning when it was overtaken by the political agenda of the NHS reforms.

Sophisticated models were also developed to allow the accurate estimate of catchment populations, to allow provider-based allocations to districts based on appropriate workloads to meet need, irrespective of where the patients flowed from. Actually the absence of contracting as we know it in the post-1991 NHS meant that the services thereby created and funded could not be guaranteed to serve the populations identified in the planning models as having the specific needs. This, however, applies to **any** system: the post-reform NHS cannot guarantee that purchasers purchase the appropriate services or, furthermore, that it is the particular subgroups of the population identified as most needy who benefit from such services. Formulae and mechanisms such as the market cannot guarantee adequate cultural and behavioural change where it is necessary.

What was promising about these models – which we can see with hindsight, following the NHS reforms – is that they sought to combine appropriate modelling of services based on populations' needs with the maintenance of free referral by general practitioners

and greater autonomy of clinical decision-making than in the post-reform NHS. Naturally there are arguments on both sides when it comes to 'planning' and 'markets' – but the intellectual argument, fruitful in the 1980s in the National Health Service, was hijacked by the political agenda of the NHS reforms. Most NHS managers in their 30s will not even have heard of such planning models and methodologies, and may be temporarily forgiven for thinking therefore that they are irrelevant! Indeed, even more astonishingly, many Directors of Finance in both purchasers and providers think that needs-based resource allocation began with *Working for Patients* in 1989 – and that 'weighted capitation' was born in a vacuum then. Such social amnesia may be useful to the Government, but it is not very helpful in promulgating liberal investigation of the most appropriate means of planning health services.

One important practical distinction between the market and planning as just described is that different means of handling the reconciliation of capital planning and revenue/reimbursement allocations are mandated. With the market, we have the phenomenon of 'capital charging' whereby trusts are supposedly businesses who go to their 'banker' (either the Department of Health or the region/regional office) to get capital based on their business plan (i.e. demonstration that they have income from purchasers). In practice, however, such capital charging is a bureaucratic exercise whereby purchasers themselves are given capital allocations in line with their intentions to fund specific providers. It is more of a paper exercise than a real motivation for efficiency.

Planning models, however, would argue that capital and revenue ought to be funded together – to the provider and not just to the purchaser. In other words, once needs-based service planning has been undertaken, capital and revenue will be allocated by the health authority to the provider. As a result of this, predicted referrals based on need will be taken into account in the revenue allocations. It may be said that this is not capable of predicting exact referrals – but of course neither is the current 'market' system, operating through block contracts and cost per volume contracts. Only cost per case reimbursement can give the provider exactly what is supplied in workload, and this is avoided by the Government of course on the grounds that it is too expensive. A full 'cost per case' NHS would expose the underfunding in the system.

The planning alternative cannot magically solve this problem either! What it can, however, do is make the process less bureaucratic (contrary to much pro-market rhetoric) and also perhaps build in an incentive for efficiency or extra productivity, whereby 'top-up' payments are available for provider units that do more work than expected. In a cash-limited system, such top-up payments would have to be a relatively small part of the system – and would be the analogy for reimbursed extracontractual referrals in the market system. The simplification and diminution of bureaucracy is important at a policy level as well as in saving management costs: there simply is not enough money in the National Health Service to allow the luxury of competing providers shopping around their 'bankers' for capital in order to compete and either succeed or fail. The money has to be targeted through a surreptitious if not an overt planning process – otherwise it is wasted through a process of winners and losers. That is why the capital charging policy is in fact a centralist and bureaucratic policy rather than a lubrication for a market.

The main challenges confronting the NHS involve some 'policy learning'. The word 'market' has increasingly been used in European as well as British health-care, and specific lessons of relevance to the UK may be learned from the Netherlands (where competition between purchasers for clients and between providers for contracts from purchasers are both major objectives, although not guaranteed to be realized, in the evolving Dutch health-care system); and from Sweden where 'public markets' (Saltman and von Otter, 1992) tend to refer simply to money following the patient rather than competitive or private-sector-style markets; and from various other countries seeking to control costs while increasing consumer choice. The heyday of the market in the United States was the early and mid-1980s, when it was alleged that rationalization of the health-care system through market discipline was an alternative to the allegedly discredited planning of the 1970s. This idea itself was, however, discredited with the setting of the Reaganite sun.

The flaws of the market approach are increasingly apparent in the UK. The next part of the chapter points to these.

On 21 December 1994, the Department of Health published its new rules for the NHS market (NHS Executive, 1994). The document, *Local Freedoms, National Responsibilities*, is at heart an attempt to use the power of the state to guarantee an adequately competitive market. It is also (and this is something different) an attempt to ensure that the market does not work too well (Robinson, 1994)! In other words, instability caused by market forces is also to be monitored and regulated.

It is hoped that these new rules will (in the words of Alan Langlands, NHS Chief Executive) 'reduce uncertainty and encourage further innovation and initiative'. In themselves, the new rules reflect a 'pro-competitive' neo-classical economist's approach to market forces. No doubt borrowing on theory used in the UK by the Monopolies and Mergers Commission (in its heyday) and in America by anti-trust (anti-monopoly) legislation, the idea is to stimulate competition where it does not exist.

The new approach can be interpreted in different ways – and often by the same commentators! For example, in reporting the unveiling of the new rules, the *Guardian*

(13.12.94; p. 2) entitled its report 'New NHS rules to encourage market forces'. Yet the text underneath the subheading states that 'the moves signal a determination by ministers to keep the NHS market in check'.

This is not confused journalism so much as a reflection of the nature of such rules. For the nature of the health-care (and especially hospital) market is such that attempts to make it more 'competitive' may be even more regulatory than planning systems.

Add to this the fact that other thrusts of Government policy are to rein in the market rather than make it more competitive, and you have the irony that – despite the pro-competitive goodwill of the authors of the new rules – attempts at reducing uncertainty may in fact produce the opposite. Let me illustrate.

An important and growing trend in many NHS regions is towards the promotion of euphemistically entitled 'market meetings', whereby purchasers are brought together to render their plans consistent, and subsequently providers are apprised of the consequences of future purchasing decisions.

In essence, this is a means whereby regions can (euphemism again) 'manage the market'. In reality, there is more management than market – as the first half of the oxymoron takes over.

Next, an important thrust of Government policy (and an essential one, as pointed out by Philip Hunt, Director of NAHAT, in his response to the new document) is to ensure appropriate cooperation between trusts – both hospital/hospital and hospital/community. Without the former, specialist services may be undermined (to name but one problem); and without the latter, locally seamless services may be rendered impossible as hospital and community trusts compete for contracts rather than collaborate. (Ironically the latter form of competition is being officially encouraged, through yet another policy strand.)

So even if the new set of rules is internally consistent, it may run into conflict with other central planks of policy.

But is the new approach internally consistent? At one level, yes – the new approach reflects a tacit recognition that (in health services to an even greater extent than in other sectors of the economy) competitive markets do not occur naturally and have to be constantly stimulated and re-stimulated.

At another level however, no – for the new approach reflects the limitations of competitive market theory in itself. Most markets, and certainly the hospital market, have an inbuilt tendency to monopoly: even if there is adequate competition in the short run, the winners have a tendency to put their rivals out of business or to take them over (sometimes euphemistically known as 'merger'). As a result short-term competition leads to long-term monopoly or oligopoly (domination of the market by the few).

At this point the pro-competitive analyst would argue that intervention is necessary (by some kind of regulatory agency) to reassert the competitive content of the market. As well as being extremely costly, however, such a regulatory approach may subvert other desirable policy objectives. Are we now saying that those providers who 'win' in the market place do not deserve to? Are we saying that a large market share – surely what is supposed to motivate your average 'competitive' hospital – is to be regulated away as soon as it is achieved? Are we saying that, although the Government has the objective of closing huge quantities of hospital beds and hospitals themselves over the next few years, surplus beds are to be maintained by the stroke of the regulatory pen in order to allow the theoretical existence of a competitive market in each locality?

Is normal market behaviour to be discouraged – for example, loss-leading in order to gain long term advantage; or generation of surplus through a pricing policy geared to protecting vulnerable or specialist services – or is this 'unjustifiable support of inefficient heath units', to quote the new rules?

At the end of the day it is a question of horses for courses – and a more radical criticism of the new 'market rules' is that they are seeking to flog a dying horse over increasingly complex fences at the end of a tiring race. A more fundamental question would ask: when the market has a persistent tendency to break down, why not acknowledge that there is a more appropriate means of allocating resources to health-care providers than maintaining an ideological or naive adherence to the concept of the competitive market and therefore being forced to 'intervene before breakfast, before lunch, before dinner, and then before breakfast again the next day' (to paraphrase Michael Heseltine).

If the aim is to ensure appropriate prices, 'market share' and local provision of services, then a planning mechanism that takes account of local choice and appropriate costs is the more direct means of achieving desirable objectives. Indeed, the perfectly planned market and the perfect planning system may appear as ideological or theoretical opposites, but may indeed involve similar 'planning' – with the exception that the former (the market route) is ironically more bureaucratic in its attempt to combine 'local freedoms with national responsibilities'.

The theory of the 'quasi-market' (and the research behind the new approach reflects the belief of its authors in the quasi-market) is often misunderstood as an attempt to restrict the market in pursuit of public objectives within the public sector. But quasi-market theory is in fact an attempt to make the market work in the public sector, where it has a tendency to break down if left to its own devices. Thus a pure quasi-market is a system for regulating competitive forces into existence in the public sector. Of course in practice, there are both public objectives and politically motivated interventions. Thus the new rules stipulate how central NHS Executive intervention will be triggered when trusts face unplanned losses, planned losses

and so forth. In a properly functioning market, the question would arise, why on earth should politically directed managers intervene simply because trusts face unplanned losses? – this is the market working!

And perhaps this is the greatest condemnation of the new framework. It has been designed by well-intentioned micro-economists who incredibly seem to assume that senior politicians and central managers will obey the new framework for its own sake. In practice it will of course be gerrymandered and manipulated in order to achieve politicians' objectives for the health service. For politicians, the NHS market is increasingly **a means to an end**, while this new document assumes that it is **an end in itself.**

What is the point of obsessive regulation to create or maintain a competitive market, when cooperation and strategic planning for the future are what the doctor should really be ordering? If the aim is to rationalize the hospital service and provide the appropriate facilities in the appropriate localities, what on earth is the point of then condemning such desirable arrangements on the altar of a pristine theory with little relevance to the National Health Service – namely, the theory that there ought to be expensively maintained competition to 'threaten' these appropriately located services?

The privatization of the railways was once memorably described by a Conservative MP as 'a poll tax on wheels' in terms of its popularity with the public. One can see alarming analogies between the destruction of a once fine national railway network through market dogma and the undermining of a once fine National Health Service likewise. It is an irony that, just as the Government was playing down market rhetoric and seeking in effect to plan the future of the health service, this report (commissioned many political moons, i.e. 2 years, before!) would lead to more flogging of the poor old dying horse. And if as a result the Government had made a rod for its own back, it had only itself-to blame – for it simply cannot decide which approach to follow, and this reflected the deeper vacuum in Conservative policy-making brought about by ideological conflict and a weak leadership.

This is not just a party political point. In other sectors of the economy, if markets are not adequately competitive and yet provision is private, regulation of private monopoly is necessary. It may not be **possible** simply to create more competition rather than regulate the prices of existing providers. And this is fundamentally the situation confronting the National Health Service: it is simply not efficient and sometimes not even possible to recreate competitors for successful hospitals, competitors which recently lost their place in the market. Instead it is necessary to accept the existing configuration of providers and regulate their prices. The debate elsewhere in the economy, in such situations, concerns whether it is better to regulate private provision or plan public provision. In the NHS, however, we are currently obsessed with being seen to produce an almost fictitious competition – which ironically has been rendered difficult by the operation of the market.

A real competitive market – of transparent prices derived under conditions of supply and demand – would mean providers saying to purchasers, 'here's the price – how much do you want?' Yet the NHS 'market' means purchasers saying to providers, 'here's the amount we want (we think): give it to us, for this total money, or we'll go elsewhere (if we can).'

Copying American anti-monopoly policy may be very naive indeed: such policy is often devised for relatively competitive and private sectors of the economy where sharp practice rather than the natural characteristics of the sector in question have prevented competitive forces from holding sway. And just as fundamentally, such policy only applies to the for-profit sector.

American hospitals have often been immune from such anti-monopoly policy (anti-trust legislation), simply because they are in the main non-profit institutions. If it is true that NHS trusts are not only non-profit but public (as the Government never tires of claiming), then a regulatory pro-competitive policy is simply inappropriate. Where hospital A is more appropriate for the provision of local services than say hospital B or C, let us accept that fact, plan the services and control costs through performance management – not through a rigmarole which is not only bureaucratic and expensive but sends confusing signals to providers. Are providers intended to compete for market advantage when that market advantage is to be regulated away?

The new rules would allegedly check abuses such as trusts sharing out the market in a collusive manner. Yet competing rather than colluding is likely in the long run to lead to winners and losers, and greater concentration of market share in fewer trusts. This is more likely to lead to 'price-fixing' (another abuse listed in the new rules), as the surviving and powerful few have more power over purchasers. And incidentally, what if choice of providers by purchasers leads to too much concentration in the market place, according to the new rules? Many regions are mandating such concentration, on the grounds of economies of scale and value for money, and are encouraging local purchasers to coordinate their activities to this end. That is, the dependence of the new 'pro-competitive' approach upon decentralizing purchasing (Le Grand, 1994) is neither possible nor desirable!

The political consequence of the regulations, allied to existing policy, is likely to be use of market rhetoric to justify closures of 'inefficient health units' and concentration of services, despite the fact that pro-competitive policy would argue against this. This is because of the fundamental economic fact that competition in the short run leads to monopoly in the long run. But we will have to wait longer, it seems, before the limitations of market forces are recognized in theory as well as in practice. To that extent, the new pro-competitive rules are a throwback to the naiveté of the early days of the NHS reforms.

DISCUSSION

- When discussing the 'purchaser/provider split', it is as well to be clear about what is meant. Any health-care system, whether public or private, has a mechanism for deciding when new facilities will be developed, when existing facilities will be used differently and when closures or reductions in capacity will be made. In a public system this is done through a planning process. In a private system it is done through a variety of means, including signals in the marketplace.

- Considering public planning, one can compare a good stereotype with a bad stereotype. The bad stereotype leads to the planning of facilities without adequate reference to need, without adequate involvement of key decision makers such as GPs and the public, or both. This concerns the **creation** of facilities.

  Regarding the **use** of facilities, the bad stereotype points to insensitive provision with one or more of the following: inappropriate services, inadequate quality or poor outcomes of services and poor cost-effectiveness. The good stereotype is naturally the reverse of the above.

  Before considering the NHS 'reforms' or any alternative means of financing and providing health-care, one can consider the best means of approaching the good stereotype.

  This would involve a sensitive planning process involving the right people; appropriate finance for the provision that such a planning process decided upon; and then appropriate reimbursement for these providers. The latter two elements may correspond roughly to capital planning

and revenue reimbursement. In the post-reform NHS, all of these processes are often subsumed under the title 'purchasing'.

- The key challenge in planning is to combine appropriate centralism with appropriate decentralization. Specialized services require relatively more central planning; relatively low-capital, low-technology services may benefit from more localized planning/purchasing. Appropriate planning will concern not only the nature of the service but the desired location of the service – or at least constraints upon service location. Appropriate choices should be made here before the use or otherwise of a market mechanism is contemplated. Otherwise a market mechanism may mean inappropriate resources devoted to making inappropriate choices.

- Any service planning or capital planning process within limited resources will mean that a trade-off between the desires of individual patients and either 'value for money' or cost effectiveness will sometimes be necessary. To put it bluntly, plans will not simply replicate every imaginable patient flow but will seek to steer these flows as well. The question arises, what is the best mechanism for so doing?

- If the health-care system is public, as with the NHS, even a market mechanism necessitates the planning of facilities, which are then used as marketplace providers.

  It is in the later phase of revenue reimbursement that the use or otherwise of a market is relevant. Once an appropriate configuration of services is created (which may of course involve a transitional or short-term market, which is something completely different), it is likely that contestability will be more efficient than actual market competition or repeated competitive tendering for services. The transactions costs of the latter, as well as the uncertainty for service providers, make this more than likely. The extent to which contestability simply becomes another form of performance management to meet agreed cost and quality standards is, of course, a very real one.

- The million dollar question then arises: how can providers (appropriately chosen, as above) be rewarded appropriately for the appropriate work and workload?

Without the need for increasing financial constraint, reimbursement of providers' workload – subject to efficiency guarantees – is the obvious route. In other words, GPs and patients are allowed to refer and self-refer, and providers are reimbursed. Something resembling this has occurred in Sweden until very recently – and is not a symptom of inefficiency so much as generosity in health service funding.

With cost limitations, it is likely that a mix of reimbursement and prospective contract will determine a provider's income. This, however, sets up perverse incentives. If, for example, emergency care is provided through automatic reimbursement yet non-emergency care is subject to cash-limited contracts (whether block or otherwise), then there will be an incentive to 'shift' patients and therefore costs into emergency services. This has been a significant phenomenon in the UK in 1994.

- In consequence, planning appropriate workload for providers based on desired referral patterns (within available resources) is a prerequisite of effective long-term planning. Extra reimbursement for hospitals that face unpredictable workload or for providing incentives to hospitals to do more at the margin is also desirable. To this extent it makes sense to have a 'reimbursement add-on' to prospectively contracted care. The main distinction between this and simply subsidizing inefficiency is that techniques of performance management ought to be used to ensure that the appropriate

providers are rewarded.

- This is all in fact a far cry from the mechanisms created by the NHS reforms. For in essence the system just outlined suggests a sensitive planning process; appropriate flows of capital and revenue to the providers chosen by that planning process; an appropriate mix of prospective contracting and reimbursement; and the accountability of such providers, through systems of performance management to their purchasers. This is not a purchaser/provider split so much as a purchaser/provider distinction. And furthermore this is only a market, if at all, at the edges.

If purchasing, reimbursement and accountability of providers to purchasers are to be jointly achieved, it is important to claim that more 'activist' planning (*via* what is now called purchasing) as the most positive outcome associated with the NHS reforms (although not with the market). This basically concerns the more effective commissioning of services – not just with regard to type and location, but with regard to quality and 'user-friendliness'.

While in many cases the operation of the market has led to more inappropriate services rather than more appropriate services, activist planning can actually involve providers. For example, hospitals can discuss innovations in service delivery with general practitioners, who can then advise the purchasers as to appropriate investment for the future.

It is important, within such a scenario, to avoid the duplication and waste of autonomous business planning respectively by providers and purchasers. On the other hand, it is often the provider who has the knowledge and ideas to interest general practitioners and therefore purchasers. An integrated planning system recognizing the respective roles of each is the best means to proceed, rather than resorting to the pretence of a market. There is no reason why such a process cannot be collaborative rather than competitive.

ACKNOWLEDGEMENTS

I would like to thank the School for Advanced Urban Studies for allowing me to draw on my chapter in their book Bartlett, W., Le Grand, J. and Wilson, D. (1994) *Quasi-Markets in the Welfare State*, School for Advanced Urban Studies, London. I also thank the *Health Service Journal* for allowing me to use an amended form of my article (in the concluding part of this chapter), 'Contriving Competition'.

REFERENCES

Butler, J. (1992) *Patients, Policies and Politics*, Open University Press, Buckingham.

Dekker, A. (1987) *Commissie Struktuur en Financiering*, Staatsdrukkerij, The Hague.

Department of Health (1989), Working for patients, *Cmnd 555*, HMSO, London.

Enthoven, A. (1985) *Reflections on the Management of the National Health Service*, NPHT, London.

Galbraith, J. K. (1992) *The Culture of Contentment*, Sinclair-Stevenson, London.

Le Grand, J. (1994) Internal market rules OK. *British Medical Journal*, 309, 1596.

Le Grand, J. and Bartlett, W. (1993) *Quasi-Markets in the Public Sector*, Macmillan, London.

NHS Executive (1995) *Towards a Primary Care-Led NHS* (EL 94-79), NHS Executive, Leeds

NHS Executive (1994) *The Operation of the NHS Internal Market: Local Freedoms, National Responsibilities*, NHS Executive, Leeds

Paton, C. R. (1991) Myths of competition. *Health Service Journal*, 6 May.

Paton, C. R. (1992) *Competition and Planning in the NHS*, Chapman & Hall, London.

Paton, C. R. (1995) Present dangers and future threats: some perverse incentives and paradoxes in the NHS reforms. *British Medical Journal*, 310.

Robinson, R. (1994) A good old British compromise. *Health Service Journal*, 15 Dec, 21.

Saltman, R. and von Otter, C. (1992) *Planned Markets and Public Competition*, Open University Press, Buckingham.

DEVOLUTION AND CENTRALISM IN THE NHS: CLINICAL DIRECTORATES, RESOURCE MANAGEMENT AND OTHER INITIATIVES

5

INTRODUCTION

The management reforms to the NHS following the White Paper *Working for Patients* were presented by the Conservative government as promoting devolution, defined as 'decisions...taken at the lowest possible level' by Douglas Hurd (1991) – reflecting a senior minister's interpretation of the overall policy agenda, including health. It was further claimed that such policies ('reforms in hospitals, in schools and in housing') were a way to 'empower citizens'. This approach was naturally an attempt to present the Conservatives' policy as pro-community and 'practical' rather than 'ideological' or free-market-obsessed. As such, it was rhetoric.

Nevertheless, it is worth renewing the debate about whether power and/or responsibility in management were devolved in the NHS – or, indeed, **to** the NHS from the Department of Health. Rudolf Klein, in the first edition of his *The Politics of the National Health Service* (Klein, 1983), had no sooner pointed to the 'devolution' inherent in the 1982 reorganization of the NHS (based on the document *Patients First* (Department of Health and Social Security, 1981) when the Griffiths Enquiry recommendations were accepted, introducing general management and (later) executive leadership. As a result, he was soon to observe that the pendulum

had quickly swung back to centralism, an observation reiterated after a few years when *The Politics of the National Health Service* came out in its second edition (Klein, 1989).

In other words, there may be a cycle from centralism to devolution and back, or at least an interpretation of events as such in health policy, and strategic management, which makes a current reassessment timely. Which direction did the NHS Act of 1990 and related initiatives embody?

The crucial components of the Act were:

- the creation of a split between purchasers of health care on the one hand and providers on the other;
- the institution of a contracting process between these purchasers and providers by which the latter would present tenders to the former;
- the creation of 'self-governing trusts' which, following the Conservative victory at the General Election in April 1992, would be the normal means of the provision of health care;
- various other policies, such as budgets held directly by general practitioners for certain services.

This chapter is not a discussion of the central White Paper policies (such as those discussed in Chapter 4) but is instead an examination of certain **managerial** initiatives, outlined below, which do not in themselves depend on the above 'market' conditions. It is nevertheless important to keep in mind the policy environment within which the initiatives discussed in this paper have been operating. Furthermore in moving now to our definitions of devolution, centralization and other key terms, seeking to measure NHS practice against these definitions, it is necessary to ensure that the particular managerial initiatives to be discussed are correctly localized within overall policy. For example, it is possible to have 'resource management' without the NHS Act of 1990, but understanding the functions and operations of resource management after the NHS reforms may require understanding of the reforms as a backdrop.

I am proposing to use the following framework, including the following terms.

Devolution: The handing down from either central government or the Department of Health of responsibility for determining local health objectives (to purchasers) or for defining key aspects for business (to providers). No Government responsibility for a publicly funded health service would relinquish all responsibility for setting objectives. In the pages below, we will therefore be looking for realistic benchmarks of devolution in a UK context.

Furthermore, my emphasis in this chapter is upon strategic issues rather than purely operational issues. It is now a truism that various operational responsibilities have been 'devolved' in recent years in the NHS.

Sometimes the concept of decentralization will be distinguished from that of devolution, especially when (for example) discussing political constitutions. In this chapter, I am not using any significant distinction between the two, as by devolution we mean the transfer of significant powers from the centre.

Centralism: In the light of the above observations, centralism means the location of power for strategic decisions at the centre of the policy-making system; in this case, it would mean that the central government in one form or another, the Department of Health and/or NHS policy board and management executive, would still be controlling the important decisions. In the context of this chapter, where we are debating whether or not centralism has been diminished by devolution we will be asking whether examples of supposed devolution are in fact misleading.

Responsibility and power: It is important for my argument to consider the difference between these two concepts (Bachrach and Baratz, 1970). This is because I argue below that in certain instances responsibility but not power has been devolved. Briefly, power may consist in any or all of the following:

- the ability to mobilize resources to achieve ends;
- the ability to win victories in situations of conflict or characterized by alternative objectives sought by different actors (Dahl, 1961);
- the ability to control an agenda, for example to prevent issues being raised which are likely to diminish the attainment of one's objectives (Bachrach and Baratz, 1970);
- the ability to control the terms of debate or even the concepts employed (Lukes, 1974).

Responsibility, on the other hand, means being beholden to a higher authority, whether constitutionally, formally or otherwise, for the achievement of objectives which may well be defined externally to the responsible agency. The implication therefore is that responsibility is delegated. Otherwise it would not be meaningful to use the concept at all. Nevertheless, responsibility may be delegated in the absence of any, or adequate, power being likewise delegated.

In the NHS for example, the delegation of responsibility without power would in essence mean that general managers are really only administrators. In the NHS before general management, administrators were, of course, *de facto* managers but the word administration implied a passivity in simply 'running the system'. In the sense that we have just developed, the passivity would consist in 'running the system' at a high level. That is, we are noting that to be a general manager as opposed to an administrator implies a certain autonomy in the setting of objectives and the mobilization of resources to achieve these objectives. It is certainly part of the rhetoric concerning the new NHS 'chief executive' that such a freedom exists. It is part of the objective of this chapter to debate this issue.

Pluralism: This implies that power over decisions is held, at the very least, at more than one level or in more than one location (Dahl, 1961). Pluralism is not the same as decentralization. One can have a centralized pluralist system – where the decision-making arena is centralized but where different actors jostle for power, or have inputs in that arena. A decentralized pluralist system is one where decisions are taken at various levels and where either these different levels are competing for turf or there are different sources of power within different levels, or both.

Similarly, one can have decentralization without pluralism in that the decentralized locations of power are controlled by single or unitary institutions. The health authority prior to the NHS reforms, in its quasi-representative form, sought to represent different viewpoints or interests. This type of pluralism has been overtly abolished in the Government's decision to create health authorities on the lines of business boards.

The market: Refers to an economic relationship in which there are buyers and sellers – or at least one buyer and at least one seller. A market, of course, may be characterized by competition (perfect, imperfect or monopolistic), oligopoly or monopoly on the supply side. On the demand side, a similar taxonomy

of purchasers exists in theory, from the many to the one (monopsony).

This chapter does not debate whether or not there is a real market in health care as a result of the NHS reforms. This has, of course, been done (Paton, 1992). What is important here is to distinguish between the operation of an economic market (whether private or public; whether 'internal' or not) and a system involving managerial decentralization. There is an assumption frequently made by NHS managers as well as Conservative politicians, in the absence of analysis, that the market and decentralization go together. This may not be the case as, for example, centralization of power to create the conditions of a market may be necessary. Alternatively, one can argue that a centralization of decision-making is a symptom of the absence of a market. That is, a market – to work properly – may require certain operational types of decentralization of decision-making in health care. This is, of course, not the same as pluralism. For example, who makes decisions as to what health care is purchased? Who makes decisions within providers as to business, employee relations and/or operating procedures? A market in which the patients are not the purchasers may well not represent pluralism in the prescriptive or appealing sense of that word.

Within the context of the above definitions and observations, I seek to ask whether devolution has indeed occurred within the NHS in the manner often assumed, by considering a number of issues on the management agenda in the post-reform NHS, which in some cases have spawned specific management tasks on a nationally understood agenda (such as resource management and medical audit). To repeat, it is not the task of this chapter to assess the NHS reforms in a wider sense. I hope, however, that by taking some tangible issues, we can shed light on the continuing debate about the nature of the post-reform NHS. The succeeding section take specific topics (such as audit, resource management and human resource management) and address their content and inherent methodology in detail.

THE POLICY ENVIRONMENT

THE AGENDA OF THE WHITE PAPER

The broader ideological agenda of the White Paper is one issue (Paton, 1990, 1992; Part Three of this book). This agenda includes, for example, whether a market ought to be developed for the provision of health care; and indeed what sort of market, if any, is currently developing in the NHS. In this chapter, however, the focus is primarily upon the particular managerial initiatives (which do not themselves require a market) promulgated broadly as part of the wider 'White Paper agenda', and how they link to national policy objectives.

Particular management initiatives considered are:

- the establishment of 'clinical directorates' (CD);
- the comprehensive adoption of 'resource management' (RM);
- the universal introduction of medical audit (MA).

More general trends in policy have been signalled by:

- methodologies for rationing resources;
- new approaches to managing human resources;
- the Patient's Charter;
- the regulation of providers by 'zonal outposts' of the NHS Management Executive on the one hand and purchasers by regions on the other hand.

This is not to say that the ideological agenda of the White Paper is not relevant to these initiatives in policy and management. It is merely to assert that the latter may have a life of their own without the White Paper's ideological baggage. The White Paper, after all, was a mixed bag, pulling together the Thatcher government's impulsive, pro-competitive objectives, yet also the various departmental initiatives (such as medical audit) that had been simmering in one form or another throughout the 1980s. Furthermore, resource management predated the White Paper and was not overtly part of its agenda. Clinical directorates and overall information strategy are 'formally' separate initiatives. The Patient's Charter is a later attempt to give the consumer a voice.

Yet in practice, the White Paper was the mechanism through which clinical directorates have been given an operational rationale. Clinical directorates themselves are not formally part of the White Paper's agenda. But, as an expression of devolved management, they are part of the philosophy and practical agenda which is now being used in an attempt to legitimize a substantial part of the NHS reforms.

Separation of the ideological and 'practical' agenda may therefore be a ticklishly difficult task in practice. This is all the truer when one considers that, even if the pro-market thrust of the White Paper is stymied by central politics and regional regulation or planning, there was still an ideological agenda behind the proclamation of devolution. This agenda was indeed integral to the whole of the White Paper. Mrs Thatcher announced the review in 1988 in an attempt to diminish expectations that central government was responsible for 'finding extra money' for the NHS every time problems – in particular, shortages – surfaced. It was hoped that devolved management responsibilities would, firstly, focus attention on efficient provision rather than demands for 'more money' and, secondly (and less explicitly), force local management to do the Government's 'dirty work' in rationing care. This may be called Reaganism rather than Thatcherism, borrowing as it did from the former US President's attempts to decentralize budgets and responsibilities in social policy from national to state and local governments (often while cutting these budgets at the same time).

On this interpretation, devolution is passing the buck.

THE MARKET, PLURALISM AND DEVOLVED MANAGEMENT

One thing is clear. Despite governmental rhetoric, devolution is not about giving democratic control over the NHS to local communities. Health authorities, following the White Paper, became executive boards and were no longer even quasi-representative. Ironically, this may have removed a local tier of decision-making perceived to be susceptible to popular or interest-group pressure – the old health authority – and therefore led to a perception that 'the centre' was more responsible than ever for local decisions – for example, to close hospitals. There was no local board other than the managers, in other words. Even a locally concerned Conservative MP might have to lobby the Conservative Secretary of State directly rather than seeking to work through the health authority. This is because the health board became a united team of Chairman, non-executive directors and executive directors (the former 'officers'), rather than a quasi-representative authority separate from its officers.

If political control for health boards becomes more blatant – as it unequivocally did throughout the 1980s – then supposedly devolved responsibilities (whether or not power accompanies them) are increasingly seen as centrally mandated.

In other words, pluralism in policy-making – central as well as local – is subjugated to 'tight management'. This may have advantages. After all, log-rolling (vote-trading, or deals between interests at the expense of 'the rest') and gerrymandering by rather ill-informed health authority members had become infamous in various parts of the country. But if log-rolling and gerrymandering are merely transferred to 'the centre' (i.e. to ministers and the Department of Health), then not much has been gained except secrecy.

There is some evidence that this happened. For example, local Conservative MPs 'did deals' with ministers on the extent and form of 'opting out' to protect their local interests. In one example, a health district's providers were to be allowed to 'opt out' of health authority control as one integrated trust, to prevent fragmentation of district planning and to prevent the dominant Regional Chairman (one noted for doing ministers' bidding rather than asserting an independent role) from sequentially merging or closing different providers in the district. In other words, the centre (the Minister) was forced to resolve a dispute that in earlier days could have been handled by a stronger local health authority.

Devolution in practice is often, of course, a political 'hurrah word' used to cloak an economic 'boo word' in health care – the market. This is true especially now that mainstream Conservatives avoid talk of the market in health care, having created a Frankenstein's monster. Devolution of management responsibility to 'self-governing trusts' **removes** local control of such providers and instead makes them responsible to the Department of Health directly. The devolution consists in allowing them to set their own priorities (within limits); raise capital and set prices more freely than directly-managed providers and – most importantly in practice – to 'reprofile their workforces' i.e. hire and fire with less regard than hitherto to 'fair employment' norms or national criteria for justice in the employment relationship.

That is, market forces – to the extent they are salient; and only time will really tell – are most strongly expressed in trusts, on what economists would call the 'supply side' of health care. Market forces may, of course, involve devolved management. But it is not devolution in the political sense alluded to by Douglas Hurd (had he examined the reality of trusts, his convenient assimilation would have been torn asunder). The introduction of a market to a service previously operating through planned provision in fact requires a heavy dose of centralism, as the new economies of old Eastern Europe are finding. NHS trusts have been created against the opposition of their local communities and staff, almost without exception.

The Government diminished pluralism in health policy-making at the centre (as professional inputs to the Department of Health were diminished); diminished pluralism on health authorities/boards; devolved responsibility (to a much greater extent than power) to management within providers; and encouraged market forces, but only to the extent that they did not produce politically embarrassing outcomes. These market forces have nothing to do with devolving accountability or extending local democracy, whether democracy means majority rule or merely a pluralistic means of making policy.

SPECIFIC MANAGERIAL INITIATIVES

CLINICAL DIRECTORATES (CDs)

The idea of clinical directorates is that doctors repatriate the management clout they had before 1974, but in the context of accountability for resources. A core definition of strategic management – setting objectives, and achieving them within given or mobilized resources – applies almost classically to the idea of the clinical directorate.

Some proponents of the idea argue that, in the old days of the NHS before 1974, a Medical Superintendent was 'boss' of the hospital; that the 1974 reorganization took planning and management away from the doctors and the 'grass roots'; and that doctors ought now to be 'brought back' into general management.

Arguably, the Griffiths Enquiry report was the first major national report to argue for 'clinical directorates' (Griffiths, 1983). However, the thrust of Government policy, in seeking to implement the Griffiths Report, was to seek clinicians to manage at regional and district level. This policy was a clear failure except on a small scale and is now expunged from official history. The reasons are clear: doctors did not want to give up clinical work to 'do administration', and certainly not for a combination of (what they saw as) low salaries and short-term contracts.

Later on, and especially following the White Paper *Working for Patients*, it was sensibly argued that it was at the level of the clinical specialty that doctors could best be induced to take on a management role. Post-White-Paper, doctors would manage on the **provider** side, in any case. This could be quite radical. If resources were devolved to specialties in (what used to be called) clinical budgets, then traditional 'lay' management would lose one of its major roles – that of agreeing to, or denying, resources to clinicians item-by-item; project-by-project. That is, as well as being a challenge to doctors' 'cultural' attitudes, the idea of clinical directorates managing their own resources would be a shock to certain managers' systems as well.

By matching resources against outputs, it was argued, cost-effectiveness could be pursued (defined as meeting objectives, perhaps at stipulated quality, for minimum resources; or, alternatively, as maximizing objective-attainment given resources). Budgets would no longer be **functional**, i.e. line items, divorced from activity, let alone outputs. Instead, resources and objectives would be part of the same equation.

The policy could be radical in other ways too. If clinical directorates involved real devolution of power and responsibility, they would become 'firms' in their own right, with the hospital merely a loose conglomerate or 'warehouse'.

Three alternative models of the clinical directorate are, respectively, advocating or embodying:

- autonomous units within the hospital (directorates/divisions);
- managed devolution;
- central control.
- **Model 1: Full devolution**
  - The directorate determines its products
  - The directorate raises its own resources (both capital and revenue)
  - The directorate seeks a surplus; retains surplus
  - Resource management is not anyone else's business: it is a means of business management within the directorate
  - The directorate has full hiring and firing rights, which are (only) bound by national legislation
  - The directorate would develop an aggressive marketing strategy (hence)
  - The directorate would develop a commercial business plan, in an attempt to flourish in the marketplace.
- **Model 2: Managed devolution**
  - 'Products' are determined by or agreed with the overall hospital board, which may include the clinical directors *en masse*. This is an increasing trend in hospitals. Doctors thus have a big role in managing themselves corporately as well as individually.
  - Resources are (mostly) allocated by the hospital (but with local/firm/directorate **control**)
  - Any surplus is partly retained by the hospital
  - Resource management monitored and regulated by the hospital
  - Employment policy is regulated and/or negotiated
  - Marketing is in line with hospital strategy (hence)
  - A quasi-commercial business plan would be developed.
- **Model 3: 'Central control'**
  - The hospital's business is regulated by the purchaser, the region and also by the Department of Health (DOH)

- Resource flows in line with regional and DOH regulation, who control how and where contracts can be placed
- There is no such thing as surplus to individual directorates
- Resource management is a tool for accountability upwards, not for local freedom
- Employment policy is (still) (mostly) national, with (at most) a local spine of flexibility within national pay bargaining or perhaps 'local bargaining' in a framework of national stipulations (hence)
- The business plan is in essence a service plan re-named.

The degree of devolution of financial and management responsibility involved in clinical directorates depends, therefore, upon which model is adopted. The above alternatives may be seen as just that – alternatives – or as different staging-posts on a route from centralism to devolution. But the latter scenario is only possible – whether or not it is judged desirable – if national policy-makers, regional and district managers and hospital boards are willing to give up traditional modes of health service politics, planning and management. This seems unlikely, in a centralized political system where the NHS is accountable to Parliament via ministers.

THE POLITICAL ENVIRONMENT

Doctors, often with justification, see CDs as an attempt to make them directly responsible for unpalatable rationing decisions, or for implementing cuts. Professor Cyril Chantler of Guy's Hospital (who may have coined the phrase 'clinical directorate' originally) quotes the Chief Executive who said, 'Give them the money, and they'll make the cuts' (THS, 1994). In other words, CDs will 'divide and rule' among doctors, setting the clinical director against his colleagues and directorate against directorate, instead of – as before – 'doctors against management'.

If this is true, CDs will fail. If it is not, and CDs are 'an opportunity, not a problem', then the Government would have been sensible to be more up-front in the debate. It should be acknowledged that quality improvement and cost-control are often straining in opposite directions. Not always – for example, reducing preoperative stays in hospital can improve quality **and** reduce costs. But often there is a 'quantity/quality' trade off. While clinical care is per se of a high standard in the UK, overall quality of care is often low, as the price of a high-quantity, low-cost NHS.

Simply relying on resource management (to be discussed below) to 'sort this out' is facile. It may, of course, systematize rationing, as well as allowing clinicians the opportunity to set out just what can and what cannot be done efficiently. In other words, rationing can be done rationally and/or indeed a case for more resources can be made more convincingly.

Resource management, in other words, is worth doing. CDs may be the best way of doing it. But, if so, we need to know what sort of CD, for what purpose, is required. Are doctors to market services or to plan them in line with higher authority? Are non-clinical managers in effect to devolve – or give up – their traditional power? This has been often a negative power – of forbidding new procedures on grounds of cost; of closing wards towards the end of the financial year. But it has been a power nonetheless. Are managers sufficiently aware of this? What type of CD can allow clinical managers and non-clinical managers to decide priorities, e.g. to shelve the least valuable of current activities in order to take on the most valuable of currently unavailable services?

In other words, how can the new market-leaning NHS preserve the best forms of strategic planning – the forms which indeed every large private enterprise must undertake? A modern planning framework calls for:

- external environmental scanning (for example, what effect upon the labour force is registered by economic trends);
- internal environmental scanning (for example, what is the current cost and quality of a department of surgery's services);
- interrelations in the above;
- objective setting;
- business planning;
  and then
- operational planning.

To what extent are CDs about strategic as opposed to operational planning? Doctors have always been involved in professionally or clinically-based planning and management. Are they to share in **general** strategic planning and management or only operational?

Are they engaged purely as planners within providers (whether in CDs or at overall board level), or are they to make inputs to the definition of need of use to purchasers?

The White Paper *Working for Patients* sought to address questions of provision of care in order to divert attention from the financing debate. Yet forbidden fruit is more delicious. Doctors prefer to talk of inadequate funding than to manage diminishing budgets.

The funding level of the NHS is one debate. There is a perfectly rational debate as to whether CDs are a good idea (and, if so, of what type), which is not a debate about overall funding. But if CDs are a mechanism for control and blame rather than opportunity, if the market is rhetoric rather than reality and CDs cannot market themselves, is it surprising that disillusionment spreads?

Merging responsibility for weighing up the benefits and costs of alternative services is the best argument for CDs. If doctors are addressed with critical insight rather than merely evangelism and jargon, then the benefits of devolution can be discussed at the same time as the costs, and decisions can be made rationally.

RESOURCE MANAGEMENT

Resource management became the NHS's variant of the Government's policy for maximizing output from constrained public sector budgets – a policy that arguably began in the Department of the Environment in 1980.

Resource management can, of course, be used as a reason for establishing clinical directorates – ensuring that resources are managed by those whose decisions are the most significant in committing resources. It is important, however, to ask exactly what power and responsibility 'resource managers' are to have. If district health boards are to set priorities for health-care provision, this may require subjective needs assessment and other 'worm's eye' views, from the consumer's viewpoint, as well as formulae or at least methodologies from the expert's or manager's viewpoint. Once priorities have been established, contracts will be placed with providers – or service plans agreed, if the paraphernalia of contracting is eventually simplified.

Resource management, then, would be the delivery within a contract or service agreement of an agreed quantity (and quality) of services at agreed costs (or prices). In other words, it is not up to the provider (clinical directorate, within the hospital or community unit) to decide what to do, i.e. how to use an available resource. Providers were not simply taking a sum of money and going off to 'do their own thing', only regulated at the margin by a variety of carrots and sticks to respond to national waiting list initiatives and the like.

However, a radical 'devolved' model of the clinical directorate would argue that marketing the provider's desired product or mix of activities to the purchaser would soon become a salient feature; just as, in conventional markets, purchasers' tastes are manipulated by providers. The balance of power between provider and purchaser (based on configuration of supply and demand, and also on the degree of competition in provision and in purchasing) is also something that cannot be predicted in advance, or as an axiom.

In such a 'market' model, resource management consists in setting objectives as well as meeting them within a given resource. The Department of Health and the NHS Management Executive were fundamentally unclear as to which version was sought – the latter 'market' version or the former 'bureaucratic' version. The latter involves devolution – but to the provider – and the former involves accountability upwards, within the hospital, which is itself accountable to the purchaser's wishes.

The problem with resource management, as with clinical directorates, is that it has been vigorously promoted as 'all things to all men'. Thus, one finds regional Resource Management Directors variously claiming that there is no quality/quantity trade-off; that resource management is a behavioural mechanism for encouraging dialogue between the various health-care professions; and that, in the time-dishonoured management cliche, it is 'an opportunity, not a problem' (a phrase which ought to be to management ears as 'over the moon' is to football ears). All these things may be true **sometimes**. But they may equally be false at other times.

More realistically, resource management can clarify what mix of quantity and quality is possible at what cost, and can therefore be a mechanism for helping providers negotiate contracts or agree service plans. But it must be used as a technical backdrop to blunt choices. For example, there may be the hard choice as to whether to do more at less quality or less at higher quality. This is not to deny that quality improvements can be sought that do not cost money, or which even save money (such as reducing an over-long preoperative assessment time in hospital, which is frustrating for the patients as well as wasteful). But, like efficiency savings, there is a diminishing marginal return of quality improvements at existing costs.

At a professional and behavioural level, resource management may be interpreted as a means of getting different professions to agree locally on clinical care protocols. For example, the West Midlands region promoted 'collaborative care planning' (West Midlands Health Region, 1991) (like so many recent initiatives, born in the USA) as a means of getting doctors, nurses, physiotherapists and others to agree on the appropriate mix and timing of their activity in treating given conditions. The aim is to provide a service which is of high quality for the patient. This may hold out a false prospectus, however, if the purchaser has a desired quantity and quality of services in mind in the context of a constrained budget. To put it bluntly, the purchaser may be tempted, but unable to reach for the wallet; so the provider has to compromise on the products or lose contracts. Where, of course, better-quality care, with collaboratively agreed protocols, is cheaper, this will not be the case. Certainly, negotiation will be possible – indeed necessary, for the purchaser will need to know from the provider what is possible. This is incidentally an aspect of contracting little noticed by market enthusiasts at the time of the White Paper's launch. Often, the doctors and financial experts advising the purchaser were also working for the provider. Indeed, as noted above, the doctor works as the provider's key employee, yet was employed formally by the region and has his contract 'managed' by the district. It is therefore unlikely that collaborative care planning will take place without tailoring plans to available budgets.

But, at the end of the day, something like 'collaborative care planning' is about defining a homogeneous product **at an agreed cost/price** – otherwise it is not 'resource management' so much as a talking shop of professionals. To 'sell' it as local autonomy (in other words, care plans produced as a result of local interprofessional collaboration and agreement) is therefore misleading. It is only local to the extent that the market is local. In the NHS, of course, if 'markets' are subjugated to regional plans managed according to national priorities, it is actually about fulfilling national expectations as to product and price, with the jargon of 'local ownership' as a soft soap.

Devolution of operational responsibility, again, may have masked a centralism based on the political need to ensure local services are available to meet national expectations. Furthermore, if clinical protocols are to be 'policed' by purchasers, we will have a situation in which the purchaser is concerned with the care process as well as clinical outcomes – and therefore concerned to have a very close relationship with the provider. Ironically, this may mean closer 'management' of providers than before the NHS reforms.

MEDICAL AUDIT

Medical audit is also a policy frequently presented as allowing local determination of priorities. At its most straightforward, it is simply a means of quality assessment or quality control, extended to produce improvements in the medical 'product' by the setting of standards and the creation of mechanisms to maintain these. If such a policy has few resource implications, or if the opportunity cost of doctors' time is at least equalled by savings due to improved procedures averting readmissions or medical complications, then it is surely uncontroversial. A full outline and discussion of medical audit is made in Chapter 9. For now, its bearing on the current topic, managerial power, is discussed.

The more interesting aspects of the policy concern its effect upon clinical standardization. Is there a 'best' way of treating particular conditions? If there is unequivocally a 'best' way – by which no patient is worse off yet at least some are better off in terms of outcome – then whether or not it is adopted will depend purely on resource availability. If the 'best' cure or care regime is no more costly than alternatives, then again adopting it is uncontroversial. If it is more expensive, then there may be a choice or trade-off between quantity and quality.

If, however, different cure or care regimes have outcomes which mean that values have to be brought to bear in choosing, then medical audit may be pulled into a difficult arena. Let us imagine that Regime X produces, in a sample of 100 patients, 99 good outcomes and one death, whereas Regime Y – for treating the same symptoms – produces 50 good outcomes, 40 marginally good outcomes and 10 patients unaffected.

Which is better? There is obviously no answer in the abstract. If one is a crude utilitarian, possibly the former. If one is risk-averse, or operating on the principle of 'do least harm', possibly the latter.

The question arises, does medical audit have anything to say about such a choice, or is it confined simply to ensuring that – whatever the individual clinician's choice – the best 'processes' are used within the best available 'structure' of care, in the hope of achieving the best outcome? If the latter, then (again) it is reasonably uncontroversial. If the former, then it may herald the end of (individual) clinical autonomy for the sake of either 'local consensus' or 'national consensus' or resource control – say, within a clinical directorate. (That is, the choice of regime is at least partly dictated by resources.)

The above scenario is all the more likely when one considers that, in many cases, symptoms are not unequivocal, or indeed unequivocal signals of a specific disease. Thus, despite, or because of, the resulting uncertainty, 'standard care protocols', perhaps even aided by 'computer-aided diagnosis', may be one destination on a route away from (current) individual clinical freedom.

It may be asked, to what extent should national standards of care be introduced? Obviously, if there is a 'best' regime, with no difficult value-laden choices, then the Royal Colleges can advocate the best regime and

best practice to achieve it. If there are value-laden choices – or choices where local factors affect management or clinical outcomes – a national approach seems inappropriate, but local (or clinical-directorate-based) practice may eventually become 'mandatory' for clinicians. Alternatively, individual clinical freedom is preserved.

At the end of the day, standard protocols *versus* individual freedom may simply be rule utilitarianism *versus* act utilitarianism (Lyons, 1964), before and unless financial considerations also intrude. This will be so especially if – in the above hypothetical example involving regions X and Y – clinicians can increasingly determine which patient might die under Regime X, and which fall into the various categories of outcome from Regime Y, Then 'the best' might again become less controversial – but subject to 'local intuition'; or at least to clinical choice in the context of adequate resources to 'do the best for each patient' assessed individually or by group/age/severity of illness and so forth.

In the situation where clinical knowledge is good enough to allow choice of care regime (e.g. X or Y, in the above example) for different patients or categories of patient, then it is, of course, the (provider) management's responsibility to ensure that clinicians produce the best possible outcome (subject to resources). That is, clinical audit can feed into management audit/control.

Where outcomes are agreed between managers and clinicians in providers (and 'contracted' for with purchasers), audit will be about ensuring their achievement, perhaps by advising on better 'structures' and 'process' for delivering care. Where outcomes are not agreed – or cannot be, because of value variance or simply lack of information on the effects of medical care, audit will be about setting process standards for different hypothetical outcomes.

In the USA, 'clinical directorates', as in their original home at Johns Hopkins Hospital, Baltimore, MD, are increasingly

presiding over ultra-standardized care protocols, imposed on individual doctors primarily
for reasons of financial control. (There is a
saying that, in the UK, doctors have traded
money for freedom, whereas in the USA they
have traded freedom for money.) The trouble
with such a policy is that doctors are saying
increasingly: if bureaucratic control is going
to be so persuasive, let managers and administrators do it. In the UK, by retaining individual clinical freedom, we have allowed a
creative compromise whereby doctors are
thereby more willing to help out with the
informal rationing of care that is a consequence of the UK's relatively low level of
spending on health care.

If medical audit becomes either a national
or local basis for standardization, it may have
unintended if not adverse side-effects, as well
as becoming an adjunct to resource management (possibly within clinical directorates) –
which spells centralism rather than devolution, or at least centralism away from clinical
choice.

MEDICAL AUDIT: A BUREAUCRATIC PROCESS?

The means of introducing medical audit
suggest that it is seen as a system of bureaucratic regulation rather than as a suggestion
as to how autonomous providers might incorporate quality assurance into their 'production function' or process.

Firstly, although medical audit was part of
Working for Patients, as described in Working
Paper 6, it was implemented before most
hospitals became trusts and before the
contracting process between purchasers and
providers had been properly developed. In
consequence, a new model of bureaucracy
was grafted on to the structure of the NHS
that existed prior to the reforms. Thus, for
example, every district created a district
Medical Audit Committee (DMAC) – now
based in providers, as local Medical Audit
Committees – on which the representatives
included the Director of Public Health (as

representative of both the patient and the
District General Manager) and a general practitioner, as well as clinicians from the
provider units.

As trusts grew in number the purchaser/
provider split became at least more of a reality than when districts were still responsible
for their own directly managed providers.
Thinking logically, if medical audit is a
specialized contribution to the process of
overall quality assurance then it is clearly a
provider function. In a proper market, it is up
to the purchaser to choose among providers
on a number of criteria, one of which may be
whether or not there is a formal quality assurance as part of the production process (good
quality may be judged by outcome and not
process, and no assumptions may necessarily
be made about whether quality assurance,
total quality management or any other
process is formally used). In the post-reform
NHS, it could be argued that quality assurance should not be a mandatory activity
monitored by the Department of Health, but
a possible provider activity dependent upon
both purchaser's demands and provider's
approaches to contracting.

Yet in the NHS, medical audit is a mandatory activity. Moreover, the specific monies
allocated for medical audit have continued to
be distributed without adequate regard to the
purchaser/provider split, with the result that
in many cases joint committees of purchasers
and providers have been allocating medical
audit monies.

This may not be so significant at the end of
the day, as the total monies involved may not
be salient. Nevertheless as an example of
either governmental confusion or governmental unwillingness to devolve, or indeed to
free up proper market relations within the
NHS, it is quite a striking one. Let us again
consider the logic. In a market, one might
expect that among the criteria by which
purchasers select providers is the question of
how the provider assures quality. If the state
is determined to stand at the shoulder of

providers and tell them how to do their quality assurance, then this would hopefully be compatible with the spirit of devolved responsibility – but it would at least be recognized that quality assurance was a provider function. If however, health authority purchasers, and above them regions, are involved in Medical Audit Committees, they are in effect controlling or at least regulating the quality assurance function in providers with whom they are contracting, rather than contracting with them on the basis of, *inter alia*, quality. This will make sense if purchasers are seeking to ensure quality in a stable and long-term relationship with 'their' providers. But if this is the case, the NHS reforms are about better planning and monitoring, not markets.

As with so much of the NHS reforms, incompatibilities in practice have had to be worked out 'on the hoof'. Medical audit is changing in orientation for this reason.

RESOURCE ALLOCATION (AND RATIONING) (CH. 10)

Methodologies for allocating resources to districts and GP fundholders, and for making contracts within constrained resources, raise questions as to how centrally or locally priorities are decided. National and regional resource allocation, originally by the RAWP formula and regional variants from 1976–1990 and then by the White Paper's 'Son of RAWP' (whereby RAWP was formally abolished yet partly retained), has given money to health authorities on the basis of 'need'. Measures of need have been based on attempts to measure morbidity, either by surrogates such as mortality and/or by social measures that can be linked to usage of health services once adjustments have been made for variations in existing supply of care (e.g. location of hospitals).

It may be noticed that there is no attempt to assess **directly** the ability of services successfully to meet such need. In our view,

that is sensible, at the level of aggregate resource allocation. Need implies a need for care, research or concern, even if cure is not possible.

At the level of actual services, however, if 'rationing' is necessary, it is argued by proponents of methodologies such as the quality adjusted life year (QALY) that outcomes (either in terms of life saved or quality of life gained, or both) must be taken into account and related to costs. (Some proponents of this type of view argue that aggregate (national or regional) resource allocation ought also to take account of QALYs, to ensure that allocations match the purchase of actual 'effective' services).

If QALYs or QALY-type procedures are used to allocate resources or make contracts for care, or both, then centralism in priorities is reinforced – unless local public opinion is used to put the 'Q' into QALY, i.e. to determine local priorities under the guise of adjustments to the formula based on local opinions as to quality. The trouble then is that there is no objective basis for allocating resources (say) to districts with different priorities – unless national formulae use traditional means of morbidity, or national judgements as to the QALY. And then, again, national and local criteria for resource allocation may be out of synchronism. If localism in determining the criteria of effective provision is allowed, the corollary would seem to be local revenue-raising, balanced by national revenue-equalization to allow for variations in local tax base (as occurs to some extent in the USA, in funding education). This is an argument which may be considered to be a corollary of local choice whether or not a QALY-style approach is adopted. Thus, a real 'devolution' would apply.

The trend, however, seems to be to disseminate 'national' data on outcomes and 'expect' local purchasers to take account of such. The culmination of this process is, of course, the White Paper *The Health of the Nation*. This, again, is a likely consequence of a system that can occasion political embarrassment if people in different localities face different criteria for access to services. Again, devolution may be rhetoric rather than reality, in policy trends. Experts – for which, read national experts – may define health gain and how to achieve it. Only then, if at all, will local 'consumerism' or 'democracy' come into play, constrained by national priorities incumbent upon purchasers. Again, this may be fine, but it is not devolution.

The question is, will centralization increase in the field of 'rationing'? After the pre-election period in 1992 in which the Government provided extra funds for the NHS, harder times to follow meant that rationing was increasingly prominent when considering priorities within the NHS.

If the distribution of income in the UK continues to become more unequal, we can expect the private sector in health care to grow – even if the percentage of the national income going on public expenditure and the percentage within that going on health care remains the same. This is because there is more after-tax disposable income in the hands of the better-off. A static public sector, unlike in Europe, where health budgets have been growing much more significantly throughout the 1980s, means in any case that the private sector will grow as people generally spend their disposable income on newly available forms of health care. It can therefore be argued that the correct term ought to be not rationing but denial of care, as the 'rationing' is inflicted upon those who cannot exit into the private sector.

Nevertheless it is clear that, whatever nomenclature is used, decisions about what can and cannot be provided on the NHS are going to be taken increasingly stringently over the next few years. If such decisions are not taken centrally, the Government will lose the ability to control the terms of the health service debate, with potentially disastrous consequences opening up. In this connection, extremely hard decisions have to be taken about the forms of social care, as opposed to health care, which are affordable 'on the NHS'. In this connection, we might see a resolution to the argument between those who defend the purchaser/provider split as a source of movement from acute to community care and those who defend it as a source of more and better high-technology medicine. Such decisions may be considered too important to be left to the 'decentralized purchaser in the market place'. If decisions as to purchasing priorities are in effect handed to purchasers by government, then centralization rather than devolution will have occurred. This is an important area in which to seek evidence in the longer term.

THE MANAGEMENT OF HUMAN RESOURCES (CH. 8)

An area where there has seemingly been a large shift in policy from centralism to devolution has been in the management of human resources and industrial relations generally. While the Conservative government did not wish – at first – formally to abolish the Whitley system of pay bargaining for various staff groups in the NHS, it was widely believed that it would be Conservative policy in a fourth term to abolish centralized pay bargaining altogether. There were different noises coming from the Department of Health, with the Secretary of State equivocating on plans to abolish Whitley and the then Director of Personnel on the NHS Management Executive, Mr (now Professor) Eric Caines, advocating the abolition of Whitley. The argument was that devolution of pay bargaining, and devolved responsibility to provider units for the management of human resources generally, would lead to greater flexibility in the workforce. In a context of market competition where, for example, self-governing trusts were seeking to respond to market forces more quickly, ability to manage one's own workforce was said to be of paramount importance. As well as issues of pay, issues of demarcation of work responsibilities between different staff groups has naturally been placed at the top of the agenda.

'Reprofiling the workforce' has become a vogue phrase. The argument is that the outcomes expected from the 'health-care production function' should be quantified and related to specific outputs expected from specific employees. In other words, staff groups are not simply functionally ascribed to units, by some central mechanism for managing human resources, but are employed in direct relationship to their contribution to output. In practice, this raises questions such as the following: what do doctors currently do that could better be done by others (for example, scientific officers or radiographers)? can the time 'freed up' in the doctor's working day therefore lead to a greater medical or clinical workload, or ability to 'get by' with fewer doctors? what do nurses currently do that could be done by 'care assistants'? and – generally – how can greater efficiency be achieved from the workforce, in the sense of minimizing the cost of inputs and maximizing output?

In some cases, senior professionals may be induced to take on extra, less professional tasks to save on employment costs of more junior staff. In other cases, junior staff may obviate the need for so many senior staff by doing work currently done only by the seniors.

That is, 'reprofiling' may mean senior staff extending 'downwards' or junior staff extending 'upwards'. This, of course, sounds democratic and flexible. The logic – and reality – may be somewhat less benign.

On one interpretation, the new approach to the management of human resources was an attempt to deepen the division of labour. On another interpretation, it lessens the division of labour in that 'people do whatever needs to be done' within the organization. There are, of course, attempts to make it 'worker-friendly', in that a more flexible

workforce can be allied to demographic and social trends which (for example) produce interest by employees in part-time working, flexible hours, and so forth. But – as in the economy as a whole – part-time jobs may be inferior jobs dressed up as 'flexibility'!

Allied to local pay bargaining, such an approach, of course, means in practice better pay and conditions for professions and workers whose skills are scarce (whether nationally or locally), and worse pay and conditions for others. Naturally, 'scarcity' or abundance of a particular skill, professional or more unskilled worker can only be determined once demand for particular staff groups has been readjusted according to the reprofiling exercise.

There is no doubt that such an approach **could** represent genuine devolution to management at the level of the provider within the health service. The question is, are the criteria to be used when deciding upon skill mixes and employment policy locally (wherein the genuine devolution arises) to be national ones or local ones? Given the financial constraints confronting the NHS and the level of unemployment in the economy as a whole, it is likely that lower-paid workers will be net losers on such an approach, looking at the nation as a whole.

Equally, 'reprofiling' **could** simply mean that the existing labour force, with the current skill-mix, could be better utilized: doctors, nurses, technicians and others could use their days more productively by doing different things in different ways, without adverse effects upon working conditions. This, however, would mean that, unless changed productivity or changed practice was proportionately the same for all cadres, bottlenecks based on the least productive cadre would arise. In turn, more productive cadres would probably require less manpower as the full potential of the existing staff complement of these more productive cadres would not be realizable. In a proper market environment, such staff might be a resource for other business, to meet potentially unrestricted demand for a desirable product. In the NHS, however, aggregate demand is static, except as part of the electoral cycle. It is fair to make the hypothesis that 'reprofiling' is about increased control of a slimmed-down workforce, where possible.

The management of human resources is, of course, a general prerequisite for health service and other 'industries', whereas there are particular schools of thought on how best to achieve this, ranging from scientific management through to a whole range of behavioural approaches of which 'human resource management' is one. The basic norm underpinning human resource management (HRM) is that the maximum fulfilment of the employee compatible with the objectives of the organization should be sought. This, of course, raises questions as to whether the interests of the employee and the interests of the organization are compatible, or to what extent they are compatible.

Allied to a new and deliberate focus on the importance of 'leadership' in the National Health Service, mirroring similar approaches in industry, it was in effect being argued by the Conservative government that the organization (in this case, let us say, the provider unit in the health service) is a unitary organization all of whose employees share interests. This approach, therefore, is partisan in terms of industrial relations theory, as it adopts a unitary approach as opposed to the pluralistic approach on the one hand (which argues that different groups have different interests) and the radical, or Marxist, approach on the other hand (which argues that there is a fundamental class conflict or employer/employee conflict in the organization).

If one subscribes to one or other of the latter approaches, the question arises, is leadership about persuading individuals that their interests lie with strategies devised by management, irrespective of alternative viewpoints or a so-called 'objective reality'? This confronts one of the most basic debates in political science and industrial relations. Are

workers who do not distinguish their interests from those of the company as a whole 'falsely conscious', as Marxists used to have it? Or are they simply being pragmatic, in realizing that – in the absence of radical social reorganization – they will be harming their own interests by harming the interests of the company or organization for which they work, as defined by management? We cannot answer such a fundamental question here. It is, however, important to note that a new strategy for human resources combined with a stress on leadership, in the National Health Service, is in effect an approach which **prescribes** the importance of the unitary organization – whether it exists or not – and seeks to unite all employees around generally shared objectives. These may be expressed in the mission statement, or the statement of 'core values', which provider units – as well as health authorities themselves – are increasingly encouraged to develop. A cynical perspective on such phenomena is, of course, possible: 'patients. . .need a bed and get a mission statement' (Widgery, 1991). In practice, it is quite possible that devolution in the realm of policy for human resources will in fact mean devolution of operational responsibility for fulfilling national objectives concerning efficiency in 'production'. In other words, Government policy allied to monitoring exercises by the Committee on Public Accounts and the Audit Commission will ensure that norms for employment policy arise which give a centralist edge to devolution!

Furthermore, localized pay bargaining with all staff groups is, in fact, a mammoth exercise for local management. Norms are likely to develop that relate pay scales for different professions locally, and indeed relate such scales to national norms, conceivably, given the centrally funded, cash-limited nature of the NHS. In other words, given the fact that there is accountability for service mix and service priorities, and also for employment policy, to a central level, devolution may not be all that it seems.

THE PATIENT'S CHARTER

The application of the Citizens' Charter to the health service by the Conservatives, in the form of the Patients' Charter, perhaps provides a clear example of the tension between centralism and devolution. The objectives of a 'patients' charter' at the broadest level are, of course, admirable. They are an attempt to provide a better and more consumer-friendly service for patients.

As well as seven allegedly existing rights, the Patients' Charter in early 1992 embraced three new rights, which were allegedly applicable from 1 April 1992, of which the two most important are:

- the right to be guaranteed admission for virtually all treatments by a specific date no later than 2 years to the day when the consultant places you on a waiting list;
- the right to have any complaint about NHS services investigated and the right to a reply from the chief executive of the health authority or general manager of the hospital (as before, the Health Service Commissioner was a further port of call if necessary) (Department of Health, 1991).

As well as the national charter standards, there were to be local charter standards that reflected local policy on outpatient appointments, waiting times and various more superficial yet still useful elements, such as better signposting in hospitals and more identifiable staff in hospitals and units. More recently, dictates on outpatient waiting have become more centralized (see Chs 6 and 8 for more direct 'performance management').

Subsequently, 'charter standards' have been extended gradually to primary care, as well as to new targets in inpatient and outpatient hospital care.

At first, the unambitious nature of national charter standards must be acknowledged. What was interesting about this Charter was that in effect it set out central priorities for the spending of scarce resources (for example, in order to meet standards on waiting times, whether for inpatient care or in outpatient departments). Reaction to the Patient's Charter pointed out that such 'rights' for 'consumers' may involve hospital and other departments in difficulties as to efficiency. For example, a 'consumer-friendly' appointments system may mean objectively more 'waste of time' by the doctor; allegedly 'doctor-friendly' appointment systems were often based on the need to ensure that it was patients rather than doctors who waited, given the scarcity of the doctor's time. This is not simply to endorse antediluvian and consumer-unfriendly systems, but to point to a trade-off that must be acknowledged if a sensible approach is to be devised.

More centrally, waiting-list priorities led directly to longer waits for many waiting less than a year for treatment for more serious conditions.

In practice, central regulation to achieve central mandates – or local regulation to interpret central mandates – means that not only is centralism asserted over devolved responsibility for the setting of priorities, but that the alleged philosophy of the White Paper *Working for Patients* is in fact undermined. The seven existing rights reiterated through the Patient's Charter included, for example, the right 'to be referred to a consultant, acceptable to you, when your GP thinks it necessary, and to be referred for a second opinion if you and your GP agree this is desirable'. If taken literally, this removed (desirably, in the present author's view) the restrictions which were imposed by *Working for Patients* upon referral, in order to make these compatible with contracts. In other words, under the guise of 'the money following the patient', the White Paper instituted a system whereby 'the patient followed the money'. Unless there was a contract, special arrangements had to be made through extra-contractual payments. Whenever these seemed not to be forthcoming, prior to the general election of 1992, scandals ensured that patients' rights rather than the logic of the White Paper won. In other words, the Government was in effect saying to health authorities 'We have ordered you to implement the White Paper *Working for Patients*. But the political consequences of this are embarrassing, so now we order you to ignore the logic of the White Paper, to save our political bacon.'

As well as being messy, this was hardly the means to persuade health service managers that devolution in order to promote local definition of priorities and local management to achieve these was a policy taken seriously by the Government. There is an analogy here with alleged devolution in the realm of education, to a system of locally managed schools. Coinciding with the establishment of a national curriculum, locally managed schools, in practice, meant local management of fairly nitty-gritty domestic issues in the context of budget constraints, and is not devolution of the type to excite strategic planners and managers.

Ironically, 'freedom' for trusts has coincided with greater control of their product, by purchasers on behalf of the Government.

REGIONS AND 'THE MARKET'

Let us consider evolving plans to 'police the market'. When the Conservatives won their fourth term, self-governing trusts became the order of the day throughout the NHS, and the question became: who will manage and regulate the effects of this increasingly mainstream form of provision? The Department of Health – the centre itself— naturally has overall responsibility. It would be peculiar, however, to pretend that control by the central department represented decentralization and devolution of strategic management responsibility. Nevertheless, while trusts are granted operational devolution to a large extent, some regulatory body is necessary to

represent the Department of Health on a region-wide basis.

Outposts (a lovely frontier word) were until 1994 responsible for certain aspects of trusts' activity. It was clear, from an NHS Management Executive paper of June 1992, that the outposts were to be directly responsible for trusts' 'strategic plans'. But which body – the outpost or the region (or the district) – would furnish 'autonomous' providers with capital? If this is only done in coordination with purchasers' plans, the purchaser/provider split is in fact a myth. In fact, responsibility for planning will have been centralized, not devolved.

If a purchaser/provider split does not occur formally at the regional level, it could be argued that it does not really matter – as the purchaser/provider split occurs at district and subdistrict level in its operational form. If, however, it is right to make the argument that central regulation will be increasingly important, the absence of a purchaser/ provider split at regional level would mean the absence of a purchaser/provider split at a key level where decisions as to criteria for purchasing are taken (or at least constrained severely.) The NHSME, in other words, may have been seeking to manage both provision and purchasing in an increasingly centralized way. This may be sensible. But clearer demarcation of 'roles and functions' – of the NHS Executive, regions and outposts – was necessary. To this end, a review of the 'roles and functions' of these structures (above district level) was established (known as 'the Langlands Review') – which on paper was an investigation of structure (albeit with overtones of yet another reorganization!), yet had far-reaching policy implications. For example, centralizing all 'regulatory' functions in one 'regional' tier might mean a 'market' much more tightly managed than envisaged earlier. For such a body would regulate both purchasers and providers – and their links and relationships.

CONCLUSION

The management of the NHS is allegedly less political, now that it has its own executive (formerly the ME) and is no longer 'governed' by the 'traditional' top civil servants whose priorities allegedly lie in servicing ministers. However, the Management Executive was itself born from the post-Griffiths Management Board, seemingly in recognition that the ME would not be as independent from politics as the Management Board's first chairman had attempted (and failed) to be. It is the Policy Board (dominated by ministers) which gives the ME its marching orders. And now the ME is the E, as the Government's tinkering with names continues.

Political appointment of health board chairmen and members means also direct, central political control. It is in this context that the Select Committee on Health saw its role for 1991–92, at least in part, as counter-manding political and managerial centralism (both sides of the same coin) and unthinking acceptance of current priorities. In a contrary direction, where trusts achieved indepen-dence to some degree, the Committee inversely saw its role as the provision of a national perspective, i.e. to countermand destructive competition (or wasteful, duplica-tive investment on a large scale in informa-tion technology by competitors, to take just one example).

Central priorities are often encouraged via neutral-sounding exhortations to phenomena such as 'leadership' and 'total quality management' (TQM) which, if not merely examples of rhetorical vacuousness, consist in a central agenda for practices and services. When TQM is linked to medical audit, it becomes a mechanism for management control by promulgation of standard practices under the guise of 'local ownership'.

When the Management Executive invested heavily in 'leadership' in 1991, one can be sure it was not in a pluralistic desire to see one hundred flowers bloom in the thousand units of the service, but to find leaders to carry out national policy and persuade local interests within their 'corporation' that they can benefit from 'following my leader'.

It might be argued that the whole structure of the post-1989 NHS represented devolution. For example, self-governing trusts were to be responsible for their own business, at least to a greater extent than provider units had previously been. Furthermore, trusts had their own 'local' governing boards, with non-executive directors separate from those of health authorities. In practice, however, it was easy to interpret this as central control under the guise of local 'ownership', espe-cially since the chairmen of such boards were appointed by the Secretary of State and the other members not appointed by local communities but representing (under the Conservatives) local business and private interests to a large extent.

One thing that is clear is that such a devolved structure made it more difficult for a Labour government to reintegrate the health service as a politically neutral, planned organization. If it is true that the Conservatives were pursuing their central objectives through local placement, Labour had the choice of doing the same or of abol-ishing the newly 'pluralized' structures. This may have been quite a deliberate policy on the part of the Conservative government. One of the greatest difficulties in rationalizing the US health-care system is the variety of plural interests that would have to be appeased or 'bought off' in order to imple-ment anything resembling a strategic plan which went against the interests of (for exam-ple) the insurance industry, local providers and local doctors.

It might be argued that deliberate central-ism in health policy, planning and manage-ment was in fact an attempt to embody the benefits of so-called 'rational planning' as opposed to incrementalism. This therefore broaches a long-standing debate in public policy and organizational theory.

'Incrementalists' argue that society or the organization is an aggregate of individuals and groups in pluralistic activity or, indeed, economic competition. It is not necessarily a market-based model, but it is a model on which many small decisions are taken with a view to individual or group advantage. Such incrementalism may be psychologically based (in that the 'big picture' is not available to decision-makers for cognitive reasons) or politically-based in that, in effect, a prescriptive argument for small-scale change pursued at the local level is being made. Incrementalism has, of course, been criticized for having a conservative bias in that, in the absence of the 'rational planners', the strong interests prevail in the social free-for-all. It could be argued that the Government was using an incrementalist **philosophy** as the justification for policy which was nevertheless centralist and indeed 'rationalist' in its **framework**. To this extent, it could be argued that *Working for Patients* was a move away from incremental policy development for the first time in the NHS.

Nevertheless, generalization is difficult. After all, the NHS Act of 1946, leading to the creation of the NHS in 1948, could be seen on one view as an example of rationalist planning in that it created a whole new publicly funded and publicly provided health service. Another interpretation, however, would see this episode as simply the summation of a series of trends and the gathering together of a number of policy strands into an overall framework.

Similarly, the White Paper *Working for Patients* could be seen as a rationalist and almost utopian attempt to transform the health-care system, or simply as a collection of initiatives which individually grew from different sources. When incrementalism becomes rationalism is a difficult question. One thing is, however, clear. Compared to the US, where any significant policies for reform tend to be 'watered down' by the ultra-pluralistic and decentralized structure of policy-making and social implementation of policy, the UK has a centralized framework which allows rational planning – if it is cognitively possible – to be at least attempted. A bias to centralism by international standards is therefore hardly surprising.

This may be no bad thing. Mobilizing 'autonomy' (Nordlinger, 1982) for the state in the US for example, is difficult, owing to social and state structure as well as to dominant ideology and the absence of salient public financing and provision in health care.

Nor is it therefore surprising that centralism allied to Conservative philosophy, under a Conservative government, leads to a style of planning which is convenient for the economic system as a whole, and which views both 'consuming' citizens and workers alike as human capital. Central planning under the guise of devolution, allied to a Conservative agenda, is not the same as the planning beloved of liberals and radicals in varying degrees, in various senses.

On this interpretation, decentralization and devolution may be strategies to pass responsibility for the management of limited resources to those providers responsible for using them. This has been an interpretation by some sceptical doctors of the policy to establish clinical directorates. It is in effect an attenuated example from the developed world of a phenomenon rife in health-care systems within the developing world – decentralization to communities as a means of admitting that resources do not exist at the central level to allow a nationally planned system.

To return to Douglas Hurd's assertion that Conservative policy was geared to 'empowering citizens', it is perhaps instructive to remember that community participation can be a double-edged sword: on the one hand, it is, of course, a means of promoting collaboration and participation; on the other hand, it is a means of leaving to the interest group and pressure group maelstrom the making of decisions that ought to be made on the basis of equity. If, on the other hand, community participation is merely a rhetoric, it is likely to mean in practice central determination of objectives with limited devolution locally to achieve them (normally, directed locally by those sympathetic to the centre's agenda.

My conclusion is that, whatever the merits or demerits of devolution, there was a significant centralist strand to much of British health policy surrounding the management agenda of the White Paper. It cannot be denied that there has been significant operational decentralization within the NHS. To conflate this with a claim that we had devolution as, for example, political theorists would understand it, would, however, be suspect. For on many strategic issues, centralism was increased in the late 1980s and beginning of the 1990s, not diminished, in that the norms formulated by Government within which strategic managers had to operate were now clearer than ever before.

The following chapters consider the internal content of the key policies addressed by management in a variety of 'managerial initiatives'.

DISCUSSION

- Devolution means the handing down of power from a higher to a lower level within a system. It should be distinguished from deconcentration, which means the dispersal of power from a central point or agency to a number of other agencies – but perhaps still at the centre. Thus, for example, the dispersal of power from the Permanent Secretary in the Department of Health to the NHS Management Board (the forerunner of the NHS Executive) in 1984 arguably represented a kind of deconcentration rather than devolution.
- One must distinguish between devolution of policy-making powers and devolution of management. Policy-making, if anything, has been centralized in the NHS

as a result of, firstly, the creation of general management and, secondly and more fundamentally, the NHS reforms. Strategic management norms have also, arguably, been centralized, although responsibility for resource management – and now, in the 1990s, human resource management – have been decentralized.

- One must distinguish between power and responsibility. Arguably power has been centralized and yet responsibility has been decentralized. At the level of management theory, devolution of responsibility, accompanied by accountability upwards, may make sense for the achievement targets. It may, however, be accompanied by a political devolution of responsibility – which may in turn be tied up with the political desire to devolve blame.

  Ironically this creates a culture whereby there is an attempt to have decisions approved at a higher level. In other words, a more creative devolution is thwarted, as managers fear the consequences of 'making the wrong decision' or displeasing their political masters.
- Examples of different types of devolution in an operational sense are provided through the operation of clinical directorates: responsibility for resource management; and responsibility for human resource management at a more local level. The chapter has explored consequences in these areas.

ACKNOWLEDGEMENTS

I would like to thank the editor and publishers of *Social Policy and Administration* for allowing me to reproduce much of my article 'Devolution and centralism in the NHS' from volume 27, no. 2, June 1993.

REFERENCES

Bachrach P. and Baratz, M. (1970) *Power and Poverty. Theory and Practice*, Oxford University Press, New York.

Dahl, R. (1961) A critique of the ruling elite model. *American Political Science Review*, **52**, 463-469.

Department of Health (1991) *The Patient's Charter*, HMSO, London.

Department of Health and Social Security (1981) *Patients First*, HMSO, London.

Griffiths, E. R. (1983) Letter to the Secretary of State, Department of Health and Social Security, London (6 Oct).

Hurd, D. (1991) Annual lecture, Blackpool, Conservative Political Centre (9 Oct)

Klein, R. (1983) *The Politics of the National Health Service*, Longman, Harlow.

Klein, R. (1989) *The Politics of the National Health Service*, 2nd edn, Longman, Harlow.

Lyons, D. (1964) *Forms and Limits of Utilitarianism*, Clarendon Press, Oxford.

Lukes, S. (1974) *Power: A Radical View*, Macmillan, London.

Nordlinger, E. (1982) *On the Autonomy of the Democratic State*, Harvard University Press, Cambridge, MA.

Paton, C. R. (1990) The Prime Minister's Review of the National Health Service and the White Paper *Working for Patients*. *Social Policy Review 1989-90*, Longman, Harlow.

Paton, C. R. (1992) *Competition and Planning in the National Health Service: The Danger of Unplanned Markets*, Chapman & Hall, London.

Secretaries of State for England, Scotland and Wales (1989) *Working for Patients*, Department of Health, London.

THS (1994) Editorial. *The Health Services*, **December**, 1.

West Midlands Regional Health Authority Resource Management Support Group (1991) *Collaborative Care Planning*, West Midlands Regional Health Authority, Birmingham.

Widgery D (1991) Broadside. *Weekend Guardian*, 14–15 Dec, 7.

PART TWO

MANAGEMENT ISSUES

THE CHANGING CONTEXT OF GENERAL MANAGEMENT

6

INTRODUCTION

AIMS AND OBJECTIVES

It is important to establish more precise definitions for various types of health-care management at the outset of this chapter. In this context, management overall involves a wide-ranging understanding of health policy and a practical approach to the achievement of policy objectives through successful implementation of policy. In other words, management as common sense – the meeting of objectives, coherently organized – is the best way of proceeding initially.

Next, a distinction can be made between strategic management and operational management. Strategy deals with steering towards long-term or overall goals. One can also distinguish between general management on the one hand and either professional or functional management on the other hand, with the former concerning the management of the whole institution and the latter concerning (for example) medical management, nursing management, property management or catering management.

It seems important at the outset that management ought to involve people from different professional backgrounds. As well as overtly trained managers, doctors, nurses, finance people, general administrators and others, all ought to provide the 'raw material' for the managers of tomorrow, whether within their own professional domains or as potential general managers. At the national level, politicians ought to be aware of the management agenda; and bureaucrats ought to be imbued with management skills to add to the other skills they have (whether political, diplomatic or organizational).

A key element of successful management is to institute management development. Training one's successor, goes the cliche, is the best means of ensuring good management in the future. And management development ought to be part of an overall management strategy, so that 'the right people' are located in the right places in the right systems (**structural features** of management), doing the right thing in the right way, and in the right relationships with other people (aspects of **management process**).

CONTENT

This chapter outlines the concepts relevant to health-care management; the balance between national and local responsibilities; the move to general management in health care and its theoretical underpinnings; distinctions between policy, planning and management; the political environment and political structures surrounding the domain of strategic management in health care; the distinction between public administration and management; and various political issues stemming from the 'rise' of strategic management in health care. A critical view of the nature and role of management is provided, with reference to health care in particular.

CONCEPTS IN MANAGEMENT

GENERAL MANAGEMENT AND STRATEGIC MANAGEMENT

General management of a health-care agency such as a hospital concerns the management of the whole with a view to achieving strategic objectives. The strategic objectives in turn may be defined as the outputs (whether particular services, treatments or programmes) that help to achieve the overall aims of the enterprise. Aims, in other words, are the broadest level of achievement: achieving one's aims may be restated as achieving the desired outcomes.

Examples of outcomes in health care are: a better health status of the population as a whole or for targeted groups within the population; more 'consumer-friendly' health services; and/or, greater equality in health status. The achievement of strategic objectives may be considered to be the achievement of outputs (such as the construction of appropriate facilities or operation of appropriate services) which have been analysed as contributing to, or likely to contribute to, one's desired outcomes.

Functional management is management within a particular function, such as: the medical profession or its specialties; the nursing profession; the catering function; or the estates and buildings function. In other words, there seems to be a strong overlap in theory between functions and professions: it might be appropriate to say that all professions have a function or 'are' a function. Alternatively, functions are support services for professionally delivered 'outputs' from the whole system.

Strategic management may be used synonymously with general management. However, it is possible for strategic issues to be managed within a functional context: for example, a manpower strategy for the medical profession may be considered to be a strategic issue but may be discussed within the remit of the medical 'function'. Strategic management can best be given meaning by distinguishing it from its opposite, **operational management**. The latter concerns the day-to-day working and servicing of services and support services required to provide health care. Strategic management can also be distinguished from **tactical management**. This is another contrast, on another dimension, which distinguishes between 'rational planning' and 'opportunism' in making management decisions. Generally, tactics are at a lower level of operation within an enterprise or institution – but not necessarily!

It is the job of strategic management to formulate plans to help to achieve strategic objectives – whether management is at the national level or at the level of the enterprise, institution or agency. One often reads articles that seek to elaborate the vague distinction between strategic management and strategic planning. Strategic management is geared to achieving strategic plans – whether these plans involve the full public provision of facilities or merely the scanning of the environment to seek to identify trends and needs and to seek by one means or another to ensure that these needs are met. The former may be considered to be 'full-blooded' planning; and the latter is often described as **indicative planning**.

Indicative planning can use a variety of techniques, such as **network planning**. This sets out a series of variables that influence and are influenced by other variables in the 'environment'. A table can be set up to investigate key participants' or actors' judgements as to influence (Figure 6.1). The variables may well include external 'environmental' ones, but also significant strategic factors affecting the internal operation of the organization.

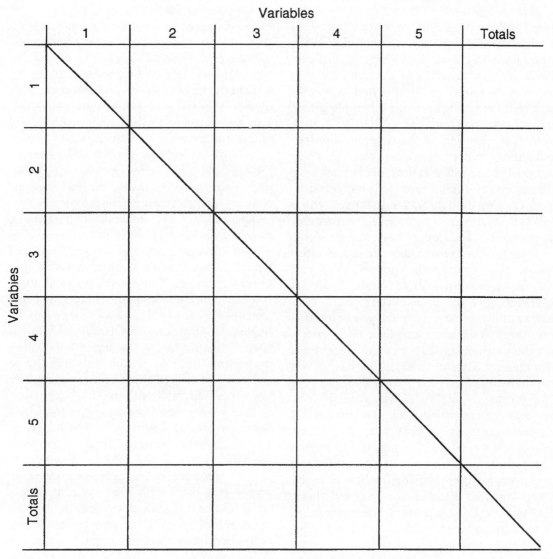

Figure 6.1 Network planning – a table showing how different variables interact

The horizontal totals show how each variable influences others, in total, and assesses their overall significance in so doing. The vertical totals show, from the same variables, each variable's tendency to be influenced by others.

Four types of variable emerge:

- strongly influencing (high horizontal totals);
- strongly influenced (high vertical totals);
- 'critical' (i.e. both);
- 'inert' (i.e. neither).

Such judgements help to scan the environment and are not definitive so much as an aid to decision-making (Gomez and Probst, 1987). The aim is to create strategic plans that rely on significant variables to achieve outcomes yet seek to minimize 'unintended' outcomes as a result of failing to detect other influences, or counteracting influences. A 'critical' variable, for example, is capable of affecting outcomes (other variables) but is easily affected itself, and therefore plans may have side-effects as a chain-reaction is mobilized.

Such a methodology has analogies with a 'SWOT' analysis, of strengths, weaknesses, opportunities and threats, but is not the same.

Strengths and weaknesses are factors internal to the organization; opportunities and threats are external 'environmental' factors (Argenti, 1980). If one uses the 'SWOT' variables not just to do a static analysis of internal and external variables and their likely effects on the product but also to predict and trace interlocking dynamic trends, one has moved to a network plan.

For example, a SWOT analysis might look at the competitiveness of a company. A network analysis would seek to portray, perhaps, how economic trends, labour market trends and so forth might affect the long-term prospects for the company; tracing how the listed variables affect each other, and therefore how desired outcomes (chosen variables) may be influenced, as well as setting up influences of their own.

THE DEVELOPMENT OF GENERAL MANAGEMENT IN HEALTH CARE

In the UK and other countries in the 1980s, there was a move away from professional management and functional management towards what is known as general management. This has applied particularly in public sector enterprises such as health services in the UK, where such an approach had previously either not been considered or ruled unsuitable for public services. Now, we see such a trend in the health service.

The essence of professional management is that, in an institution such as an hospital, the medical profession has its own hierarchy, the top of which cannot be countermanded by somebody from another profession or from outside the realm of professions altogether. The same applies to the nursing profession, and if one moves from career grades known as professions to those known as functions – for example other types of personnel, catering, X-ray, and so forth, in the hospital context – one can trace a similar logic.

The logic of general management, however, is that at each operational – or indeed strategic – level of the enterprise, all top professional officers are responsible to a general manager. Thus, in the hospital, there is an overall Unit General Manager or Chief Executive; below this, there are general managers who are the heads of clinical specialties, normally doctors; and other professions have to accept responsibility to the chiefs of each of these units, who may be known as General Managers.

It obviously confuses the issue that, in a world of clinical directors, in which doctors are in fact the general managers of their specialty, what is in essence a move to general management is perceived by other professions, often with some logic, as simply subservience to another profession, i.e. the medical profession. There may be arguments as to why this is a sensible thing, but that is a different story.

The essence of general management as described above is that professional and functional hierarchies may cease to exist altogether. Thus, not only is the overall general manager responsible both for his own board (Director of Finance, Director of Personnel, and so forth) and for the heads of the professions and functions (horizontally), but he is also responsible for lower level general managers within the organization (vertically). Thus, the lower tiers of the professional and functional hierarchies, for example the heads of clinical specialties and below them individual doctors, may be responsible to general managers for each of the hospital's divisions or specialties. These heads of divisions are then in turn responsible to the general manager. However, there is, for example, no medical responsibility up the medical hierarchy to the Chief Medical Officer.

This causes problems, in some people's minds and in reality. For example, there may well be an advisory professional relationship between a designated Chief Medical Officer and clinical specialists. But this is not the same thing as a managerial relationship, which has been abolished. Often, a confusion between the two leads to great anxiety in reorganizations informed by such principles.

Just as a general management-based chain of responsibility seems to have replaced other chains, what of the top management board (of the hospital or institution generally) comprising the Director of Finance, Director of Personnel, Director of Planning, and whoever else? Obviously, these are responsible to the overall boss, the general manager or the chief executive of the whole institution. However, it may be asked whether they have responsibilities for their own managerial lines or hierarchies. For example, are there Directors of Finance lower down the organization, for example within clinical specialties or departments, who are responsible to the Director of Finance as well as, or instead of, to their local general manager? The answer in a full general management model would have to be no. The Director of Finance, Director of Personnel, Director of Planning at the top of the organization are in fact 'advisory' rather than executive *vis-à-vis* their own functions lower down the organization. Just as the Chief Medical Officer is advisory for his professional matters to do with doctors. In other words, a Director of Finance can advise on policy for the organization but not be an operational manager, or indeed a strategic manager. He may be a strategic planner but not a strategic manager.

This raises a new distinction. Planning is

the gearing of the organization to meeting its objectives. In other words, strategic management has the responsibility for meeting strategic plans, which in turn will meet the organization's objectives *vis-à-vis* the health status of its local population, patients treated, and so forth.

General management in a hospital may be construed as a vertical chain to which former vertical chains such as professional and functional management have been subsumed. For example, different medical specialties may be responsible to general management in a hospital. Within each specialty, professions and functions generally may be responsible to a 'general manager', who is likely to be a 'clinical director' – whether or not supported by a non-medical manager/administrator.

General management is on a different dimension from professional and functional management. Obviously, general management may be concerned with operational matters concerning the servicing and continuation of functions within its own organization. However, the higher one goes within general management, the more general management is concerned with strategic matters: in other words, the meeting of objectives and the gearing of the organization, or redesign of the organization, to meet objectives. Indeed, the questioning of objectives is also a strategic matter, given that objectives may no longer be consonant with overall aims. Better strategic plans, to meet objectives, may have to be changed as objectives are changed, in line with a need to pursue aims differently. Aims are concerned with the overall mission of the organization – for example, the improvement of the health status of selected groups within the population in health care. The particular objectives by which this may be achieved may change as the environment changes, as causes of ill health change and new diseases come on the horizon.

Thus, mission equals overall aims. Strategic plan is geared to meeting objectives, which may change even though aims have not changed. Business plans within the organization are geared to providing a range of activities, and resourcing them, within the organization in order to contribute to the overall task of the organization: in other words, to meet objectives.

NATIONAL OR LOCAL?

It always seems a long distance from the articulation of the objectives of the health-care system to improvement within a particular specialty, within a particular ward or in a particular community. The emerging orthodoxy in Western management circles in the 1980s has been based on the distinction between the articulation of central objectives (which may be national objectives in the case of the health-care system) and local responsibility for achieving these objectives. In other words, one ought to be 'tight' about stated objectives – and certainly about aims at the broadest level – but one ought to devolve responsibility for achievement to particular agencies, with as much operational and financial devolution as possible. A number of 'Western' countries have seen such trends in their health-care systems, often aligned to the introduction of general management. In the UK, the Ibbs Report, *The Next Steps* (Ibbs Report, 1988), advocated that agencies responsible for delivering services within Government or through Government-funded programmes ought to be as independent as possible. In New Zealand, the introduction of board level management within the health-care system was accompanied by an attempt to devolve responsibility away from the centre. In the Netherlands, the introduction of greater competition in both the financing and provision of health care has been accompanied by greater autonomy for financiers and providers within the context of national regulation. These are but examples. However, they represent a discernible trend across national boundaries.

In order to 'develop' managers capable of

acting within their own budgets and guidelines received from 'above' as independently as possible, awareness of national policy objectives and awareness of skills required in order to operate at the local level are equally necessary. Hence, a management development programme ought not to make any artificial distinctions between 'policy' and 'management' on the one hand or 'strategy' and 'operations' on the other hand. Instead, they ought to be seen as a continuum, different parts of which are relevant for different people at different times.

Both at the national level and at the level of the providing institution, overall aims ought to be set out in what has come to be known as the 'mission statement'. Whether one likes the type of language or not, a statement of aims is essential. It is also essential that this is shared with staff and communicated, indeed developed, as democratically as possible. Objectives can be set out in the strategic plan, which again is necessary at both national and other levels. How particular components of the system (at the national level, the different regions or providers within them; at the level of the institution, the different specialties and supporting functions) may be mobilized to achieving objectives within the strategic plan is addressed by what may be known as the business plan, if one wishes to use private sector language. This links proposed activities of 'parts' within the system to the objectives of the whole system (whether the hospital or the health-care system as a whole). For example, objectives may be translated into particular targets for provision for specialties within a hospital. This may be part of a publicly planned system or part of a private sector system which is gearing anticipated demand in the marketplace to supply to be offered through the hospital's specialties. As a result, a business plan will link resources for investment and recurring costs across different specialties and functions in order to render the plan operational and in order to allow the plan to be compatible with budgetary and other constraints and opportunities. Below the level of the business plan, one is then into the realm of operational management, seeking to 'grease the wheels' of the system and to ensure that it is routinely operational.

MANAGEMENT AND ADMINISTRATION, POLICY AND PLANNING

MANAGEMENT AND ADMINISTRATION

There are many differing perspectives on the scientific status of management studies. Some would even deny that management can be studied scientifically at all, and that it is a subjective 'art'. Others would argue that management principles are geared to the achievement of ends, and that quantitative measures can be derived to monitor the success or otherwise of management tasks with given ends in mind.

One may make a distinction between **management studies** and **management science**. Management studies concerns the broad area of enquiry that looks at the overall objectives of management; the different schools of management; the political, economic and social environments within which management operates; and perspectives on organizations. (Naturally, this definition is illustrative rather than exhaustive.) Management science, on the other hand, focuses on the empirical and quantitative skills, and the analytical methods, that can be used by managers or commissioned from professionals, scientists and statisticians by managers, as tools geared to the achievement of ends in an organization. Studying management generally will, therefore, be a broader engagement than studying management science, which is a component of the task of management.

A number of distinctions made in the previous section need to be developed further. Firstly, there is **general management**. This concerns the level and type of management responsible for the overall direction of an organization or a unit within an organization (such as a district health authority). General management involves the setting of goals for an organization or unit, the mobilization of resources, manpower and planning systems to achieve these goals and the monitoring of progress en route to these goals, involving the management of the components of the enterprise. These specialized components may be dominated, as in the National Health Service, by different professions. This brings us on to a second type of management, **professional management**. This concerns the internal management of the responsibilities and workload of a profession – for example, the management of pathology services in a district health authority. Clinicians have many management concerns within their own specialty before even considering the wider territory of resource management.

Thirdly, there is **operations management**. This concerns the management of operations or functions necessary to service or support an organization. Support services have to be managed to achieve the subgoals within an enterprise or organization that allow the meeting of overall goals as defined by general management. As we will see later, a relevant question in the UK today when considering the merits of centralization and decentralization within organizations is whether the management of support functions is centralized and fairly autonomous within an organization or whether each unit manager within an organization is responsible for determining the level and nature of his own support services.

Management is often contrasted with administration. Administration refers to the servicing of an organization's needs given an acceptance of its current course – an often legalistic 'hand on the tiller' – as opposed to management's concern with determining and reassessing objectives and steering the organization (with all that implies for changed internal practices where necessary) – 'changing course' when necessary.

British public life, naturally, is peppered with references to administration and management which reflect either overt or hidden assumptions as to the style of operation of an organization. The term 'the administrative class' of the Civil Service points to the original ethos of administration as opposed to general or professional management. Until the Griffiths Enquiry reported in October 1983 and was accepted by the Government, the National Health Service did not have a system of general management to steer its components, but was serviced by a system of administration reflected in the titles Regional Administrator, District Administrator, and so forth. An important question then is 'what has instituted and formalized a change from "the age of administration" to the "age of management"?' It would be dangerous to see such (contemporary) historical trends as inevitable or indeed automatically rational. However, there have been compelling forces behind such change in the UK recently, and it is important to understand them.

POLICY AND IMPLEMENTATION

One can consider a policy at two levels. Firstly, there is Government policy, which affects the management of the organization and, secondly, there is the internal policy devised by and for the organization. It is important to distinguish policy-making in both those senses from implementation. Policy is – on its own – mere intention; implementation affects results and outcomes.

It is important at this stage to identify some key terms. In policy and organizational analysis, three central terms are **inputs**, **outputs** and **outcomes**, as introduced in Chapter 1. At the political level of making policy – for example, through passing legislation – inputs refer to the factors that affect the policy-making process: for example, the relative strength of political parties in a legislature, the effect of interest groups and the contribu-

tion of academics or think tanks to the realm of ideas are all likely to provide examples of inputs to policy-making. At the political level, the key output is the accomplished legislation or regulation. However, it is when thinking of outcomes that one realizes the effective implementation.

Laws may achieve unintended results, or little result at all. Regulations may not work as expected. The way in which policy is implemented determines what might be called social outcome. Using the terms in a different context, one can apply the language of inputs, outputs and outcomes within an organization, for example in a private firm or a service.

In the manufacturing process, inputs are the factors of production – primarily capital and labour. Outputs are the products made, and outcomes can be considered to be the longer-term results either for the company (for example, in terms of the profits and incomes received) or for the public (in terms of the availability of goods and their ability to satisfy preferences and live a certain lifestyle).

In the National Health Service, inputs to the 'production' process are also reducible to labour and capital: in this case, we are talking about doctors, nurses and similar professions, and every form of labour within the National Health Service; at the level of money, we are talking not just of capital investment but of revenue budgets, as indeed in private firms. Outputs refer to the services delivered – for example, the number of operations, number of home visits by district nurses in a community setting, number of cervical smears carried out. Outputs, however, are not the same as outcomes here either; outcomes refer to the effect upon the health status of the population which the provision of a health service has (notoriously a difficult thing to measure, when one considers the many effects upon the health of populations, groups and individuals that have to be disentangled).

Just as the implementation of policy affects how outputs are transformed into outcomes at a political level in society, how services are delivered affects outcomes in an 'industry' like the National Health Service and how products are marketed affects outcomes both for the firm and for society in the private enterprise.

THE DEPARTMENT OF HEALTH – PLANNING AND MANAGEMENT

It is naturally the case that, in the public sector, the political aspect of strategic management is more important – or at least is more direct and often more visible. That is, in an arena such as the National Health Service, the influence of the Government and politicians upon the delivery of services is more direct. This is not to deny the influence of politics in setting the constraints within which private enterprises operate, but the Department of Trade and Industry in the early 1990s, for example, is very much a 'bare bones' partner which sets the framework and offers relatively minimal restraints within which industry operates, by comparison with the 'corporatism' of the 1970s.

Public enterprises and public corporations in the business world have generally copied the management structures of private enterprises, at least at a formal level. The large corporations in the public sector, like their parallels in the private sector, have a corporate board with a chief executive, whatever the exact form of the title is. In many cases, the chief executive will be entitled the Chairman of the Board or Company (for example, Michael Edwardes became Chairman of the publicly-owned British Leyland in October 1977). This corporate board will have as its key members a Director of Finance, Director of Corporate Affairs/Corporate Planning, and Director of Personnel – whatever exact forms these titles take.

Service industries or services in the public sector have not traditionally had a similar form of strategic management. It is only recently, for example, that the National Health Service has been given first a Management Board (in 1983/84) and subsequently a Management Executive (following the White Paper of 1989, *Working for Patients* – Department of Health, 1989) to direct and oversee the service. The analogy here is with the public or private corporate board, which is the 'apex' of the company or service and which is responsible for managing the achievement of corporate goals and priorities. As with the public or private corporation, such a board has its Director of Personnel, its Director of Corporate Planning and Information and its Director of Finance. The Management Board was, however, dogged with the reality of alleged political interference. The first Chairman of the Board, Mr Victor Paige, resigned because he felt he was not free to manage without a tight political agenda. Some see this an inevitable in a publicly financed NHS which is responsible to ministers, themselves responsible to Parliament (at least in the UK's informal constitutional theory).

The NHS Management Board and Executive sit uneasily with traditional Civil Service control or 'administration' of the National Health Service. Prior to the Griffiths Enquiry and its acceptance in 1983, there was no apex for strategic management of the National Health Service. There was a Secretary of State responsible to Parliament, with the 'top of the office' of DHSS civil servants (on the Department of Health side of what was then the Department of Health and Social Security) responsible to the Minister for the administration of the department first and the NHS second. In the opinion of many, there was a basic lacuna where strategic management was lacking. This, of course, went to the heart of the distinction between 'traditional' administration and 'modern' general management.

There were various professional lines of control linking the Department of Health with lower tiers of the National Health Service. For example, the Chief Medical

Officer had his hierarchy, the Chief Nursing Officer hers (the gender reflecting empirical reality rather than sexist assumptions), and various other professions likewise sent their tentacles down into the National Health Service. However, at the administrative level, ministers and civil servants had no clear lines of control to regional and district administrators. District management teams were responsible to district health authorities, which were not, however (at this time), necessarily responsible to regional health authorities. Regional management teams were responsible to regional health authorities which were only loosely responsible to the Department of Health on certain key parameters.

It should be observed that, even when managerial relationships have been tidied up and developed to parallel general management in private corporations, the fundamental problem remains: what role are the politicians going to play? Does the establishment of a professional management structure for a service mean that 'politics' is removed from the operation of that service? In theory, this was what the Griffiths Report was seeking to achieve. In practice, however, it was not achieved – in that politicians, and indeed civil servants, were unable to 'keep their fingers out of the pie'. The White Paper *Working for Patients* called for (in an important clause tucked in behind the advocacy of a provider market for health care) the establishment of a Management Executive which would recognize the inevitability of political control (hence the – renamed – 'Policy Board' which would oversee it) yet which would be responsible for better management within a (tacitly admitted) more limited sphere than that granted the Management Board in the Griffiths Report of 1983.

This is understandable. Politicians are responsible to Parliament; the National Health Service is a politically very visible and popular service; and there is no way that individual MPs, let alone the Secretary of State for Health, are suddenly going to be silent – even on matters of health detail, let alone broad policy. The ambulance dispute of 1989/90 showed a lack of clarity as to whether – on operational and tactical matters – the NHS is 'neutrally' managed by a Chief Executive or 'politically' by the Secretary of State for Health.

The interaction of policy, planning and management is crucial. **Policy** may well be set by politicians. **Planning** means many things. In the provision of public services, it may mean the derivation of need on a geographical basis, the provision of services to meet them and the development of plans to provide these services. This is the sort of planning that the National Health Service has traditionally gone in for (whether or not it remains after the White Paper of 1989 is a point open to question). Naturally more detailed policy may have to be developed in practice by strategic managers, as they seek to implement broad policy guidelines.

Some form of planning will, of course, take place in any large-scale corporation. Even if it is not geographical need-based planning for populations, it will be organizational planning to meet targets – what one might term 'internal' planning. In the late 1980s, following the trend in the private corporate world, large-scale strategic planning even of this latter sort, especially in a centralized form, has fell into disrepute. By the early 1990s, 'planning' was undergoing something of a revival, both for and in the private sector (respectively, by governmental and by industry itself), in the Western world and especially in the USA (if less so in the UK), and in the NHS in particular.

ASSESSING THE TRANSFORMATION: ABANDONING THE CULT OF THE AMATEUR

In the middle of the 19th century, the North–Trevelyan Report of 1853 had called for the professionalization of the Civil Service and its recruitment by open and meritocratic methods. This led to a reformed Civil Service in 1870 which Anthony Sampson described as 'the first great British meritocracy' (Sampson, 1983).

The essence of the reform was that the recruited civil servants should be 'a profession of amateurs'. The rationale for this is now more than well known: it was argued that generalists could provide lay advice to ministers and lay administration of their departments, while relying upon technical and specialist advice where necessary.

It is fair to say that this approach has been perceived, rightly or wrongly, as increasingly anachronistic throughout the latter part of the 20th century. As the economy has become more specialized and the responsibilities of the Civil Service have increased dramatically, the ethos of lay administration has become increasingly unsuitable. In consequence, the Wilson government in the 1960s set up the Fulton Committee to make proposals for reform of the Civil Service. When it reported in 1968, it confirmed the belief that the Civil Service structure and the education of its senior officers were geared to the needs of the 19th century. As Sampson says, 'they insisted that the "amateur" or "generalist" was "obsolete at all levels and in all parts of the service"'. The Fulton Committee proposed that the multifarious separate classes of the Civil Service be removed and be replaced by a simplified structure. Secondly, it was thought vital that specialists should have more responsibility and a more central role in the administration and management. The Fulton reforms included a new college for civil servants and a new Civil Service Department, independent from the Treasury, to manage the Civil Service itself. Of course, this Civil Service Department has subsequently been abolished.

As with many significant reforms affecting the Civil Service in individual departments, this overall reform affecting the whole Civil Service was – perhaps inevitably, yet astonishingly – put in the hands of the civil servants. In consequence, many people believed that the essence of the reforms proposed was ignored. A traditional Civil Service stalling job was accomplished.

Even the supplementary aspects of the Fulton Committee's recommendations did not necessarily achieve the effect intended. The French ENA (Ecole Nationale d'Administration) had been the model for a Civil Service College, which was set up at Sunningdale. This college never lived up to the ENA-style pretensions.

More recently (in 1991), plans for a 'National Health Service staff college' were developed by the then Secretary of State for Health, William Waldegrave. Again the follow-up was minimal.

It is no surprise that Prime Minister Thatcher had little respect for the traditional norms of the Civil Service. Her attitude to government was that, however much she might enjoy an argument on selected occasions, business had to be conducted by people who could individually be described as 'one of us'. In the same way as left-wingers feared the stalling influence upon left-wing governments of the Civil Service, Mrs. Thatcher and her right-wing supporters feared the influence of the Civil Service in moderating or reducing the impact of her proposed policy reforms. Nevertheless, the Thatcher governments steered clear of large-scale institutional reorganization in the Civil Service, instead stressing behavioural change. Although the Civil Service Department was abolished and its functions transferred to the Cabinet Office, Thatcher governments attempted to limit any imagined Civil Service opposition to policy by judicious appointments, rather than by formal reorganization, and indeed by the politicization of the senior Civil Service. New permanent secretaries were generally 'one of us' – or had to pretend to be such.

CIVIL SERVICE REFORMS AND HEALTH SERVICE REFORMS

Initiatives throughout the 1980s to improve management of the Civil Service have had direct implications for the health service. One of the first such initiatives involved the return of Sir Derek Rayner (later Lord Rayner) to Whitehall (he had previously come from Marks & Spencer to report on waste and extravagance in the Ministry of Defence), to work as the Prime Minister's personal adviser on efficiency. It is not unfair to say that Rayner set the ground rules for subsequent changes in Civil Service and then health service practice.

The former Permanent Secretary at the Department of Health and Social Security, Sir Patrick Nairne, subsequently observed that a key task of the Permanent Secretary up to the 1980s was to **administer his department**, not to **manage the services his department was responsible for providing**. Sampson points out, referring to Rayner, that 'he soon observed that the mandarins who were running the nation's biggest organizations were far more interested in writing minutes on policy questions – which was how they got promoted – than in the workaday problems of management.' That is, civil servants at the 'top of the office' dealt in general policy and advice to ministers, while at lower levels administration was internal and not related to efficient management of services.

The Rayner Scrutinies were devised to investigate cost savings achievable in specific programmes within departments. This technical approach soon became identified with profound implications for the Civil Service. It became implicit that skill in the realms of programme management and efficiency ought to be a criteria for most civil servants, so that such skills would feed through to the top. A corollary of this was that administrative class civil servants of tradition were not necessarily the best people to reach the top – the implication now was that provincial civil servants 'running local offices' might be just as suitable, if not more so. The trouble was, no middle ground between 'policy papers' and 'cost savings' was identified: managerially based policy analysis was ignored for shorter-term savings.

Subsequently, various initiatives known by their acronyms VFM and FMI ('value for money' and 'financial management initiative') reinforced the ethos of Rayner and were implemented in the NHS, as elsewhere in Government departments and the public sector branches for which they were responsible. Sir Derek Rayner, who had returned as Lord Rayner to Marks & Spencer, was succeeded by Sir Robin Ibbs. The Ibbs Report, discussed above, advocated the diminution of large, functional, 'direct labour' departments within the Civil Service and their replacement by contracting and providing agencies. Often the agenda was simply to change terms and conditions of employment. These became known as '*Next Steps*' agencies and it was argued that the NHS Management Board (succeeded by the Executive) become one. It remains, however, a hybrid; formally, it is within the Department of Health yet it is encouraged to be independent when it suits politicians!

Specific initiatives in specific departments have also come broadly from the same stable. The whole ethos of the Griffiths Report was to instil effective management into the National Health Service.

The essence of the Griffiths Report was that general management should be introduced at the apex of the National Health Service, to provide a management board with corporate direction for the service, as other private and public industries had. The implications were quite radical. The key civil servants in the Department of Health (separated from Social Security in 1988) would now have to be general managers and not generalist policy advisers and administrators. The Permanent Secretary would still play this role, but he would no longer be the 'bureaucrat running the health service'. The Chairman of the NHS Management Board – and subsequently the Chief Executive of the NHS Management Executive, following the 1989 White Paper – would now play the direct managerial role.

Thus, the generalist policy advice to ministers and the 'administration of the office' continues but can be interpreted as either being somewhat sidelined or as only one of a number of major activities at the centre of the Department.

One implication of Griffiths to many was that 'the administrative staff' of the Department of Health be diminished. In the early days of the Griffiths inquiry, when it was thought that Griffiths was going to succeed – not only in the service but also at the centre – with his 'brave new world', with severe implications for the Department of Health, it was envisaged by some commentators that two-thirds of the civil servants would have to be removed from the Department. This, of course, never came about, due to effective rearguard actions, Fulton-style, by the Permanent Secretary and some of his senior staff.

Indeed, the initial logic of the situation was that the new management executive or board for the National Health Service would not be based in the Department of Health at all. The idea was that a management board ought to be outside it. In other words, one should distinguish between the executive management board of a particular service, such as the National Health Service, and civil servants, however management-minded, who are not directly responsible for running particular services. One can, for example, distinguish between management-minded civil servants in the Department of Trade and Industry, who are not after all responsible for running industry, and the management board of an actual industry. (Of course, most such industries – such as telecommunications, gas and electricity – were privatized in the 1980s and early 1990s.) Such industries were generally in the realm of transport (British Rail), communications, utilities or strategic primary production (Coal, Steel).

Nonetheless, in the case of a publicly provided public service like the National Health Service, the distinction between the manager and the civil servant may be some-

what blurred. In the end, the Griffiths recommendations for a management board for the National Health Service were accepted, but the management board was placed within the department: its Chief Executive and Chairman was to be a civil servant with the rank, indeed, of Second Permanent Secretary. He was now to be the Accounting officer for the National Health Service.

In practice, there has been 'turf fighting' between traditional civil servants and management board appointments. Following the White Paper of 1989 and the subsequent legislation, the National Health Service Act of 1990, it seemed likely that some of the more awkward managerial relationships would be ironed out, on paper at least. The Secretary of State would now work closely with the management executive, while still relying on 'advisory' policy inputs from the traditional civil servants, headed by the Permanent Secretary. Unfortunately these changes were accompanied by a blatant politicization of NHS chairmanships and senior managerial appointments, leading to a new 'quangocracy' whereby quangos ran the public service rather than accountable politicians or managers.

Regarding a number of departments, including Health (but also Education and Social Security, for example), the cabinet, which in the Thatcher administrations was very much dominated by the Prime Minister, relied on advice from external think tanks, and in particular, the Prime Minister's 'No. 10 Policy Unit', to a much greater extent than previously. The Central Policy Review Staff (the 'think tank') had been set up in the Heath government of the early 1970s to provide outside advice to shed new light on policy questions. In Mrs Thatcher's first administration, this think tank was abolished, and the No. 10 Policy Unit was probably more directly under the personal control of the Prime Minister (although the first head of the original think tank, Lord Rothschild, had also had a particularly close relationship with the Prime Minister of the day).

More importantly, the No. 10 Policy Unit dealt much more in partisan advice, in the field of health care. Supplemented by advice from other think tanks (such as the Adam Smith Institute, the Institute of Economic Affairs Health Unit and especially the Centre for Policy Studies), traditional civil servants were initially surprised to find their advice often being ignored in favour of prescriptions which only a few years before would have been seen as coming from the impractical wing of quasi-academia. Under the subsequent Major administration, the 'new right' think tanks diminished somewhat in import, owing not least to turf fighting within them between 'Thatcherite true believers' and 'pragmatists' who were ambitious for influence in the post-Thatcher Conservative Party. Nevertheless an obsession with 'privatization for efficiency' – even when private provision is more expensive – came to dominate NHS debates, especially concerning the provision of new **capital** for the NHS. In this realm, the public sector was hamstrung by regulations which called for 'private capital as a first resort'. This resulted from an unholy alliance between the Treasury, keen to restrict public investment for short-termist reasons, and more ideological privatizers.

To summarize, although the Civil Service has not been substantially cut and conditions of service have not been substantially altered by reorganization, the significant changes which have occurred can be listed as follows:

- the diminution of the centrality of traditional lay advice on policy matters;
- the diminution in the functional provision of services through direct labour in Civil Service departments in favour of agency relationships;
- the infusion of private sector techniques via management efficiency studies within the departments which led to new criteria for 'successful' departmental management;

- the increased role of private sector individuals in advising politicians through secondments (working alongside official civil servants);
- the involvement of the private sector in administering and managing particular projects (for example, the Training and Enterprise Council in the field of training and enterprise; regional development through the Manpower Services Commission; and involvement in the Education Department's Technical and Vocational Education Initiative (TVEI).

Private sector techniques and advice were imported into health care through increased 'businessmen's' involvement on slimmer, corporate-style health authorities.

Following the 'NHS reforms' instigated by the 1989 White Paper, all health authorities were to have eleven members, including a chairman, five non-executive members and five executive officers. Self-governing trusts were to have similar representation, on the 'provider' side. Likewise, family practitioner committees were replaced by supposedly more 'businesslike' family health service authorities.

'MODERN' APPROACHES TO MANAGEMENT

THE DECLINE OF STRATEGIC BUSINESS PLANNING

In the private sector, both in the USA and in the UK, a conventional wisdom developed in the 1980s that centralization of planning and control within large companies does not make for effective management or good outcome. In consequence, decentralization into units within companies, with separate responsibilities or separate markets, has been the developing norm. Centralized planning, for example, with a divisional structure, with all divisions responsible upwards to a central board, has not been considered flexible enough to meet the needs of increasingly competitive markets.

'Strategic planning has been born in a flurry of optimism and industrial growth in the 1960s and early 1970s.' Every business aspired to have a strategic planning staff and every business had a planning curriculum. But by the 1980s, the fashion had shifted. The new buzzwords were 'corporate culture', 'quality', 'implementation', 'just in time' management. Japanese companies, it was observed, did not prepare corporate plans. Criticism of strategic planning may have been deserved; such planning had not, in most companies, contributed to strategic thinking.

The decline of strategic planning was not, however, based on some sort of theoretical inadequacy that it might be considered to have, but on its failure to operate in practice. Similarly, in public services, or public industries meeting populations' needs, it may be considered that strategic planning has often failed not because it has theoretical shortcomings in the abstract but because in practice its pretensions have been belied. A service such as the National Health Service attempts to plan to meet the needs of populations. Public enterprises attempt to 'plan' to meet needs which consumers are likely to demand in the marketplace.

One ought to separate public or private ownership of provision, and public or private purchasing. The traditional nationalized utilities in the UK, for example, were publicly owned but sold to consumers in the marketplace. On the other hand, the National Health Service, while by and large publicly provided, is also publicly financed – the Government is the surrogate consumer on behalf of the public and there is no direct provider/consumer relationship in the same way.

Corporate planning, however, has fallen into disrepair in public services for general ideological reasons. When related to its decline in favour in the private business world, a political momentum against it is strengthened. As the above quotation shows, the new buzzwords become corporate culture, quality, devolution and implementa-

tion. 'Buzzword' is an appropriately chosen term, for the transition from large-scale strategic planning towards decentralized forms of operation was not based on scientific research so much as evolving trends in the business world. These are often the most determinate factors leading to changing policy (indeed internationally, let alone from sector to sector within one country). If we therefore turn to the question of devolution, we have to ask ourselves: what is devolution all about?

DEVOLUTION AND DECENTRALIZATION

Firstly, it is about financial decentralization. If units are to be given operational control for their production of services or products within the overall company responsibility and market, financial decentralization has to be given to allow them a flexibility to invest and finance their revenue budgets as required. If every budget functionally ascribed from the top of the company, then decentralization is a myth and the decentralized unit has responsibility but not power. Therefore, flexibility in decisions over finance, over personnel, over product mix and over particular operational systems of control in order to meet output goals are necessary.

This may therefore mean that financial decentralization is accompanied by decentralization of decision-making about how much labour to employ, what type of labour to employ and indeed at what rates to employ labour. Most typically, such decisions will not be wholly free but within a 'spine' or system of constraints imposed by the central company. Just as national wage bargaining and centralized wage bargaining within firms have fallen into ideological disrepair (Chapter 8), centralized decision-making, including decisions about employment and wages within public industries and public services, have also been sharply questioned increasingly. One sees this in the National Health Service. That later chapter on the management of human resources discusses this issue.

The theory is that decentralization downwards is accompanied by accountability upwards. Decentralized units may well have targets for performance (based on performance indicators); overall criteria within which they have to manage their resources (systems of resource management or norms for efficiency); overall norms for achieving planning goals (despite the demise of planning) and other obligations. That is, one can question for any one enterprise how the mix of devolution downwards and accountability upwards works in practice. Is it closet centralism? Or is it a creative relationship, or creative tension, between centralism and devolution?

Interestingly, as overall operations have been decentralized according to the prevailing trend, or one might say fad, conventional wisdom is also emerging that education and training of workforces ought to be centralized. There are perhaps two reasons for this. Firstly, there is a reason based on economic theory: if individual units are responsible for their own training needs, economies of scale will not be realized and a unit may train important staff merely to see them poached by other units.

Thus, for example, if, in the National Health Service, districts or trusts are responsible for their own training, they may simply be training to benefit other districts than themselves. Therefore, there is no incentive to do so. The other reason is not so narrowly economic, but is concerned with the importance of career development, especially when it comes to more significant staff within a company organization. To be effective, systems of long-term career development have to be developed company-wide, or even industry-wide, to ensure that meaningful career progression is possible. Naturally, such systems could not be developed within the constraints of small intracompany units.

MISSION AND CORE VALUES

Public enterprise and public service have followed private corporations in developing and refining what are known as 'mission' statements and statements of 'core values'. The objective here is to integrate different professions engaged in the design, production, and delivery of products into meeting overall company objectives to a greater extent. At the end of the day, the aim is to improve market share, improve quality, and – through integration of activity – improve efficiency also. Thus, in the public sector, organizations that were not well known for having a 'corporate culture' are often seeking to develop such in order to copy, once again, what seems to be an accepted criterion for success in private industry.

In the Health Service, for example, health managers are seen increasingly as part 'corporate loyalists' and part 'obedient civil servants' rather than (in the former caricature) semi-detached lay administrators who were responsible for their patch but were not directly or corporately responsible in a line of command upwards to the central apex of the service. One might argue that such accountability is a necessary analogue for decentralization of operational responsibility. Nevertheless, the new regional directors are responsible for 'managing the market' (if that is not a contradiction in terms) and have a lot of unaccountable power. The personal integrity of many NHS regional directors is high. But the Government's agenda is generally tight, and a system of 'checks and balances' to prevent hasty implementation (say, of hospital closures, in the absence of adequate community care) is generally absent.

QUALITY *VERSUS* QUANTITY: 'NEW' MANAGEMENT *VERSUS* 'OLD' PLANNING

In the National Health Service as elsewhere, there has developed a not-quite-tongue-in-cheek aphorism which goes, 'quantity is now a quality issue'. This goes to the heart of the tension between reconciling quantity of output and quality of output in any cash-limited service.

If we are talking about the private market, the firm or corporation's incentives will generally involve the production of maximum profit within given organizational constraints, and given trade-offs, for example between short-term and long-term. A company may seem to maximize profits by producing a smaller output of higher quality at higher prices, or, as in the 'mass production', through maximizing quantity given a minimum definition of quality at a lower level than in a 'high quality' market. Indeed, finding one's 'market niche' may mean an overt decision as to what level of quality – is one seeking to be Safeway or Waitrose?

If we are talking about a public service or public corporation operating within budget constraints, there may be expectations of a certain quantity to be produced and, likewise, expectations as to quality. It may be that the stated objectives as to both quantity and quality are unrealistic. Efficiency improvements will always, albeit with diminishing marginal returns, make the reconciliation of quantity and quality easier, yet there is obviously a limit as to what can be achieved within given resources.

A health service, for example, may have an implicit or explicit obligation to deliver a quantum of services – acute hospital services, mental health services, community services, general practitioner services, and so forth – to a population or a whole country. If the resources within which these services are provided are limited, then there will be corresponding limits on what quality can be produced. Furthermore, by quality, do we mean something intrinsic to the output or outcome (for example, a higher quality operation leading to greater quality of life or longer life for a patient) or do we mean quality in support services (for example a pleasant room and good food when one is in hospital)? The later chapter on quality analyses the concept more rigorously.

One supposed distinction between the 'old' planning and the 'new' management (seen as marking the divide between the 1970s and the 1980s) is the former's concentration upon norms defined in quantity terms and the latter's alleged ability to make more subtle distinctions in defining corporate objectives. Centralized planning naturally often has to deal with the provision of norms, whether to be obeyed or merely used for guidance, in the provision of services. The new corporate management approach, however, is geared to allowing leeway to decentralized managers to determine their product mix and therefore implicitly the trade-off between quantity and quality. Naturally, especially in public services, simply to state this is to gloss over the complexity and political difficulty of managing freely. Politicians may impose impossible constraints upon management as to quantity expectations as well as to quality expectations. For example, in the National Health Service, although by international standards we have areas of high quality in core medical care, the overall quality of the product is often seen as inevitably taking a back seat to the need to squeeze the maximum out of limited resources, which adversely affects the 'glossy' side of quality.

Another question might ask, to what relative extent is 'secondary' (glossy) quality important in the NHS, *vis-à-vis* 'primary quality', i.e. safe, effective medical treatment with a good outcome? The answer might be, less than on an airline. Virgin Atlantic is genuinely good quality, arguably, because one expects safety and ability to arrive from all 747s, and therefore appreciates an individual TV on the back of the seat in front. But medical care is more variable and more 'complex'. It is more important to 'get the core products right'. Despite its hitherto standardized or 'Fordist' hospitals, medical care is a highly differentiated product, and one moreover undergoing constant change and 'post Fordist' modernization. (Witness, for example, the slow but noticeable decline in the centrality of traditional secondary care *vis-à-vis* primary and tertiary care.)

SOME CURRENT ISSUES IN STRATEGIC MANAGEMENT IN HEALTH CARE

AGENCY STATUS: THE CONSEQUENCES FOR THE NHS

A fundamental institutional change running through the public sector in the UK, and also in many countries abroad at the present time – as noted above – is the movement from centrally controlled functional divisions of corporations and organizations to contractual relationships with autonomous agencies.

In other words, a distinction is made between strategic or corporate management and support services or operational management; the latter are hived off from the central enterprise and the services for which they were responsible are contracted as necessary by a central board of the enterprise or organization. To give some examples: unit management boards in the health services (for example, of hospitals or of community service units) buy in nursing and physiotherapy services in accordance with the specific goal-related tasks they are pursuing, rather than using the nurses and physiotherapists who are on the payroll according to some centrally planned norm which determines their numbers, grades, and so forth.

In the Civil Service generally, the Ibbs Report drew attention to a perceived need to distinguish between top-level policy advisers and top-level general managers on the one hand, who together comprise the core staff of Civil Service departments, and the staff responsible for providing operational services on the other hand – who, in a radical interpretation of the report, would no longer be functionally employed by a large central organization (like in this case, the Civil Service), but would be 'hived off' to autonomous agencies who would sink or swim according to their ability to sell their services to their former departments, in a competitive environment.

In the event, the idea was implemented slowly in the UK. The Employment Service and the NHS Estates Department were, however, granted agency status, and there were proposals that the whole of the NHS Management Executive should become an agency, responsible for health authorities and therefore the provision of health care. It is interesting to note that in New Zealand, a similar strategy has been carried out much more universally and radically. Nevertheless, the 1993/1994 reviews of the Department of Health (the Banks Review) and of the supra-district NHS (the Manpower and Functions Reviews, supervised by Langlands) have stopped short of this option. Arguably there has been instead fairly incremental tinkering – which may, of course, be the right approach.

THE PRINCIPLE OF CONTRACTING

The essential aim of creating management agencies to replace functional divisions of large administrative departments is that greater cost-effectiveness (or economy) should be achieved in meeting certain goals. If one starts with large, centrally planned, functionally organized departments, it is alleged that there is a tendency to 'make the work fit the inputs' rather than 'hiring inputs to do the job'. In other words, if one defines cost-effectiveness as achieving a given output or outcome with minimum cost inputs, it is not sensible to start with already determined, centrally ascribed or functionally ascribed inputs. Instead, a principle of competitive tendering ought to inform purchasing of inputs.

Note that this assumes a given set of objectives to be translated into outputs or outcomes. If one has a given quantum of inputs (for example, direct labour employed by a department, fixed financial resources and fixed use of these resources, i.e. with little virement between alternative uses), then a definition of cost-effectiveness incorporating the notion of efficiency would argue that the maximum output ought to be achieved from given inputs. However, it seems to make sense that, given that it is up to the policy-makers to take responsibility for the goals, it is then up to the strategic managers – who may, of course, help to determine these goals – to devise the best strategy for meeting those goals efficiently.

THE SPLIT BETWEEN PURCHASING AND PROVIDING

The essence of the reform promulgated in the health sector as a result of the White Paper *Working for Patients* had as its rationale a split between purchasing and providing in the National Health Service. The purchasing/providing split and agency status are linked. The former calls for more flexible providers, who can be seen as types of agency rather than centrally administered arms of the organization. In the political debate about whether 'self-governing' trusts are 'opting out', use of the term 'agency' might have diffused some of the row, if it had been made clear the agencies were publicly owned.

TARGETS FOR HEALTH AND 'FUTURES'

It is not just in the pro-competitive policy and structural changes inherent in the post-1991 NHS that strategic management faces significant challenges. Allegedly, a desire to concentrate on outcomes – the health status of individuals, groups, classes and the population as a whole – led to the 'White Paper' of 1992, *The Health of the Nation*, which set targets for achieving reductions in mortality and morbidity from specific diseases. Of course, such an agenda is a convenient 'motherhood and apple pie' means of diffusing the row over more controversial health policy.

The achievement of quantified outcomes is perhaps the touchstone of 'scientific manage-

ment'. In health care, effective management therefore requires a similar approach in theory, even if the practice is infinitely more complex than in (say) a one-product industry.

One means of bringing about better outcomes is by scanning the environment to identify likely trends, alternative possibilities and therefore alternative 'futures', i.e. future outcomes when trends are mediated by appropriate health-care interventions. The Department of Health has recently shown signs of learning from established programmes in the Dutch Ministry of Welfare, in this regard. Nevertheless, many of the *Health of the Nation* targets are simply projections of already-existing trends.

Value judgements, here as elsewhere, are important in deciding priorities even when or if trends are known. The QALY (quality adjusted life year) – as discussed in Chapter 3 – is perhaps the best known methodology for helping senior policy-makers and strategic managers at least to evaluate 'hard choices'. In this respect, it is a tool which nevertheless involves value-judgement. QALY may be a good servant, but is a bad master. Policy analysis (in the sense of devising good policy) and strategic management are arts as well as sciences.

MARKETING

Marketing has long been a basic concern for private companies, for which the rationale is naturally to sell a product. At its simplest definition, marketing is about how to do this best. In public organizations that do not sell a traditional product in a traditional manner, the concept of marketing has also been applied much more in recent years.

It is clear that the word 'marketing' will have a slightly different connotation in this context. While it may involve the promotion of services for the public (social marketing), the fact that there are surrogate purchasers (health authorities) in an industry such as the National Health Service means that providers are not (necessarily) marketing themselves directly to their customers.

LEARNING FROM THE PRIVATE SECTOR

The message from Handy (1989) seems to be one of 'permanent revolution' based on both changing markets and manipulation of markets by providers. Decentralization is the great theme of the business and management world of the future. Even in the realm of ideology, both the political left wing and political right-wing now build manifestos on decentralization, albeit with different connotations. But this may simply be a rationalization of modern capitalism. Handy (1989) refers to 'half the people working twice as hard while the other half have not enough to do'. He goes on to say that 'the new rich will not have the time or the energy to enjoy their riches; the leisure class will be those at the bottom of the heap rather than those at the top. An upside-down world.' Thus is a great management guru persuaded of what critical theorists have been arguing for decades.

Arguably, 'post-Fordism' in industry – the passing of the traditional industrial 'production line' – finds a mirror in health care, as flexible techniques and new services change the nature of provision.

One of the fastest growing cottage industries of recent years has been development of personalized prescriptions for business success – guides for strategic and general managers to re-order their whole mode of management in order to achieve better results. While useful prescriptions certainly may exist, two caveats must be recorded. Firstly, prescriptions may not be generalizable – we may not be talking about universal science so much as anecdote and case history, however important or valuable. Secondly, the charlatan promoting the fad is always a danger. This is translated into 'contingency theory' (or lack of it!) in management textbooks. Often, the fad may not be something wholly disreputable so much as 'the obvious' translated into management technique; or, alternatively, the unjustified attribution of 'cause' to 'effect'. One is reminded, when facing the airport bookstall groaning with prescriptions for 'how to succeed in business', 'make a million' or promote 'outrageous quality', of the old aphorism: 'Your thesis is both true and original. Unfortunately, what is true is not original; and what is original is not true'!

NHS MARKETING AND BUSINESS PLANNING: FROM OLD TO NEW

Strategic management of and within the provider (the hospital and other service units) has become more central since the NHS 'reforms'. In a context of 'managed competition', the provider is also managed from outside – by the region or regional office; through central regulation; and in effect through the dictates of various purchasers of health care. Strategic management within the provider is also, however, more important. Indeed one of the less directly political aspects of the NHS changes is the move towards greater self-management by providers – whether or not in a market context; whether or not in the context of an institutional purchaser/provider split.

Prior to 1974, NHS hospitals were managed by boards, and managed separately from community services. It was only after the 1974 reorganization that areas and districts (in England) took over responsibility for services – with areas responsible for planning and districts responsible for operational management. Following the 1982 reorganization, areas were abolished in England (subsequently, similar changes were made elsewhere in the UK) and districts became responsible for local planning and provision. Prior to 1974, doctors and indeed nurses had greater managerial clout in hospitals than they did after 1974 – the medical superintendent or equivalent post and the matron were powerful figures. In a sense therefore the changes introduced through clinical directorates within hospitals and self-governing boards for hospitals are a return to the past rather than a new policy.

The major difference, however, is that self-government is now in the context of strict financial regimes, and (possibly) a market of competing providers. Rather than returning to the hospital as portrayed in a sepia-tinted picture, characterized by local community values, therefore, we are returning to physician self-management in a context of sink or swim.

This discussion focuses on the hospital. Some of the points made are, however, equally valid for community services – and indeed areas where the responsibilities of the hospital and community unit or trust overlap are identified.

Having considered marketing, the discussion goes on to consider what business planning consists in – drawing to some extent on the brief framework introduced in Chapter 5 (under Clinical directorates).

Given the political and central managerial control of the NHS today, despite rhetoric about devolution, performance management is heavily regulated from the centre. This is because criteria for good performance – and therefore for contracts, in the centrally managed NHS – are laid down at the centre; means for achieving the relevant standards in line with these criteria are also mandated heavily from the centre, albeit via different purchasers; and therefore performance management of the hospital, even if formally carried out 'by itself', is very much a standard affair.

One can trace a continuum of strategic activities within the hospital which runs logically as follows: strategic business planning, answering questions such as, 'what sort of business are we in' and 'what do our purchasers expect of us'; marketing within such constraints to specific purchasers; agreeing contracts for specific services at specific prices at specific levels of quality with purchasers; operational business planning, within clinical directorates and other departments of the hospital, to ensure that contracts are met; indication of performance through various performance indicators to ensure that agreed standards (whether agreed externally or internally) are being met; and corrective performance management where necessary. Such corrective performance management then provides part of the 'feedback' which leads to internal awareness (within the clinical directorate or within the hospital) as to what is possible in the next round of strategic business planning and marketing.

In consequence, marketing is an activity sandwiched between two different types of business planning, **strategic** and **operational**. The reality, of course, is that many hospitals know what business they are in – they are in the business of pleasing the local purchaser, who is seeking a wide range of services with a fixed and increasingly squeezed sum of money available for them. Contracts can be placed by the local purchaser in a variety of ways. Firstly there is the block contract, under which the purchaser seeks a range of services, which are not fully enumerated or quantified, and makes a sum of money available. The contract may be amended through a system of thresholds and rewards or penalties, whereby extra work is rewarded (normally on a diminishing sliding scale) and either 'underwork' or under-achievement is met by financial clawback by the purchaser. A second system is the cost per volume contract, which is self-explanatory in that a volume of services is provided in return for an agreed reimbursement. The cost per case contract – used heavily but not exclusively by GP fundholding purchasers – rewards individual procedures for individual patients at an agreed 'cost per case'.

One of the first decisions in marketing services is therefore how to balance possible financial reward with the hospital's clinical activity. Are senior doctors – and in particular, clinical directors – willing to pursue a 'corporate' strategy that stresses the maximization of income rather than treatment on the basis of clinical need? There are national regulations, agreed hurriedly in Spring 1993 in response to concern expressed by various parts of the medical profession that finance was dominating clinical freedom and indeed equity for patients. These regulations are, however, weak. In practice, many trusts – especially those facing financial instability, merger or closure – are increasingly able to persuade senior doctors that survival itself depends on following a 'maximizing' (or survival-oriented!) financial strategy. As a result, such hospitals may well give priority to GP-fundholding purchasers, for example, if workload is increasing under a block contract with a district purchaser but finance is not increasing to compensate for such workload.

Doctors often find themselves in a difficult position in such situations. They may argue that they will not amend their clinical practice to suit such organizational or financial objectives. They may indeed be ethically justified in so deciding. Nevertheless if it really is the case that the alternative is the closure of their specialty due to financial insolvency, they often decide tactically it is better to 'bide their time' and ensure a financial survival in the short term by undertaking whatever strategy this requires. The only alternative, after all, is a more overtly political campaign against the NHS changes, and their effect on the local provider, which is not guaranteed success by any means.

The different types of contract have different types of incentives attached to them. Chapter 7 explores some of these, in discussing purchaser/provider relationships in practice. Chapter 14 summarizes them at a broader political level. Meanwhile, it is important to point out that block contracts encourage the purchaser to stipulate a wide range of services with unpredictable quantity, and to 'pass the buck' to the provider in terms of meeting such requirements within a fixed sum of money. Thus the purchaser/provider split is used to pass the buck rather than to

run an effective market. On the other hand, it can be argued that such a system does not allow the purchaser to specify sensitively which services ought to be prioritized. To that extent some operational decision-making is handed over to the provider.

A cost per volume, or indeed some forms of heavily modified block contracts, may seek to get round the problem of unreasonable expectations from the provider. However two different agendas clash here. Firstly, there is the market agenda, which in effect calls for increasing specification of workload and financial reward. Secondly, there is the national agenda of 'cost cutting' and 'tipping the balance' from hospitals altogether to community services of one sort or another. As a result, bringing pressure to bear on providers is more important than operating an elegant market. The latter situation is currently dominant in the NHS. There is a national 'push' to what is called primary care, but what is often in effect merely secondary care in community or GP surgery settings.

Is marketing new, then?

Without turning to general theories of marketing outside health services altogether, it is worth tracing what marketing means in a health service context, in order to distinguish what is new following the NHS reforms. Firstly, new diseases and health-care problems generally arise, and new cures or regimes of care may become available for these. Secondly, new cures may become available to existing diseases. Marketing in this context may mean the development of appropriate procedures which are then offered to the financiers of health care (in a post-reform NHS, the purchaser) – acting under regulations from central government. Next, new techniques become available for existing 'cure and care regimes' – in other words, improved or different procedures may apply. All of these can be 'marketed' in one form or another. All of these naturally are 'marketed' in any type of health-care system.

In the pre-reform NHS, for example, such procedures might be adopted within available budgets by clinicians, as and when they were able to do so (either in terms of their interest, their expertise or the available resources agreed with local management in a unified national health service). In the new NHS, such services may have to be sold overtly to purchasers or to central regulators (the NHS Executive and regional offices).

There is a variety of purchasers to which the provider can market itself (whether acting as a unified body or whether individual specialties market themselves through autonomous clinical directorates). There is the local district health authority, or commissioning authority comprising the family health services authority as well; there are other district health authorities whether local or non-local; and there are GP fundholders. There is also the private financier, generally the private insurance company.

In the old NHS, finance was made available by local districts for revenue (recurrent) expenditure on the basis of a formula (the RAWP formula), which was intended to measure the relative need of regions and districts. From this budget, districts as 'purchasers' had to allocate to their local 'providers' sums of money which ideally would relate to workload and would cover local services. It should be noted that regions were responsible for working with districts to plan and identify the need for capital projects, i.e. regions were – in part – purchasers, which naturally affected which hospitals got which revenue budgets in the long run, if the system worked smoothly. Where patients travelled outside the district to care, this was at the behest of the GP referrer. Such referrals were made either in line with the GP's wishes or simply because of the situation of services as planned by regions – which itself ought to take account of GPs' and other actors' wishes.

Such 'cross-boundary flows' were reimbursed under the old system by affecting the RAWP formula's target, which adjusted districts' allocations according to how many outflows and inflows they had. Firstly it should be pointed out that this target was not the actual allocation. While regions eventually reached a target under the RAWP system, districts might never do so – as in a context of constrained financial resources, giving districts more money to reach their target might necessitate 'robbing Peter to pay Paul', i.e. taking money from other districts.

Secondly, there was therefore a difference in the basis by which hospitals were reimbursed for local patients and for cross-boundary flow patients. Patients treated within their own district were treated at hospitals that were reimbursed from the available monies. However cross-boundary flows affected the target at actual cost, based on the national average specialty cost relevant to the relevant to the particular patient flow. This contrasted with the 'local' reimbursement – which was made simply by balancing the available local budget over the local services which were to be provided.

The just described phenomenon was in fact the major **intellectual** as opposed to **political** impetus for the NHS reforms! It was thought that, if cross-boundary flow patients were reimbursed directly from district to district in a 'cross-charging' system, providers would have more incentive to market themselves to non-local patients. Additionally, if the system were therefore to be generalized, local patients as well would have to be reimbursed directly through a contract system – and this, it was hoped, might reduce the discrepancy between local and non-local patients.

It is interesting and highly ironical to note that Alain Enthoven overtly saw his proposal for an 'internal market' as helping the great London teaching hospitals to survive by receiving direct reimbursement rather than simply having their local **districts** rewarded by a long-term-oriented formula. This was, however, based on a misconception. The problem with the London teaching hospitals was not so much inadequate reimbursement for patients flowing in to London as inadequate local recurrent monies for the range of commitments that the local districts had weighing heavily on their shoulders – namely, expensive teaching and research 'centres of excellence'; local social deprivation; locally inadequate primary care; and so on. Ironically enough, London hospitals had been situated in a part of the country which traditionally had had more reimbursement *per capita, ceteris paribus*, both for local and non-local patients, than in other parts of the country.

Enthoven's idea provided a partially intelligent solution to a partially misdiagnosed problem. For the new (RAWP-based) system of targets took account of flows into London, from neighbouring counties (and indeed all over). The fact, additionally, that targets were never wholly reached at district (and therefore provider) level, actually helped London and its teaching hospitals. For then, the population-based part of the target (which was hurting London) also had less effect. It is the reformed NHS which has hurt London most.

If the old system had worked as intended, hospitals would have been able to increase their long-term income by marketing themselves to general practitioners – all non-fund-holding, of course, in the old system. The system would then have worked if the targets which these hospitals' parent districts then were allocated through the formula were reached quickly; and, secondly, the districts used their extra money to reimburse the specific providers who had earned in the extra money – rather than simply letting the money go to other services. Within this big 'if' lay, of course, another rationale for the idea behind the NHS reforms: providers themselves would be reimbursed rather than simply the parent districts, with the danger that the 'virtuous' providers were not those to receive the extra money! Hence another idea

within the NHS reforms – not proposed by Enthoven but proposed later by the Prime Minister's review committee – consisted in the purchaser/provider split, with providers rather than parent districts allocated 'cross-charging' money.

All this may seem some way from a marketing strategy. But it is the most central element of marketing of all – who attracts which patients and what financial reward is available for so doing?

If the new system were to work in its best form, providers would seek to match their services to local need, to match their costs and quality to available resources from purchasers and then to maximize their income – in the expectation that extra work would produce extra income. Unfortunately there is not the money in the system to allow this procedure to operate. As a result, block contracts – or even certain forms of cost per volume contracts – do not give providers incentive to market themselves in the certainty that money will be available. GPs are not free to refer, in line with patients' wishes where possible, with the expectation that money will follow the patient. There is not enough money for this to happen. As a result, contracts are made between district purchasers and hospitals, which non-fund-holding GPs and patients have to accept. The patient follows the money, or the contract.

Marketing in such an environment consists in identifying those purchasers with money. GP fundholders – in the early days of the system – have often been given what might rather scurrilously be called a 'bung', to help get the GP-fundholding system off the ground. As a result, it has often been to GP fundholders that providers market themselves. It should, however, be pointed out that providers still have an incentive to market themselves to GPs of the non-fundholding variety, in the new system, if such GPs are able then to persuade their local purchasers to follow up their referrals with contracts, with money attached.

If referrals are made by non-fundholding GPs, in the new system, which are not accompanied by district contracts with money attached, these become known as extra-contractual referrals (ECRs). It then becomes a matter for negotiation between purchaser and provider as to whether such ECRs are reimbursed or not. In some cases, the provider may be able to 'bounce' the purchaser into institutionalizing these referrals as contracts. Alternatively, if the purchaser refuses to pay, pressure will be brought to bear by the hospital management board upon the admitting doctors, in all likelihood, to stop accepting unreimbursed referrals. That is, either 'provider marketing', allied to GP referral, will win; or 'purchaser strength' will win. Either way there is quite a lot of negotiation and bureaucratic procedure attached to the management of the ECR process.

It is widely believed that, in the old system before the NHS reforms, cross-boundary flows were similar to ECRs. This is not, however, the case. For flows were *part of* the system; ECRs are 'unintended'. Cross-boundary flows may have been unwelcome, if money was not attached except in a theoretical sense, through a formula which affected a future target for the district. On the other hand, especially in districts which were considered to be 'over target' and therefore had to shed resources, cross-boundary flows were often a useful way of influencing the target upwards again. The logic – if not the clinical reality – was that such cross-boundary flows might therefore be welcome.

The difficulty, of course, in the old system was that they might be welcome to the analyst or to the far-seeing strategic manager, but less welcome to the doctor. There was no mechanism in the old system to compel the doctor on commercial grounds to fall in line with corporate policy. This, of course, may have been a good thing in some respects as well as a bad thing in others!

The similarities between the old system and the post-reform 'new' system are greater than the differences in this purely analytical sense. Both systems are characterized by 'too little money' to service free referral by GP in line with patient wishes. As a result, the old system in effect restricted access through waiting times and waiting lists. The new system, however, restricts access by overt contracts. When these are block contracts, it may in effect be through the 'management of the waiting lists' that a provider can cope within the available resources. Moreover, if all care had been funded through the cross-boundary flow process in the old system, i.e. at national average specialty cost, the system would have been bankrupted. In the new system, if all required care were reimbursed through cost per case, the system would equally be bankrupted. It is simply a case of what mechanism one takes to deal with this.

Firstly, there is the choice of spending more money on the National Health Service. Secondly there is choice of allowing things to be worked out informally, as in the old system. Thirdly, there is the choice of system-atizing everything and making overt rationing decisions by purchasers. In practice, the new regional offices have to direct purchasers (whatever euphemism is used) – including GP fundholders – to make consistent contracts (consistent as between purchasers) with providers. Otherwise, cost-saving transfer of contracts by one purchaser may be undermined by another and/or the whole system may not rationalize provision and save money. The reality is that, since performance targets are so tight, money **cannot** follow the patient or the independent GP. Marketing therefore consists in selling a centralist strategy to purchasers, providers and the public!

There are, of course, different reactions to different local circumstances, in the post-reform NHS. Certainly there is not 'more money available' as an answer to the problems of the national health service. The question therefore remains, will providers 'influence' purchasers or will purchasers take autonomous action to do a combination of needs assessment and rationing? Another widespread view is that the problems of the 'new system', which we are currently witnessing are due to inadequately strong purchasing. This is, however, an over-optimistic and naive assumption. While it may be necessary to strengthen purchasing skills *vis-à-vis* provider tricks, the problems of the system are much more fundamental than that.

Needs assessment is not a magical answer – it is simply a new name for what used to be known as epidemiologically based planning. The old system had this, and had it very well at its best. Regions and districts jointly planned services in line with available resources, assumptions as to equity and effectiveness, GP desires, and so forth. Overt rationing cannot be done on a purely scientific basis, as discussed in Chapter 3. It is rather a question of 'who wins' – does provider marketing influence the public, GP fundholders, non-fundholders and therefore districts who are 'bounced' into making contracts? It should also be pointed out in this context that districts are heavily squeezed in their 'purchasing function', as national priorities (such as Health of the Nation targets, dealing with outcomes, and Patient's Charter targets, dealing with processes) constrain funds. When one adds to this the demands of local acute medicine, represented by waiting lists which are actually worse in 1994 in aggregate, there is little left for 'scientific' needs assessment, especially that with a primary care bias. Primary care and secondary care are complements, not opposites: an improved primary care strategy in fact increases the need for secondary care in the long run and the money required for an improved primary care strategy, which relies on NHS money rather than 'social policy money' generally (local authority money, Department of the Environment money and so forth), is simply not available.

In this environment, marketing by providers is an attempt to redirect referrals rather than interest purchasers in new techniques. There is some of the latter, but more marketing time in today's NHS is spent on wining GP fundholders than on eulogizing innovation. A particular feature of the NHS 'quasi-market' identified in Chapter 4 is relevant here: marketing is a zero sum game and, if a hospital is successful in marketing new techniques, it may lose money for existing procedures. It is therefore more sensible for the local hospital, given existing incentives, to seek to take a rival's business.

Marketing and business planning

At the beginning of the above section, the role of marketing and the overall strategic management of the hospital was identified. As in the old system, hospitals in effect had to market themselves to regional decision-makers – in other words they had to make what became disparagingly known as 'political bids' for expansion, more capital and the like. In the new system, it was remarkably similar. Regions, and now, we learn, regional offices following the 1993 and 1994 reviews of regional functions, are responsible for administering the system of capital charging. This may seem an arcane technical point. However under the aegis of this policy, regions are responsible for deciding which hospitals to 'lend' capital to (rather than give, in the old system) and therefore are drawn into 'advising' districts and other purchasers as to which hospitals are likely to be the winners and losers in the new system. GP fundholders might seem a million miles away from such a process. It is, however, interesting to note that reality is significantly different from rhetoric. The Government's main 'macro' objective for the health service for the coming years is to diminish the number of hospitals and acute beds – whether through overt closure or through merger, as well as through bed reductions in specialties in particular hospitals. As a result, other agendas – such as 'local choice' and the further development of GP fundholding (the rhetoric calls it 'strengthening and deepening', as there are more fundholders responsible for more services) – often have to take a back seat, or be reconciled with this overriding priority. Who can do this other than the region or regional office?

When the policy of creating self-governing trusts was being developed, the Department of Health's Management Executive handled capital policy for such trusts directly. Hospitals that remained integrated in the district system (directly managed units, as they were called) dealt with the region on capital matters. Now the system is increasingly systematized, as nearly all providers are trusts. It is systematized **and** centralized: regions are in effect the banker for that part of capital which comes from the public sector (admittedly a diminishing proportion of the total, as a squeeze is made on public investment for ideological reasons).

The most basic form of 'marketing' therefore consists in marketing one's provider, and its particular services, to the region – in general terms: and also through the strategic business plan, to attract the necessary capital investment. Capital is no longer an allocation made through a planning process and to be reconciled with revenue allocations (which would now be called contracts) also through the planning process. Instead, capital charging systems ensure that the hospital has to account for its capital, at least in a financial sense.

Capital charges have two components – depreciation and interest. A trust is responsible for managing its own depreciation: that is – in layman's terms – it has to set aside money year by year ready to replace capital (equipment and so forth) which is at the end of its useful life. In consequences, it has to cover this cost – nominally at least – in making contracts with purchasers, as income from purchasers now has to cover 'the total cost', i.e. capital as well as recurrent. Concerning the interest component of the capital charge, the hospital pays interest to its banker (now to be the region or regional office) and therefore has to recoup this component also through the contracting system. If the NHS remained wholly public, this would be a complex accounting loop which gained some efficiency advantages in theory but left it an open question as to whether the bureaucracy in practice outweighed any so called efficiency benefits.

The reality, however, is that trusts are to be encouraged to cooperate with the private sector, and have access to private capital as a result. Here the Government decided to have it both ways. It was to preach flexibility in the public sector – which would argue for allowing public hospitals to use capital markets freely. In reality, however, this is heavily regulated – the Government gives with one hand and takes away with another. Access to capital is not to be through the public sector going to the high street bank (and, on the Government's logic, why shouldn't it, if it is an efficient hospital?) but instead through attracting private investment through joint ventures and various other projects (Willetts, 1993).

The irony is that private capital is generally (much) more expensive. Private services are more expensive. This policy is pure political dogma, allied to Treasury short-termism in 'saving money'. Public investment is generally cheaper – for purchasers, and therefore the taxpayer.

The most attractive business plan, therefore, will include: an effective capital proposal; collaboration with the private sector where possible; and documented income from purchasers for future years. Thus the primary element of strategic business planning is an ability to fit in with the region's plans. Only the region can steer purchasers in line with capital policy. It is within such a context of strategic business planning that marketing must occur.

Who is responsible for marketing and business planning within the hospital? Different approaches exist, very broadly in line with the three models of the clinical directorate presented at the beginning of Chapter 5 – that is, ranging from the centralized hospital to the 'devolved hospital'. The most common model is perhaps the one where the hospital itself is responsible for marketing, perhaps through an executive director (one of the 11 board members, comprising executives and non-executives) responsible for services or marketing, perhaps aided by a marketing manager. It is then up to the individual directorates to make more operational business plans in line with the hospital's marketing. A problem arises when marketing is undertaken without adequate reference to the realities of the directorate in question. That is, markets might be acquired and then pressure brought to bear on the directorate to 'come in on line'. While any effective business will demonstrate an ability to 'come in on line', if the marketing agreement made with purchasers, soon to be translated into contracts, does not adequately involve the relevant specialty (directorate) a lot of time is spent internally within the hospital in reconciling what may at first glance seem incompatible positions.

In practice, this is where the business manager of the directorate has a pivotal role. The business manager is a 'hospital manager' on the one hand, responsible to a senior manager outside the directorate for his or her job description and indeed performance-related pay through individual performance review! On the other hand, the good business manager will be an ally of the clinical director, and will work with that clinical director to bring benefit to the directorate and to ensure that clinical services within the directorate are appropriately developed and adequately funded. There is therefore a significant conflict of interests for the effective business manager, who has to become a local politician of some skill. The reality may, of course, be

that the business manager is in effect simply an agent of central hospital administration. In such a circumstance, if the clinical director and other senior doctors in the specialty are not in tune with hospital policy or their interests diverge from hospital policy (as suggested above may often happen), then such an individual will tend to lose influence with the clinical director. Equally, a business manager may 'go native' and become a champion of the directorate as against the central administration. At this 'micro' level, personalities and related factors may therefore affect hospital policy.

HEALTH SERVICE MANAGEMENT REVIEWED

What has been identified as the trend away from 'administration' and towards 'management' has indeed been an international one. Titles such as Tom Peters's *Thriving on Chaos* (Peters, 1988) and Charles Handy's *The Age of Unreason* (Handy, 1989) imply that challenges facing both the private business world and the public management world are to do with managing change in conditions of uncertainty rather than administrating familiar structures in conditions of stability. As with all detected trends, there may be hype as well as insight here. Nevertheless, whether such a prophecy is self-fulfilling or not, there is no doubt that public managers – not least as part of the attempt to ape the culture of the private sector world – are facing ever more demanding jobs.

Perhaps the single most important change has been the move to manager as a guarantor of outputs and outcomes rather than manager as a mediator in inputs and processes. In other words (to use Stephen Harrison's phrase from his book *Managing the National Health Service* – Harrison, 1989), 'the manager as scapegoat' is an increasingly common occurrence. In a centralized political system such as the UK's, and in publicly-controlled enterprises, political rules and ambitions may determine expected policy outcomes and it is up to managers to deliver them. These may not always be outcomes of the most glorious sort. There is more than a little truth in the 'Yes, Prime Minister' ethos, whereby politicians and civil servants, for different reasons, do not wish outputs from Government departments or public agencies to be measured very carefully – for fear that political and bureaucratic shortcomings may be exposed. However, in today's NHS the push for intensified production is leading to measurement of output; and shortcomings are then blamed on the manager, not the politician. Thus NHS management today is about devolving blame!

When the achievement of policy is a political imperative (such as in the National Health Service, without significant increases in finance), then managers will often find that they are carrying a heavy responsibility for achieving much within little resources. And, indeed, much of the emphasis on 'good management' today is in effect an emphasis upon good housekeeping, and indeed more economical production.

The White Paper on the National Health Service (*Working for Patients*) was rightly diagnosed by the House of Commons Social Services Select Committee as being about 'managing the resource' rather than managing the delivery of health care. In the United States also, managers of both public and private programmes are finding the exigencies of cost control to be their most pressing problem.

Managers in the public sector are finding that the stress upon results, specifically interpreted in terms of cost-effectiveness, efficiency and pure economy, is leading increasingly to a separation of the roles of the provider and the purchaser yet close direction of the former by the latter. The budget holder for a particular Government programme is responsible for producing a product and for contracting for the inputs geared to producing that output.

That is, a process of competitive tendering in order to maximize efficiency has both nationally and internationally become 'the flavour of the age'.

In the United States, budget holders and managers of Government programmes such as Medicare and Medicaid, the health programmes for the elderly and poor respectively, find themselves increasingly given the responsibility of 'shopping around' in the market place of provision to ensure that Government money buys the most economical deal for the programme's clients. In the UK, the essence of the National Health Service and Community Care Bill of 1989/90, following the White Papers *Working for Patients* and *Caring for People*, is to separate the funder of the health care (in other words, the purchaser, still the State acting on behalf of its people) and providers of health care, in order to ensure that a process of competitive tendering guarantees an efficient result. In New Zealand, health boards constituted in line with the principles of general management, British style, are being discharged with a similar responsibility to health authorities in the UK.

Thus, although it would be foolish to generalize either across all different policy areas or across all nations, there are significant trends throughout the world towards this approach. Even in the former communist countries of Eastern Europe, the concept of the marketplace with a unified purchaser on behalf of the public, contracting with competing suppliers, is becoming dominant in the provision of goods such as health care which have traditionally been provided through social administration.

The separation of the roles of the provider and the purchaser has been the hallmark of Government policy in a number of sectors of the economy beside health care. Attempts to increase competition amongst providers, defined as a policy of 'provider markets', have been widely fostered.

- In health, such a principle is the essence of the White Paper *Working for Patients* and the Community Care White Paper *Caring for People*.
- In education, it is the basis of proposed reforms in higher education, and – to a limited extent – in education generally.
- In housing, it underlies the attempt to remove 'monopoly' rented provisions by local authorities.
- Public industries have been privatized, allegedly to allow provider competition.

What is the key argument for such policies? The theory (and ideology) underpinning these moves derives from a belief in the free market and also a belief in decentralized budgeting to achieve efficiency and to improve incentives to provide.

What is the main argument against such moves? A major problem in a number of areas has been the limited existing and potential supply in provider markets. How can hospitals compete to offer care if there is no surplus or spare capacity? How can schools compete if they cannot expand and contract freely; likewise, hospitals? Often, Government regulation prohibits fully free markets, or rather markets as free as possible. 'Market failures' often prevent the operation of effective provider markets. Chapter 4 discussed these arguments.

CORPORATISM OR INDIVIDUALISM?

The theory of public management associated with the trend towards strategic management tends to be one which identifies 'top-down' responsibility for the making of policy and 'bottom-up' responsibility for implementation, or at least decentralized responsibility for implementation – local freedom but within strict limits and along strict lines. It should be pointed out that this type of approach has implications for democratic theory. There has grown up a conventional wisdom that 'the 1970s' in the UK were char-acterized by what was known as corpo-ratism. At its most general (and often pejorative), corporatism implied the smoke-filled room wherein representatives of the strong institutions, in dealing with controversy, got around a table and hammered out some sort of compromise.

The corporate state implies a state dominated by politicians and the bureaucracy, business leaders and labour leaders. At its more precise, therefore, corporatism implied a tripartite system for making policy (for and in British industry, for example) and, indeed, a tripartite system for actually implementing and managing, not least in the sorting out of industrial disputes.

The decline of corporatism is allegedly associated with Thatcher governments. Mrs Thatcher, in a famous aside, remarked that 'there would be no more beer and sandwiches at No. 10'. This referred to what she saw as the tradition of leaders of both sides of industry getting around the table with politicians and civil servants to sort out the problems of industry – problems that she saw as the responsibility of management acting in a unified manner.

Thus, corporatism in some respects was identified with consensus. From the left, corporatism was attacked as leading to a decision-making process in which elites from both sides of industry dominated, and therefore industrial democracy was diminished or excluded. This was, of course, an idealistic view. 'Localism' in industrial relations is often merely the wolf of the market in shop stewards' sheep's clothing. Without central state action, localism may even mean devil take the hindmost. From the right, as just seen, corporatism was attacked as pandering to institutionalized interests and what one might term guilds, creating an impediment to efficiency and effectiveness. In the 1990s, the pendulum may, of course, swing back somewhat, to allow more consensus in the management of large public enterprises.

FISCAL CRISIS? THE RADICAL AND OTHER PERSPECTIVES

One of the key factors promoting general management and strategic management, as opposed to what might be termed administration, in the public sector, was the pressure brought about by the shortage of resources available through public expenditure. Analogously, one might argue, in the private sector, sharper national and international competition began to ensure that strategic management in pursuit of efficiency and profit, or even just survival, became a more pressing imperative.

In the public sector, there have been fears of what both the right and left wings in politics have dubbed a 'fiscal crisis' in financing and managing public expenditure. The argument from the right wing of politics goes as follows.

In order to provide incentives both to individuals and corporations to invest in the private sector, taxation rates must be kept to a certain minimum or below a certain level. In consequence, there is a constraint upon public expenditure if inflation is to be avoided, as the only alternatives to low taxes and high public expenditure would be budget deficit (US-style) or an inflationary printing of money. The policy agenda for right-wing governments, on this argument, is to restrict the growth of public expenditure and, indeed, where possible, to cut public expenditure. In order to do so, there may need to be a change in political culture as well as a structural weakening of certain traditional interests and interest groups in society. Trade union bargaining rights in the public sector must be reduced in this argument; the beneficiaries of social programmes must also be restricted in their access to the political system.

'Public choice' theorists (who may or may not have an ideological involvement in politics) argue that democracy itself has a bias to fiscal crisis of this sort or at least to fiscal problems. The argument here is that the operation of the free market is interfered with or distorted by the operation of a political spoils system, whereby interest groups can (in proportion to their political power), through their access to the political system, gain advantages, which may include Government spending programmes to benefit them or their members, tax incentives (in other words, back-door Government expenditure) or special rights and privileges that interfere with the operation of the free market and economy. It is argued, therefore, that restrictions on what some American political scientists call the 'democratic distemper' must be made if fiscal soundness is to be allowed. Otherwise, people will vote themselves benefits without paying the costs.

Let us now consider the so-called 'left-wing' theory of fiscal crisis. Like the right-wing version, there is a belief here that, in what such left-wingers call 'capitalist society', there is always pressure towards an imbalance between revenue (taxation) and public expenditure. The argument here is similar as regards taxation – the capitalist economy relies on incentive through low taxation to operate, both on the individual and corporate level. At the level of public expenditure, the left-wing argument is analogous but slightly different. The argument is that the natural inequality and economic class distinctions produced by capitalists have to be mediated through welfare-state activities involving substantial public expenditure. They call this the 'legitimation' of capitalist society – if you like, the price that capitalists have to pay to be allowed to run their preferred economy and society.

Public expenditure has many sources – not just to 'spend on the poor' to prevent riot or revolution or instability. The pressure is on the state also to provide significant public expenditure for what is called the infrastructure of the economy – to ensure that the conditions under which private investors in private markets can successfully operate are met. For example, public health services might be seen as investments in human capital organized by the state on behalf of the economy. Perhaps the most lucid account of this approach is found in James O'Connor's book *The Fiscal Crisis of the State* (O'Connor, 1976). The tendency, again, is to fiscal crisis. It was believed in the 1960s and 1970s by some who were termed 'neo-Marxists' that this would prove the undoing of welfare capitalism.

In considering these views, given the partial (at least) success of what such commentators call the Thatcherite ideological project (in the UK at any rate), it may be that the dominance of right-wing politics can both produce and benefit from a change in people's expectations – the state may not have to spend so much on social policy in order to 'legitimize' capitalist society. Pure free market theorists do not see a significant role for the state in what is known as capital accumulation – aiding the infrastructure of the capitalist economy, if you like. Others, however, do. Nevertheless, there is an implication that, at the end of the day, the balance between revenue and expenditure is manageable, as a result of ideological as well as economic adjustment. Just as 'beer and sandwiches at No. 10' seems a distant dream for significant trade union leaders, automatic right to social programmes and their protection against inflation (1960s- and 1970s-style) also seems a dream to various social interests, especially those at the poorer end of the social spectrum.

The fact remains that many societies that could be termed 'welfare capitalist' or even 'social democratic', but involving significant private enterprise as the engine of the economy, do not suffer so acutely from this perceived political or fiscal crisis. The Netherlands and Sweden are examples, despite their own recent fiscal problems.

The implication for the general or strategic manager in a public enterprise is that the management of resources allocated to the enterprise will have to be increasingly tighter;

that, where the enterprise is engaged in the delivery of services, rationing and choice among both types of programme and recipients or clients who benefit from programmes will have to be tighter; and that, generally, the design of programmes in the realms of education, training, and manpower development, will have to be more tightly integrated with the 'needs of the economy'.

This perspective accepts a broadly Marxist or 'radical' analysis of management, which interprets management's role as helping to meet economic demands of both the enterprise and the capitalist mode of production.

In a public National Health Service, 'surplus value' is not extracted from workers as private profit. But there may be a conflict between workers and 'consumers' if the latter expect 'free' services within the context of a parsimoniously funded service. Managers in the public sector may have to 'squeeze out' surplus value from workers in order to serve patients/consumers. In other words, the Government may manufacture a trade-off between the interests of the worker and the interest of the patient. This is further 'Marxized' if the NHS is also seen as a means of investing cheaply in a healthy workforce on behalf of the private economy.

Consider a private company, seeking profit. Traditional Marxism saw the conflict as between capitalists and workers, 'fighting' over profit.

In 'perfect competition', profit might be less, as competition reduced profit margins – but this would only help workers if they benefited from being 'in demand', as labour, by competing capitalists. Otherwise, they might be exploited even more, to try to maintain some profitability. In other words one must look not only at **market structure** but at the **security** of the overall market. Microeconomics (the structure of the market) is affected by macro-economics (the level of unemployment and therefore potential for exploitation of workers). In the 1980s the macro-economic strategy known as monetarism was used as an ideological justification for high unemployment.

In monopolistic situations, workers might benefit a little, as excess profit was partially handed on to them. Then again, they might not, if monopoly producers were monopoly buyers of labour. Galbraith has argued in the past that the 'large', even multinational corporation is the best guarantor of good working conditions (Galbraith, 1967). But it may not be the case if transfer of production to developing countries – to take advantage of 'cheap labour' without much social protection – is a significant option.

Overall, however, 'output' used to be taken as a given. Nowadays, paradoxically, in a public service within a capitalist society, management techniques may be employed to ensure that workers 'produce the maximum effort' – in what is effectively a low-wage sector of the economy, given the constraints on demand (i.e. purchasing power of the public purse). Some of these techniques are discussed in Chapter 8. It is not capitalists who are extracting 'surplus value' but the state which is acquiring investment in human capital (health) 'on the cheap'. (Alternatively, if health care is seen as 'non-productive', the state is – as in some former Marxist states – not affording health or health-care workers a high priority.) Doctors may be part of this process, increasingly squeezed; or may be relatively privileged providers whose 'class' affiliations protect them. But they are not 'capitalists', not in the NHS at any rate.

In the late century 'advanced capitalist' society where two-thirds are comfortable and one-third is poor, the consumer–worker conflict may be more severe (whether overt or not). This is because the 'affluent majority' gain more as consumers in a tightly managed society than they lose as workers. The poor third, however, including peripheral and part-time workers, lose more as 'squeezed' workers than they gain as consumers.

Overall, a 'market' NHS allows providers to make 'quasi-profit', which is increased by exploiting workers. In a non-market NHS, income to providers via health authorities is at least guaranteed to be ploughed back into patient care if a 'surplus' is made.

LEADERSHIP IN THE NHS?

One can interpret the current management agenda in the NHS as seeking to *enforce* a 'unitarist' enterprise (Chapter 8). Quality processes such as 'total quality management' and even medical audit may have as an important focus the 'bringing into line' of key providing workers. Issues in the management of human resources may involve techniques to squeeze more productivity out of workers, by bypassing or de-emphasizing collective rights. By focusing initiatives such as resource management on 'the patient', the worker–consumer trade-off may be fed. This is not to deny the possible utility of such management techniques. It is, however, to condition against their 'illegitimate' or manipulative use.

The challenge for constructive and progressive health services management, towards the year 2000, is to harness an advocacy role ('upwards') with Government, on behalf of the health service, to a leadership role ('downwards') within and of the organization. Otherwise managers become merely agents of governments, shorn of the legitimacy to carry out local dialogue with their populations as well as 'obey orders'.

Leadership, if it is not a pseudo-technical set of skills devoid of normative framework, includes prescriptive as well as descriptive elements. NHS managers can be effective leaders if they agree objectives and outcomes with staff, then take responsibility for their achievement. **A patient's charter necessitates an employee's charter**, based on non-manipulative discourse.

CONCLUDING OBSERVATION

Perhaps the most important distinction,

within the general management of the NHS, is between 'top-down' general management of a 'hierarchical' organization (1983–1991) and 'marketing management' post-1991. One problem is that not only the culture but also the tools and techniques of the former may be undermined by the latter. For example, in the hospital, the potential for 'self-management by doctors' – as in Guy's, pre-1991, when the chairman of the management board was a doctor – was replaced by the new trust boards. These became often cumbersome vehicles for political 'non-executive' appointments, which cut across efficient management linking the hospital with higher tiers of the health service.

Instead of integrating clinical management into NHS general management, the trust boards often become the source of 'anti-doctor' machismo. Additionally, local vigilante behaviour by trust chairmen – in a market environment – cut across clear management lines of control and responsibility. Was the General Manager (now Chief Executive) responsible, via various stages, to the overall NHS General Manager/Chief Executive, or to his chairman? Was the NHS Chief Executive able to deal with chairmen, or was that a role for the Secretary of State?

General management (as the late Sir Roy Griffiths observed) required to be 'bedded in' and developed rather than radically transformed at birth!

DISCUSSION

- It is important to note that the development of general management in health care has been merely one example of the development of the 'general management function' in the public sector generally. This has often stemmed from a desire to import private sector management principles into the public sector, and to replace 'public administration' with public management.
- It is important to distinguish those aspects

of management where private and public sectors may be considered to be alike and those areas where private and public sectors differ significantly. Additional to this, the complexity of the health sector may mean that it is fairly 'exceptional', even within the public sector.

- Development of general management in the health sector can be split into two types: firstly, there is the reform of the Civil Service and the creation of a central management apex for the National Health Service as a whole; and secondly, there is the creation of general management within the National Health Service, succeeded by the further differentiation between management of purchasing authorities and management of providers (hospitals and community trusts) after the NHS reforms.
- There are many different types of strategic planning. If strategic planning means central determination of services through central capital allocation processes, then overt strategic planning has declined within the National Health Service. If, however, strategic planning means more comprehensive approaches to identifying need (however these needs are to be met within the system), then it can be argued that strategic planning has increased in importance and indeed ought to increase in importance.
- There is a mixed picture as a result of the NHS reforms concerning strategic planning and its accompaniment, strategic management. (In this context strategic management may be defined as the combination of action and systems to achieve the objectives of strategic plans.) The reason the picture is mixed is because, on the one hand, there is a rhetoric and even in some cases a reality of more comprehensive needs-based planning; yet on the other hand there is a fragmentation of the planning function as a result of a fragmentation of what is known as

purchasing in the National Health Service.

- Allied to the general principle of contracting in health services, and the split of purchasing and providing, there is the general public sector phenomenon of the creation of semi-autonomous 'agencies' to replace directly managed Government departments or directly managed services within the National Health Service. There is an argument in management theory that agencies are more efficient; but the reality may be that they acquire 'quango' characteristics and become a source of patronage and a mechanism for obedience to political dictates. This produces rather the opposite of the justification from management theory.

ACKNOWLEDGEMENTS

The theory in this chapter was used as the basis for an article, to which Kenneth Lee made a separate contribution, in Burrows *et al.* (1994) *Management for Hospital Doctors*, Butterworth Heinemann, London.

REFERENCES

Argenti, J. (1980) *Practical Corporate Planning*, Allen & Unwin, London.

Department of Health (1989) *Working for Patients* (NHS White Paper), HMSO, London.

Galbraith, J. K. (1967) *The New Industrial State*, Penguin, Harmondsworth.

Gomez, P. and Probst, G. S. B. (1987) *Thinking in Networks for Management: An Integrated Problem-Solving Methodology*, International Management Institute, Geneva.

Handy, C. (1989) *The Age of Unreason*, Business Books, London.

Harrison, S. (1989) *Managing the National Health Service*, Chapman & Hall, London.

Ibbs Report (1988) *The Next Steps*, HMSO, London.

Nairne, P. (1983) *Political Quarterly*.

O' Connor, J. (1976) *The Fiscal Crisis of the State*, Harper & Row, New York.

Peters, T. (1988) *Thriving on Chaos: Handbook for a Management Revolution*, Macmillan, London.

Sampson, A. (1983) *The Changing Anatomy of the UK*, Coronet, London.

Willetts, D. (1993) *The Opportunities for Private Funding in the NHS*, Social Market Foundation, London.

INTRODUCTION

This chapter reviews the development of policy and practice in commissioning, in and for the National Health Service. After providing a background, it defines and discusses policy objectives in commissioning *per se*; goes on to discuss evolving practices, including particular approaches, structures and types of commissioning; discusses issues arising in purchaser/provider relationships as a result of the NHS market; draws attention to some international lessons and warnings; and is then concluded.

THE BACKGROUND TO COMMISSIONING

The term commissioning (in particular referring to the role of the District Health Authority) is in its present guise a relatively recent one in the National Health Service. Originally, the term commissioning (with a naval origin, it seems) referred to the bringing on stream of a hospital or other capital project. More recently, with the purchaser/ provider split in the National Health Service, commissioning is the role undertaken by purchasing authorities. These may be single health authorities in the sense in which they have existed from 1982 until the early 1990s; merged and therefore larger district health authorities; commissioning agencies comprising district health authorities and family health services authorities (soon to be formally merged as a result of the 'Langlands Review' and the NHS Act of 1995); or other evolving arrangements. GP fundholders are seen as purchasers rather than commissioners, although they may also have a commissioning role.

This begs the question as to what the difference is between purchasing and commissioning. The difference is in fact what one would expect it to be simply by looking at the terms themselves: purchasing is the act of buying something, whereas commissioning is a more ambitious process which ranges from initial assessment of need and prioritization through the formal purchase via a contract to the further purchaser/provider links and evaluation which satisfy the purchaser that the services are appropriate and effective.

Prior to the NHS reforms, there was no **overt** purchaser/provider split in the National Health Service. There are different ways of characterizing the pre-reform situation. One way is to say there was no 'purchasing' at all, and that there was simply a form of public sector third-party reimbursement, whereby patients used the services of providers and a formula sought to reimburse the health authorities responsible for the providers. In other words, the Government, acting through its health authorities as agencies, was the 'third-party reimburser' after the first two parties (the patient and the provider) had together defined the service or episode of care.

Of course the general practitioner was in most cases the gatekeeper to such a process, or rather the referrer of patients to existing services. Another – not necessarily mutually exclusive – way of characterizing the pre-reform situation is to say that in effect the region was the purchaser and that the District Health Authority was the 'catchment provider': in other words, the region was at the end of the day responsible for capital projects which led to the siting and design of services; referrals were made to these services; and money flowed to districts as the manager of these services.

Thus ironically in the pre-reform NHS, there was an attempt to make the money follow the patient. This was not a wholly successful attempt, of course, in that money arriving at districts (through a mixture of allocations to populations on the one hand and adjustments for flows from one area to another through the RAWP formula, on the other hand) was not guaranteed to be used to reimburse providers (hospitals and community services) in line with their workload. In a sense providers, in the old system, got money through what we would now call block contracts, although less systematized. Some of this money came from the local health authority, in 'block' for locally consumed services; some of it was through reimbursement for 'cross-boundary flows'. Of course such 'flows' money went to the parent district and not directly to the provider. Furthermore, capital allocations (to districts/providers) were not necessarily in line with 'recurrent' allocation.

In the old system, an imaginative approach to commissioning new services and re-designing or re-siting services would have led to the 'purchasers' (in practice both regions and districts) taking advice from general practitioners, patient and citizen desires and cost considerations to decide on future service mix – in other words there would have been a **conceptual or functional** purchaser/provider split but not an **institutional** purchaser/provider split. In practice, of course, it was not as often like this as it should have been: GPs simply referred to the services that were available and future planning decisions were not necessarily taken in a very imaginative way. Nevertheless new services were planned by the more imaginative regional management teams to fit in with what we would now consider to be **commissioning** criteria – the desires of patients; the desires of the public more generally; the opinions of

general practitioners; the opinions of a whole range of professionals, health and otherwise; and cost or cost-effectiveness considerations.

In the post-reform NHS, the overt purchaser/provider split has created an overt purchaser – still in most cases the district – which replaces the commissioning role in the old system of (at the bottom end) the general practitioner (non-fundholding of course) and (at the top end) the regional allocator. In the old system an interplay between these two forces led to the evolution of services over time.

Overt purchasing by actors other than general practitioners, therefore, means that general practitioners' referrals and desires have to be in line with 'the purchasing plan'. Already, therefore, we have an entry into what commissioning means in practice. It means agreement and consensus as to the appropriate form of services to be provided and therefore purchased.

Purchasing and commissioning jointly may be seen as a means of setting priorities and *in extremis* rationing. Prior to the reforms, waiting lists and more particularly waiting times, along with informal clinical decision-making, decided what must be prioritized and what was not to be prioritized. There was of course an assumption that a comprehensive National Health Service provided services which were required at the time of need, on an equitable basis as long as there was judged to be benefit to the patient. Measuring such benefit was of course a tricky question, and the role of clinicians and other actors in the system in so doing has also been formalized as a result of the NHS reforms. Put bluntly, however, in the old system a referral by a GP did not require ratification from a contract made by a district health authority.

A second aspect of the commissioning role is therefore to formalize (through an overt decision-making process) types, quantities and qualities of services to be commissioned – as a separate exercise from free or decentralized decision-making by the general practitioner.

POLICY OBJECTIVES IN COMMISSIONING AND PURCHASING

Assumption 1

The advantages of moving to an overt commissioning process ought to be greater than the disadvantages, as a general judgement

This calls for a clear picture of the objectives of commissioning. It is now widely accepted that creating an overt purchaser/provider split leads to significant 'transactions costs' which derive from the following process:

- decision as to overall priorities for purchasing, by certain evaluative criteria (such as the QALY at the formal end or, under consultative processes, more informally);
- assessment of specific needs within these priorities, perhaps involving choice as to groups of patients most likely to benefit and procedures most likely to produce an appropriate benefit/cost ratio (again, formally or less so);
- the translation of such needs into particular packages of care;
- the translation of such packages of care into contracts with providers;
- the commissioning (in the older sense) of services by working closely with selected providers (whether or not involving a competitive marketplace amongst providers);
- the evaluation and amendment of such services in future years.

To take an extreme example, if such a process led to a service mix and the provision of services not different from that produced through simple GP referral in the 'old system' – or a worse mix – one would have incurred a lot of cost for no benefit. Where the contracting process merely (but at great effort) formalizes and bureaucratizes what was previously done informally, the NHS has simply created a significant new bureaucracy

with little gain other than employment opportunities at high salaries for managers instead of direct patient-care professionals.

If the purchasing process (within commissioning) involves many actors – such as significant quantities of GP fundholders and the need for coordination between districts, FHSAs and such fundholders – then the transactions costs are even higher. When one adds to this the need for a regulatory process to ensure appropriate purchasing (and also appropriate provision, through, for example, an accreditation process) then one is in the business of building empires to police other empires. The working assumption must therefore be that there are specific benefits to be derived from an overt purchasing and commissioning process which were not attainable in the pre-reform NHS.

Firstly, it is hoped that more effective control of providers is enabled by an overt commissioning process. A later section of this paper deals with purchaser/provider relations in the context of a purchaser/provider split.

Secondly, the dominant rationale for an overt commissioning process is to ensure that limited resources are appropriately prioritized, and that such priorities are translated into effective services for 'the chosen populations'. Again to characterize the situation somewhat historically, in the pre-reform NHS, the assumption that GPs could refer to whatever services were available was couched implicitly (and sometimes explicitly) in the philosophical assumption that referrals should not be restricted within what would now be known as an overall purchasing plan. In the old system at its best, as stated above, services were reshaped in order to accommodate input from referrers (who might now be referred to as purchasers as well as providers – in other words general practitioners).

The challenge now, therefore, is to ensure that sensible or at least agreed priorities are better able to be implemented through an overt commissioning process, such that the costs of operating such a process are less than the additional benefit by comparison with the pre-reform NHS.

Assumption 2

Purchasing plans, in order to be translated into effective processes, must take full account of the views of the primary doctor who has first contact with the patient – in other words the general practitioner (whether fundholding or non-fundholding)

To take account of this assumption, it is helpful to point to both a similarity and a dissimilarity with the pre-reform NHS. The similarity is that the general practitioner is allowed to have a significant say in which services, in which location and in which particular provider, are made available to the patient. The difference from the old system is that general practitioners – if their views are to be integrated with an overall purchasing plan – must take account not only of the costs of the individual referral but also of the total quantum of available resources within the district health authority's purchasing budget. Indeed the need for such immediate and less immediate calculations to be combined in the referral process is one rationale for GP fundholding – fundholders can actually hold the budget and manage referrals of their patients within that budget.

Some referrals will be made to local providers; some referrals will be made across boundaries (producing what under the old RAWP system would have been known as cross-boundary flows). Contracts between district purchasers and providers, therefore, ought to reflect agreement between general practitioners and districts as to which services are to be available, and which providers are to supply these services, to use somewhat blunt business language.

Again there is a similarity and dissimilarity with the pre-reform NHS: the similarity is

that districts (now known as purchasers) will enable the provision of services within their own boundaries, and that services made available for the district's population outwith these boundaries will be adequately funded if at all possible. In the old system, the region was responsible for this through its funding formula. Now direct contracts are responsible.

And therein lies the dissimilarity: services are not funded in relation to patient flow (which was the aim of the old system, i.e. that the money should follow the patient, although this did not always work very well in practice), but only through overt contracts between purchasers and recipient providers (whether local or receiving patients across boundaries).

In both systems, there is a need for a supra-district body to ensure the viability of purchasing plans both in themselves and in order to sustain providers (thus to enable such providers to plan on a long-term basis). This is the role of the region, the regional directorate or whatever it happens to be called.

Assumption 3

Commissioning must combine the advantages of both centralization and decentralization

This somewhat paradoxical statement refers to the need to combine the advantages of economies of scale in purchasing (not least to display adequate power *vis-à-vis* providers) and also locally sensitive purchasing. If, in the pre-reform NHS, the region was a kind of purchaser and the district both purchaser (for its own residents) and provider (for its own and other residents) informally, then immediately it can be seen that the essence of the post-reform NHS is to decentralize purchasing to the district and to the GP fundholder.

This has the advantage of ensuring that particular sums of money are earmarked for particular groups of patients at a more local level. The move to locality purchasing is an attempt at decentralizing purchasing further, such that – whether localities actually hold budgets or merely are responsible for indicative budgets – the particular needs identified for particular localities can be met (rather than simply assuming, as in the old system, that services could be provided and that somehow the right patients would get to the right services). It should of course be pointed out that simply giving local budgets for specific services for specific groups still does not guarantee that the earmarked patients will receive the services. A significant amount of social and cultural, as well as managerial, challenge is involved here.

The other side of the coin is that decentralizing specifically earmarked budgets and contracting for services within these may sometimes throw out the baby with the bath water: specialized, tertiary and supra-district services of any sort may require coordination at a higher level than that of the local purchaser. There is a difference between ceasing to purchase services simply because purchasers have 'rationally' decided they are not a priority, on the one hand, and local purchasers failing to 'get their act together' to ensure that what they wish to purchase is rendered possible, on the other hand. That is, the latter case involves a 'problem of collective action'.

One solution, in the case of specialized services, has been to earmark funds for such services, but still to devolve them to local purchasers. This has, however, involved significant rigidities. For example, where it is impossible to predict statistically or otherwise where within a region the need for heart transplants (of a limited number) will emerge, simply allowing each district to purchase 'two a year' is to create a rigidity which damages patient care and both wastes money in some districts and leaves shortfalls in others.

Thus centralization of some functions is necessary, along with decentralization of others. This is a crucial part of the overall commissioning process, at the level of district policy overall – and district coordination with the regional level.

Assumption 4

Purchasers, providers and regional directorates will require to work carefully together on the provision of new services

Contracts for services ought to reflect as wide agreement as possible between: GPs (as agents of patients); patients' groups directly, where possible and sensible; local citizen opinion generally; and district purchasers' views (based on social, epidemiological and economic criteria) as to which services ought to be provided where. In consequence, the commissioning process ought to be part and parcel of a wider process whereby appropriate patient flows are 'modelled', i.e. predicted for the future, and where both new services and future contracts are therefore laid.

Again, therefore, there is both a similarity and a dissimilarity with the pre-reform NHS: the similarity lies in the fact that there is bound to be a significant supra-district role in planning capital investment and the future shape of services, to reflect both current referrals and sensitive planning of future referrals; and the dissimilarity lies in the fact that there is now a significant coordinating process to be undertaken formally between local purchasers, general practitioners (who no longer have the right of budget-free referral) and higher-tier bodies such as regions. It is a real danger that the 'post-regional' NHS will leave local purchasers 'to sort things out themselves', discover shortcomings in such a system (especially in terms of stability for providers) and then intervene with a heavy hand on a political agenda to clear up any mess that results.

Assumption 5

Effective commissioning will be a multi-agency process covering the 'soon to be merged' DHAs and FHSAs but also local government (especially departments of social services) and other Government or quasi-Government agencies whose actions affect 'health gain' generally

Thus as well as locality purchasing, the assumption is that joint commissioning with local authorities will take on a new importance – or rather a more formalized shape – and the compatibility of such approaches with (for example) the evolution of fundholding will be a serious concern in years to come.

There are two alternative scenarios concerning the roles of GP fundholding in a system in which joint commissioning and global purchasing are also seen as an objective. One scenario sees GP fundholding becoming dominant, and therefore fragmentation of the DHA and other budgets becoming a significant problem. Such a scenario would see a regulatory role rather than a fundamental global purchasing role for the DHA, and inevitably – given the political nature of the public NHS – a regulatory role for higher tiers such as regional directorates and central government (the NHSME and politicians).

The other scenario sees GP fundholding being reincorporated into the system (whether implicitly under a Conservative government or overtly under a Labour government) and the role of the general practitioner in purchasing and commissioning being retained through influence upon the overall purchasing process rather than through fragmentation by allocation to GP fundholders.

It is, however, possible to see a convergence between what seem to be two very different strategies indeed. The current conundrum in policy may illustrate this. On the one hand, the present government is encouraging the extension, and also deepening and widening, of GP fundholding, so that GP fundholding covers more and different services as well as being generalized across more general practitioners. The present government, however, also has a long-term scenario, working with regional directorates, to ensure an appropriate long-term provision of services – with what they call a 'downsizing' of the hospital sector, a concentration upon significant 'standard hospitals' of the future, spread across the regions (with assumptions already made in many cases as to which hospitals will survive and which will not!) and also assumptions about the shape and location of community services. The closeness of ministers and their regional appointees, in turn close to trust appointments, facilitates this.

To put it bluntly, if GP fundholding means what it meant to many first wave GP fundholders, this scenario is simply unattainable if GP fundholding is strengthened. Therefore one can assume either that the Government does not know what it is doing or that it has a scenario for making sure that GP fundholding does not lead to results incompatible with broader strategy. A cynic might assume that the former applies in the short-term, but that the latter will soon be forced upon the Government! The next section of this chapter looks at various options for combining joint commissioning with various means of involving GPs.

EVOLVING PRACTICE IN COMMISSIONING

THE GP/DHA RELATIONSHIP

In the post-reform NHS, GPs can now (in addition to their role as primary health-care providers) act as purchasers (fundholders) of health care and manage their own budgets. Both GPs who become fundholders and those who remain primarily as providers can have an impact upon the DHA in the sense that they influence either the size of the budget that a DHA has or the demands placed upon that budget.

Consider first the relationship of the DHA with the traditional (non-fundholding) GP. When a DHA sets out its contracts with providers, it does so with the intention that GPs within its area will make referrals in such a way that they are covered by such contracts. However if this does not occur (say, a GP refers patients to a hospital with which the local DHA does not hold a contract), then the DHA will either 'disown' them or will have to find extra funds for such referrals. These are covered by a tranche of the budget set aside for extracontractual referrals (ECRs).

This is obviously not an ideal situation for the DHA, which now faces the risk of not knowing how much to set aside for ECRs. In addition, it risks not utilizing the contracts it has made with providers. This is a particular risk if such contracts are not specific to utilization (e.g. block contracts).

GP fundholders pose a different threat to the DHA, as GP fundholding becomes more salient. In some areas, over 80% of practices have fundholding status. The size of the DHA's budget will fall when GP fundholders take on the role of purchaser for (say) large amounts of elective surgery. They will control increasing amounts of the purchasing budget and – importantly – leave the DHA with the 'residual' responsibility for emergency health care which by its nature is more prone to fluctuations. Hence greater risk will be imposed upon the DHA. While the prevalence of GP fundholding varies from area to area, in some areas it is predicted that the amount of the previous DHA budget that will now be in the hands of GP fundholders will rise to as much as 50–60%. As a result a situation arises where there are two different types of purchaser – one large single organization (the DHA) and one equally large fragmented set of GP fundholders.

Each purchaser has its own particular identity. The DHA is a commissioner for health care acting on behalf of large populations and has a sizeable administrative staff increasingly educated and trained to perform this purchasing role. The GP fundholders are acting for small sections of the population and have only a few staff devoted to the purchasing role. Owing to their direct contact with patients and providers, they are better able to acquire specific detailed information while being less able to obtain larger, population-based epidemiological data as to patients' health needs and the ability of providers to meet those needs.

If such purchasers act autonomously and even partially disregard the activities of the others, the provision of health care can be adversely affected. For example, if one purchaser does not believe in one form of treatment for a particular health condition and hence moves that element of his budget to another service, yet the other purchaser either holds a contrary position or is simply uncertain, then it is possible that either or both purchasers could be attempting (individually) to purchase services from providers at a level insufficient to cover the overheads of the provider. There may well exist a critical income level for provision of a particular service that can not be attained by either purchaser individually.

Hence the DHA must accept the impact of both GPs and GP fundholders on its role as purchaser; and, likewise, GPs/GP fundholders must realize the potential benefits to be gained by coordinating their actions with the DHA. There can be benefits to both parties from cooperation (not least, purchaser power in areas with limited provider competition). If GPs are involved within district purchasing, this should limit fragmentation and administrative overheads while still being sensitive to the needs of local communities and individuals.

Evidence suggests that the importance of GP fundholders and GPs within the internal market is becoming ever more apparent to DHAs. Thus we observe the increasing prevalence of:

- GP advisory committees;
- DHA road-shows for GPs;

- joint commissioning projects;
- the creation of GP posts on DHA purchasing boards;
- the creation of GP contact points within DHAs (and DHAs going out to visit GPs) and – in certain instances, where a locality model of health care is being pursued – the role of link GPs who act as the GP representative for each locality. A locality system occurs where the DHA subdivides its area into smaller localities based upon population or possibly other organization boundaries. Each of these localities is then allocated a notional budget.

While the above initiatives can encourage GPs to act in a way more conducive to the DHA's purchasing intentions, such is not guaranteed, and in many instances (regardless of such innovations) GPs wish to maintain their clinical freedom and refer patients to institutions that they decide upon themselves.

Alternatively, GP fundholders may not wish to relinquish the new-found power that fundholding has given them.

To solve the problem of the former and offer incentives that at least encourage the GP to consider the costs of his actions, DHAs can apportion a budget to a GP for certain activities over which he has control, and thereby give an incentive to the GP to be more discerning as to where he refers. This is obviously a kind of 'fundholding by default'.

With the latter, the difficulty in persuading GP fundholders to toe a combined purchasing line may be a short-term problem. GP fundholders have been keen to use their own budgets to exert power and may sometimes have used this power inappropriately. Yet in the long-term, such fundholders may become aware of the overall impact of their actions within the market. The DHA can aid in developing such an awareness that GP fundholders will accept the need of long-term planning (providing that they have influence upon such planning). Therefore the role of the DHA specifically with GP fundholders should be to facilitate the change from autonomous power to corporate power as a key purchaser along with the DHA.

PURCHASER/PROVIDER RELATIONSHIPS

As the DHA needs to recognize the influence of GP fundholders and hence their purchasing decisions, so it must also recognize the influence of other purchasers and the advantages to be gained from cooperation with such purchasers (and the disadvantages of not cooperating). There are two key purchasers with which a DHA may consider having a close working relationship (1) neighbouring DHAs and (2) local and neighbouring FHSAs.

The key advantage to the parties concerned of such cooperation (whether it be collaborative agreements, the merger of the functions of those organizations or actual mergers) is that it enhances capacity in terms of knowledge and power. With (1), the size of the budget and the geographical area over which the combined organizations have an influence will enable them to exert greater control over providers. With (2), a combined staff will enable an organization to benefit from a larger selection of skills (especially when such skills are in short supply). This will aid not only in the purchasing role and the setting and monitoring of contracts, but will also improve representation of the public, by enabling more comprehensive health needs assessment.

Concern, however, must be stated over firstly, the ability of such large combined organizations truly to represent the public and secondly, the lack of incentive for efficiency where there exists little or no competition to the purchaser. The former highlights the need for provider and GP involvement in the setting of health need requirements, while the latter may imply the necessity for close political accountability.

Examples of purchaser cooperation exist

across the country, with either joint working on purchasing plans (possibly via purchasing consortia) or the actual institutionalization of roles, i.e. DHAs and FHSAs (where there may be a single chief executive or a single combined budget). Obviously, once the recommendations of *Managing the New NHS* are fully implemented, DHAs and FHSAs will merge. Currently, examples of such a future exist in Wessex Region: the creation of health commissions has led to larger geographic boundaries, with a virtual merger of the DHAs and FHSAs concerned. South Derbyshire DHA and FHSA have a joint purchasing forum, in which the purchasing plans of both are combined with that of Derbyshire County Council and Social Services Department. In North Derbyshire their locality model has been duplicated by Social Services.

In addition to merging of functions, closer cooperation between neighbouring DHAs and FHSAs can also lead to benefits for all concerned. There exists the opportunity to combine funds and certain responsibilities for their resident populations, so as to spread the risk of certain low-volume, high-cost patient episodes, e.g. haemodialysis. Likewise, since separate purchasers often use the same providers, by cooperating on contractual decisions, the adverse impact of one purchaser's decision on another may be reduced.

For example, when considering the GP fundholder relationship, there may exist a critical mass as to service provision. If one purchaser reallocates certain contracts from one provider to another, the total remaining income level for a provider for a particular service may be insufficient to maintain supply. This places the remaining purchasers in (at least a short-term) problem, if gaining alternative provision for that particular service is difficult. Hence in such instances it would be preferable for purchasers to act in cooperation. A purchaser may be removing a contract from a particular provider, but if it is done in such a way as to enable other purchasers to find alternative providers, then

the actions of one DHA will not have such a detrimental effect upon the patients of another. (In Wessex, for example, such a situation did occur with regard to orthopaedic services. In this case the RHA intervened by supporting the provider concerned until purchasers could find alternative sources. Given the abolition of RHAs such intervention may not be guaranteed in the future.) This emphasizes the need for purchaser cooperation or regulation from the new regional directorates.

OTHER DHA RELATIONSHIPS

As well as the formal and informal relationships with providers and purchasers that result from a DHA creatively pursuing its role as a purchaser there is also the need for relationships with many other individuals, groups and organizations – as the DHA carries out its wider role as a commissioner of health care. Not least of these are the relationships of the DHA with other public, private and voluntary bodies.

The DHA's concern is for the health of its resident population. Given that there are many influences upon health status other than health care (e.g. social, environmental and personal factors such as housing, pollution, diet and lifestyle), it becomes imperative that, in order to ensure optimum efficiency in the use of resources, the DHA enters into negotiations and agreements with those other organizations able to influence health status. To date, the main area of emphasis with regard to such closer working has been in the area of community care, (not least owing to the Government's 'care in the community' policy). Hence we observe instances of coordination, or consultation, of purchasing between such bodies as social services, local authorities and the DHA. Alternatively 'locality' models of purchasing offer the ideal opportunity to combine health-care services to match specifically targeted population needs.

As DHAs exist to ensure that the needs of their resident populations are met, a key relationship is that with the public – specifically with regard to the assessment of health-care needs. One of the failures of the system so far has been the lack of accountability of the DHA to the public. Thus the public is either unaware of specific agencies and their responsibilities within the new NHS or unclear as to their role and hence their responsibility. It may be in the interests of DHAs to allow such ignorance to persist. On occasion DHA behaviour may have further clouded public perception. The advantage to the DHA of such a situation has been that, since providers bear the brunt of public outcry, they can try to get providers to provide extra service with no extra funding. This results in a number of problems.

Firstly, as stated, DHAs lack incentives to fulfil their role. Secondly, because of this, providers are often forced to act in the manner of a DHA, making priorities without the requisite information. Thirdly, as a result, in the long run, since providers' chief executives are answerable more for the financial viability of their trust rather than the optimal provision of health care for a resident population, the patient could lose out.

That said, there has, however, been much progress in developing the role of the DHA as commissioner and the interpretation of public needs. One problem has lain in slow movement, and the fact that purchasers could still be said to be 'following providers'. While Government intentions have been to remedy this imbalance, the question remains as to the source of the imbalance and hence the practicality of various solutions.

If the problem has been the lack of trained staff or the market manipulation by provider monopolies, then increasing purchaser power or information would be a viable solution. If, however, public accountability is the problem then increasing purchaser power is unlikely to enhance the functioning of purchasers.

SPECIFIC INITIATIVES

THE CREATION OF HEALTH AGENCIES

North West Thames is a good example of a number of regions which have sought to create an overall planning framework within which DHAs, FHSAs and GP fundholders can operate (Light, 1994). The philosophy behind such a framework is that the radical nature of the NHS reforms must be harnessed to an agenda for purchasing health and health gain, rather than simply purchasing medical services. Locality-based joint commissioning should bring together purchasers in local areas so that they can creatively develop services. The ultimate aim is to ensure that strong purchasing leads to an appropriate system that covers all types of health care – from primary (including prevention and promotion) to tertiary.

The North West Thames Region's district health authorities were made coterminous with family health services authority boundaries wherever possible, in order to create joint commissioners. Initiatives to improve the strength and salience of purchasing were taken alongside these structural reorganizations (Lane End Group, 1992). Additionally, a radical definition of primary care was made in North West Thames (embracing community services and primary care in the hospital setting as well as traditional primary care) (North West Thames Regional Health Authority, 1992) . Cooperative commissioning between NHS agencies, housing agencies, local education agencies and a variety of other services (including community care) is intended to promote primary care where relevant. This is to be done where possible using GPs as 'core managers of primary care teams within the NHS' (Light, 1994).

Such initiatives, of course, depend upon both structural reorganization and issues of personality and behaviour. Additionally, the two-edged sword of GP fundholding again raises a sharp point: how much will the often innovatory freedoms of GP fundholders be compatible with the search for 'seamless care' (Glennerster, Matsaganis and Owen, 1992).

THE DORSET HEALTH COMMISSION

An informal merger of DHAs and the FHSA into the Dorset Health Commission, perhaps to be formalized after the forthcoming national legislation, is intended to create joint decision-making binding on both legally separate authorities (the DHA and the FHSA). In effect the commission is an overarching health authority which commissions both primary and secondary care and handles the contracting process. The chief executive has identified surplus funds for pump-priming and innovation as critical success to such a venture (Carruthers, 1992). The particular initiatives which the commission has stressed are:

- a provider development programme (PDP) based on GP practices, both fund-holding and non-fundholding; practices are encouraged to carry out community health services;
- the development of community care centres covering a broader range of services than a community care or community services trust would normally provide;
- the development of GP hospitals, based on old cottage hospitals, for long-term and respite care as well as acute care where appropriate;
- a radical policy of interagency joint commissioning (embracing district health authorities, family health services authorities, providers, GP fundholders, County Council and district councils).

NORTH YORKSHIRE: LEAD AGENCY, JOINT PURCHASING AND PRAGMATIC ACTIVITY

'Local schemes and contracts are being set up within a wider framework of a county strategy and encouraged by allocation of joint finance money' (Hornby and Wistow, 1994).

The planning processes inherent in joint commissioning are to be used, with one purchaser acting as lead agency, to be responsible for needs assessment and make contracts 'in which two or more purchasers are party of the documentation' (Hornby and Wistow, 1994). It is interesting to note that the Health Service Act 1977 can be used to enable joint commissioning. There is furthermore a need to combine large-scale purchasing with, on the one hand, locality purchasing and, on the other hand, care packages for individuals and groups. Where a number of agencies are involved in joint commissioning, it is important to ensure that institutions and modes of working exist at each level to 'operationalize' joint commissioning into care plans and (where relevant) contracts, at each relevant level. The North Yorkshire approach furthermore has been to focus upon specific pilot schemes, to allow practical initiatives to be developed from which 'good practice' can be synthesized. Initial pilot schemes deal with respite care, personal care at home and support for carers.

RESEARCH ON EMERGING PRACTICE: WHERE AND WHY GPS REFER PATIENTS

The project based at Manchester University's Centre for Primary Care Research (Department of General Practice) seeks to focus on where and why GPs refer their patients, as opposed to merely rates of referral (King and Newton, unpublished).

This will in essence seek to provide a rich picture of GP referrals – especially outside their own districts. Variation among otherwise similar GPs and the range of hospitals to which they refer will, for example, be one interesting potential result. Such research will provide the basis for comparing purchasing aspirations with existing practice, and will at least indirectly allow the distillation of good practice from existing practice to inform future contracts.

HYBRID APPROACHES: PRACTICE-SENSITIVE PURCHASING AND GP INPUT TO HEALTH AUTHORITY PURCHASING

Ham and Willis (1994) have identified a continuum of options for GP involvement in purchasing ranging from GP fundholding through to traditional or developed health authority commissioning. Moving from left to right on a line representing a continuum, we find:

- **GP fundholding**, consisting in real budgets for all activity allocated to individual practices, who do all commissioning and all purchasing;
- **Practice-sensitive purchasing**, which consists in notional budgets covering a wide range of activity managed on behalf of practices by health authority or other purchasing agencies;
- **Locality purchasing** with the resources allocated to and services commissioned for localities by the health authority or other agency;
- **GP input to health authority purchasing**, consisting in surveys, practice visits, representation by colleagues and purchasing teams, and so forth;
- **Health authority commissioning**, where purchasing feeds into a health authority commissioning process done by the health authority without any GP involvement at all.

Ham and Willis emphasize that different approaches are likely to be relevant at different levels, and that none of the approaches is likely to be sufficient on its own, given that each has strengths and weaknesses.

Based on a project undertaken for Northampton, a team visited health authorities around the country where experience of different approaches to purchasing had been pioneered (Ham and Willis, 1994). Interestingly, a common thread was agreement that 'further efforts should be put into specialist liaison groups'. These mainly involved joint audit by GPs and specialists concerning the best use of resources for particular services.

KEELE UNIVERSITY (CENTRE FOR HEALTH PLANNING AND MANAGEMENT)/ STAFFORDSHIRE FAMILY HEALTH SERVICES AUTHORITY: PRIMARY/SECONDARY 'INTERFACE' AUDIT

The aim of this project, funded by the Department of Health, was to develop good practice locally in securing agreement between GPs and specialist doctors as to:

- more accurate measurement of waiting times to ensure more appropriate purchasing;
- improved communication between GPs and specialists;
- elucidation of good practice and development of better practice in patient management, especially while waiting for treatment for specified conditions (Centre for Health Planning and Management, 1994).

There are of course myriads of purchasing initiatives, with different objectives for services, value for money, and organizational development (Manning and Dunning, 1994). The further reading list at the end of this chapter documents some of these. The next section of the chapter looks at purchaser/ provider relationships. It should be stressed, of course, that the nature of these relationships is not a wholly separate issue from what might at first seem to be an issue exclusively concerned with commissioning – in other words, how to do needs assessments and how to translate these into contracts.

One study, for example, quotes a public health consultant with a purchasing authority as saying, 'about time we gave up on this notion of needs assessment...it's a joke...we should be honest and admit that we are involved in a health-care system rather than a health-needs system' (Freemantle *et al.*, 1993).

The point here is that providers may capture the marketplace and use non-economic means (political use of the media, for example) to place purchasing authorities clearly on the defensive. **Prioritization may not become more objective simply because it is explicit** (Freemantle *et al.*, 1993).

To such observations (research-based), it can be added: whether or not a provider unit is a trust might not be seminal for whether or not the market functions as intended. A trust may have the freedom to manipulate purchasers. But it may be squeezed financially by purchasers. A directly managed unit may 'bind in' the purchaser to local preference. Alternatively, it may be easier for a purchaser to close or merge a local directly managed unit. There is no one rule for all circumstances.

The essence of the internal market in the next few months and/or years is likely to consist in an attempt by purchasers to get providers to do more for less. The pressure which can be brought to bear on a trust through block contracts may be similar to the pressure that can be brought to bear on a directly managed unit (if any remain) in this regard. In the Freemantle study, a DGM remarked 'the problem is that we have no incentives to offer, we are expecting our clinicians to carry on doing the same amount of work with fewer resources'. While Freemantle *et al.* argued that therefore a directly managed unit (the DGM just quoted was responsible for such a unit) retarded the functioning of the internal market, putting trusts into such a situation of 'squeeze' may produce the same effect.

The overarching phenomenon is that trusts may have market power, in certain circumstances, that may subvert the aims of 'strong and effective purchasing'. This goes beyond the purely behavioural reasons for purchaser weakness, including the Department of Health's early obsession in developing trusts and belated recognition of the need to develop purchasers.

Ironically, in this situation, the Government is often seeking to close the purchaser/provider split, through the rhetoric of cosiness and so forth, in response to the problems it has created by opening it!

Providers furthermore have information which purchasers need in order to make purchasing decisions. In consequence 'good practice' might be best elucidated nationally, where possible, so that purchasing can take account of it in making contracts without simply being 'provider-driven' by local contracts. Implementing such good practice, however, involves a close dialogue between purchaser and provider at the local level to ensure that national criteria are translated into meaningful and manageable local standards – for the provider.

On the other hand, purchasing power increasingly lies in a scarcity of resources for a multiplicity of ends. Thus the purchaser has the money; the provider has the information and in some cases the market power. This is the greatest challenge to effective commissioning – which involves not only effective definition of needs and the translation of these into contract aspirations, but the commissioning of services as a result of contracts and their improvement over time.

We have in effect seen a cycle from the pre-reform NHS (with no purchaser/provider split), through a 'steady state' or cautious beginnings of the purchaser/provider split, through aggressive and 'macho' marketing based on the assumption of a significant split, back to the desire for a 'cosy' relationship between purchasers and providers – promulgated at the national level. Whether or not such a cosy relationship enables a market to bring its advantages or not, of course, is a very relevant question.

There is a great different between the text book market and the 'quasi-market' of the public services and of the NHS in particular. Whether the quasi-market improves or destroys the market is very much an open question at this point in time. Nevertheless it is important to realize that closing the purchaser/provider splits to some extent, through long-term and stable relationships between purchasers and providers, may be driven by the desire for cost savings (not the same as cost-effectiveness or even efficiency). That is, there may be an attempt to learn from the industrial model of contractors and subcontractors, whereby purchasers 'sit heavily' or 'lean heavily' on providers using modern management techniques such as 'just in time' delivery and total quality management. That is, on this interpretation of evolving events (based more on conspiracy than cock-up), the purchaser/provider split was deliberately opened to create pressure on costs and labour force costs in particular, and then partially closed again – but in a new environment.

The next section considers more overtly the effect of purchaser/provider relationships upon commissioning.

THE PURCHASER/PROVIDER RELATIONSHIP

In the post reform NHS where the DHA acts as the 'champion of the people', a major element of its commissioning role is as a purchaser of health care. By the mechanism of contracts with provider units, the DHA should be able to ensure that those health needs of the population that it has identified are met by the provision of appropriate health care. As a result a key relationship within the NHS internal market is that which exists between the DHA and the providers with which it contracts.

The explicit element of the purchaser/provider relationship is that of the contract i.e. the written agreement between the purchaser, the DHA, in this case, and the provider unit. Therefore, in commenting upon the features of the purchaser/provider relationship, the intention is to use the contract as the cornerstone. What can one conclude about the nature of the purchaser/provider relationship from the nature of the

contract; and, likewise, what can be learnt about the purchaser/provider relationship from observation of the process of contracting and the process of monitoring those contracts?

TYPES OF CONTRACT

Firstly let us consider the implications of different forms of contract. Taking the original three forms of contract described by the Government (Department of Health, 1989) of block, cost and volume, and cost per case, we can observe the following features.

The **block contract**, where the provider receives a fixed sum of money for a predicted activity, but with no additional funding if such activity is greater than anticipated, can be of great advantage to the purchaser with regard to the burden of risk. If demand for a service (and hence cost) is greater than anticipated, rather than the purchaser having to find extra funding, it is the provider who must accommodate the excess. This effect is enhanced by the provider 'facing the music' with the public on a daily basis. However the disadvantage of such contracts for the purchaser is that, due to their content being general rather than specific, it is difficult for the purchaser to exert control over the process by which the contract is fulfilled. As a result it is possible for (say) case-mix to be manipulated. Thus the health-care needs met by the provider are not those necessarily intended by the purchaser.

At the other extreme of contract specification is the **cost per case contract**; these enable the purchaser to exert greater control over the actual health care that is provided to the resident population (assuming the purchaser is able adequately to monitor such health-care provision). However, with greater specification in provision comes greater specification in cost, i.e. once the nature of the service provided can be detailed so can its cost structure. As a result it is now the purchaser who faces the financial risks from unanticipated demand, i.e. the provider can insist upon extra funding for the provision of additional care. The only alternative for the purchaser is to deny such funds and justify itself publicly. In addition, since the provider has no incentive to minimize on cases treated, it can be potentially difficult for the purchaser to control costs. In between these two extremes of contracts, there is the **cost/volume contract** possessing the compromise characteristics of both extremes.

The intention of the Government has been to move away from block contracts to contracts with greater specification. 'Block contracts are necessary building blocks; but as reliable information on costs and prices becomes more readily available, I am sure there will be, and should be, more concerted moves towards "cost and volume" and "cost per case" contracts' (NHSME 1993). While the incentives to the provider of specified contracts may be perverse, hopefully since the purchaser will have both the incentive to prioritize with greater clarity and monitor contracts more rigorously, both allocative and technical efficiency will hopefully be enhanced by the use of cost per case contracts.

There are some reservations, however. Firstly, to what extent can information sources be advanced to enable the DHA to perform this role successfully, i.e. incentives may be a necessary condition for improving efficiency but are not sufficient. Secondly, to what extent is there an incentive for the DHA to exert such tight control, i.e. given that the purchaser/provider split is not well understood by the public, can the DHA be said to be truly accountable?

Thus, even though the DHA may be accountable to the Department of Health, is this for the same requirements and on the same basis to the public? Indeed on occasion DHAs have fed false information to the public as to their responsibility, e.g. blaming hospitals for a contract rather than detailing their involvement.

While there is evidence that changes have occurred (with a movement towards cost and volume contracts) for the majority of contracts placed by DHA, the block contract is still the preferred or at least accepted type. When surveying and interviewing in trusts concerning the nature of their DHA contracts, figures of 70–100% were cited as the proportion of DHA income within block contracts.

This said, however, there are instances of trusts whose DHA income is almost entirely contained within cost and volume contracts. In many cases contracts are at a transitional stage between block and cost and volume (sometimes referred to as sophisticated block contracts). As a result the nature of contracts are open to a certain degree of interpretation, this being dependent upon whether agreements upon volume are implicit or explicit. When volume agreements are made explicit it is not always by the setting of stated workloads and agreed remuneration but can also be by the use of 'trigger points' which signify the need for reassessment but still permit substantial flexibility.

What can be observed quite clearly is that there is a lack of movement towards cost per case contracts which are only observed in particular high cost specialties and in the contracts of GP fundholders.

Observing the current situation, it would appear that DHAs are avoiding many of the financial risks imposed by the market by placing the burden upon their providers. In certain respects this was the original **intention** of the purchaser/provider split, such that a purchaser (the DHA), rather than pursuing cosy relationships with providers, should select purely on grounds of price, thereby encouraging competition and hence technical efficiency. However as the post-reform NHS has progressed, opinion as to how the purchaser/provider relationship should operate has changed. Hence, observations from the private sector have led to the conclusion that, while contracts with suppliers may be short, relationships are ongoing and hence an adversarial purchasing stance may not be conducive to the optimal organization of health care (see *Health Service Journal*, 27/1/94, 27–29).

While providers would generally prefer more specific contracts, and purchasers (especially capitation losers) have an incentive to place the greater burden of risk upon the providers, it does appear that many DHAs are still acting in an adversarial manner, and in many ways are avoiding the requirements of their own position (e.g. priority setting). However, this situation may not be the result of the DHA trying to pursue its own 'selfish' agenda, but rather the result of the practical difficulties of the commissioning role. To be able to specify contracts at the level required for cost per case, there is a necessity for large amounts of high quality data on both population need and service specification, in addition to which it must also be possible to monitor those contracts (once set).

While in certain instances (such as GP fundholder contracts) these criteria are met and specific contracts can be set, on many occasions this is not possible – particularly with DHAs, where the large populations for which they are responsible can be subject to a multitude of health conditions with often an array of potential treatments.

Of greater concern than either the current contract or data situation is the predicted scenario for the future. While there is general acceptance that data within the NHS is still inadequate to achieve widespread use of specific contracts, there is a certain degree of doubt as to whether this situation will continue. In the case of certain DHAs, there appears to be a reluctance to move towards more specific contracts on the grounds that the information upon which those contracts are based (however good) is the wrong information.

That is, contracts are input-based rather than output-based. This may be true. (Indeed since health gain is the goal, outcome should be the relevant feature of contracts.) But this does not excuse a DHA from pursuing such information and moving towards more specific contracts. The excuse of the DHAs concerned seems to be that pursuing such output information is even more difficult than the current pursuit of input information. Using the difficulty of the former and the inadequacy of the latter as an excuse for doing nothing, however, hardly seems a respectable reaction.

INTRA-CONTRACTING BEHAVIOUR

The contract itself is only part of the structured relationship that should exist between the provider and the purchaser. In addition to this there is both the negotiation period that occurs prior to the signing of the contract and the monitoring that occurs during the period with which the contract is concerned. The nature of the relationship between the purchaser and the provider during negotiation can be judged by the influence that each has upon the final contract and the process by which such influence occurs.

While purchasers are tending towards a more far sighted outlook, with the production of 5-year purchasing plans and strategic direction documents, these cases are fairly generalized and do not have the detailed content from which one can specify individual contracts. Thus while targets and general processes are specified which may aid providers in organizing the structure of their own organizations, the details of how targets shall be met and what the specifics of the processes will be are left very much to the individual contracting rounds.

As a result of this and also owing to information problems, it may come as no surprise that (currently) contracts are very much being led by providers who have better access to the information necessary to specify the details of contracts and often the salient indicators that should be monitored. Such a situation is of concern since it leaves the purchaser open to exploitation by the provider. That is, the provider, acting as the agent for information to the purchaser, can encourage the setting of a contract that is to its own benefit rather than to that of the purchaser and the population that it represents.

The provider may well be an ideal source for information, and providers may not always intend to hoodwink the DHA but to aid it in the contracting process. Because of the above perverse incentives, however, the DHA is likely to be untrusting of the information it receives. A solution for the DHA might be to contract for information as it would for services, i.e. to contract with providers in other regions over the information necessary to produce and monitor contracts successfully. This approach may, however, be subject to the difficulty that different regions experience different conditions and therefore may not possess the required information. Also, the transactions cost of such an approach may be great.

National data sources, moderated locally, may be the answer. But these would require governmental regulation to force competitive providers (and purchasers perhaps) to provide appropriate, and appropriately standardized, information. What would this do to the market?

Many trusts have complained that DHAs act in a 'God-like' manner, contracting on the basis that the information they possess is correct regardless of providers' statements to the contrary. Provider information may be acted upon only when it validates the DHAs opinions. As a result contracts can be produced which are at worst unattainable or at best inappropriate. When purchasers do not take such a stance but rather are willing to be informed by providers, the result can be a long-drawn-out negotiation, taking a lot of time and resources and leading to frustration for both parties. Thus, rather than quarterly contract meetings being used for ironing out disagreements and trying to achieve mutual compromise, what actually occurs is the provider having to explain to the purchaser in great detail why certain conditions cannot be attained (with often the DHA taking a opposing stance, more on grounds of image than of opposing opinion).

An alternative problem can arise when the DHA and the provider do have a good relationship. For example, while one or other may be at a particular advantage or disadvantage with regard to particular aspects of information, they cooperate to the extent that (while not deliberately colluding) neither is clear as to their true role.

As a result, the DHA can find itself in a position where it has effectively handed over the management of its budget to provider units or is itself acting as the management for such units.

In addition, if collusion is deliberate, the result could be detrimental to the provision of health care. For example purchasers may place a high priority on waiting lists and times due to their high public profile and Government interest through Charters and the like. Yet the provider (because of internal structure and consultant influence) will not be so interested in the same interpretation of waiting times unless those people on the lists are clinically urgent. The result can then be the creation of secondary unstated waiting lists i.e. delaying in putting a person on a waiting list. Or, if the purchaser has his way, waiting times may be reduced overall at the expense of 'sensible clinical priorities'.

MONITORING

The third element of the contractual relationship between the purchaser and the provider is that of monitoring. Superficially, major problems in terms of providers failing to meet contracts are rare. But this must be set against a backdrop of information still in short supply. Hence contracts in many cases are either not difficult to fulfil or (if unfulfilled) failures are difficult to identify.

The problems of contract monitoring are complicated further when one considers that the various types of information available are not necessarily of equal importance, and information is prioritized for the attainment of short-term goals rather than long-term objectives. Therefore one must be careful to ensure that contract targets are set so as to achieve what is desirable rather than what is measurable.

For example, as a result of such directives as the Patient's Charter, there is a tendency to put greater emphasis upon such features as waiting times and hospital facilities (car parking, surgery design, etc.). While these are quite valid quality indicators, especially in so far as they are based upon patient preferences, one must ensure that these are not used at the expense of other equally (if not more) valid indicators of quality and contract attainment, e.g. morbidity and mortality! Likewise, mortality and morbidity rates should not be used as crude performance indicators.

One approach to monitoring providers is to use information acquired by GPs, who possess both direct indicators of provider competence (e.g. promptness of discharge letters) and indirect indicators (e.g. patient feedback). As a result GPs often have a far greater understanding of the operation of provider units, even down to the competence of individual staff members.

Finally, the DHA, as well as being a participant within the NHS internal market, can, because of its size and nature, also influence the operation of that market. While a DHA may encourage an ongoing relationship between itself and provider units, it may also have to act as arbiter so as to encourage similar relationships among the providers themselves. This may seem contradictory to the NHS reforms, where provider competition is allegedly the backdrop to the attainment of technical efficiency. As a result of the particular structure of the NHS market, not to encourage provider collaboration can lead to perverse incentives.

To take an example, consider the common

situation in which community services and acute care are provided by separate trusts. Quite often, when a person requires a total episode of health care, it will be from both these sources, e.g. a person who needs a hip replacement and is admitted to an acute unit for such treatment will (following discharge) require the attentions of a physiotherapist. It could be that delaying discharge from the acute unit would reduce the need for such community services and as a result would reduce total costs. However the acute provider has no incentive to pursue such an approach, since their concern is only with minimizing their element of total cost regardless of the impact on other providers.

Likewise, for the community care provider, it might be the case that suitable interventions performed earlier could have reduced the need for such a hip replacement.

Hence the purchaser has a role to play in resolving these conflicting and potentially cost-increasing incentives. In this case solutions could involve:

- having combined contracting arrangements with all providers;
- a 'lead provider' model, where the DHA contracts with one provider and then mandates it to subcontract for additional services.

There are other options as well.

Indeed in one health authority a number of solutions were being tried in different situations so as to ascertain which would yield the best results: e.g. for mental health, a lead provider model; for child health, a coordination of purchasing; for elderly care, separate contracts were still in operation. (In contrast, the neighbouring health authority was not making any arrangements to deal with such perverse incentives and was content to 'wait and see'.)

Prior to the NHS reforms, hospital and community services were not, of course, separate trusts. The problem then was that pressure on high-visibility hospital services often led to the 'swallowing up' of the community budget. A countervailing problem, post-reform, may be that separate trusts have an incentive to 'cost-shift' and 'patient-shift' to each other. Only tight regulation, with high transactions costs, or assumptions of altruism incompatible with market competition, can solve this problem.

One answer is, of course, combined hospital and community trusts. But this can again 'swallow' the community budget. Another answer is to give the budget to the community trust, in line with the philosophy of 'primary' care as the future.

The problem here is that, by primary care, the Government often means simply acute care in a community setting. If contracts for acute care of whatever sort are to be given to community units, subcontracting to acute doctors, it is important not to undermine the hospital. For example, some community trusts are contracting session-by-session or even privately with hospital consultants to provide certain types of acute care in a community setting (whether in a GP fundholder's surgery, or small local hospital owned by a community unit, or whatever). These may pay only the marginal costs of services for which the infrastructure costs are paid by the hospital – but not reimbursed to the hospital. Perverse incentives – or rather short-termism, threatening the viability of overall services in the long-term – have to be carefully monitored in this realm.

LESSONS FROM ABROAD: A BRIEF POINTER

In one sense the NHS reforms are quite unique. The only other part of the world in which fully socialized health-care systems (on paper) are now being transformed in a market direction is in the former Eastern Europe and former Soviet Union. There, of course, the situation was radically different from that of the successful British National Health Service.

The creation of a purchaser/provider split, and therefore the development of a full overt commissioning function, within a system of still (mainly) public financing and provision, is, however, a new departure.

To that extent lessons from abroad are likely to be less at the level of the overall system than at the level of the individual initiative, as from various types of successful health maintenance organization in the United States, for example, or from light shed on how best to consider commissioning and purchasing *vis-à-vis* providers from other public systems (such as that in Sweden). This does not, of course, preclude insights from other systems, especially where public financing is strong (such as the Netherlands). Nor does it preclude careful negative lessons (i.e. warnings) from around the world in general!

GENERAL LESSONS ON COMMISSIONING

Commissioning, and particularly joint commissioning between different agencies, is a process geared to translating the needs of populations into a strategy for provision of services at the required quality. A major challenge for commissioning in the UK is to overcome forces for fragmentation inherent in aspects of the NHS reforms – principally, the split between GP fundholding on the one hand and needs-based purchasing by district health authorities on the other hand. To that extent, lessons are available from other countries where the unification of formerly separate sources of finance, in order to indulge in global commissioning, is necessary. Unified commissioning is necessary to increase equity as well as to increase efficiency and decrease the bureaucratic costs of fragmented purchasing and fragmented contracting.

A general lesson from abroad concerning commissioning centres on the need for stability for both purchasers and providers. Ability to spread risk (by both purchasers and providers) would imply that both should be of adequate size, and that failures (or bankruptcies, as in the US) can thereby be more easily avoided.

More specific lessons, generally from abroad are:

- the difficulty of ensuring a desired level of budget for primary care and community services, and of focusing upon a 'health' strategy as opposed to a health services strategy;
- the need for a global budget for purchasing;
- the limited relevance of health reform in other countries, where such countries are often moving from private, third-party reimbursed health care in the direction of the 'internal market' and the purchaser/ provider split as a move towards socialization (not a move away from socialization, as is arguably occurring in the UK); such countries may be wise to do so, the UK, however, may be 'beyond' such a need;
- the dominance of US advice and US literature in European health-care reform especially 'English-speaking health-care reform' (which would include English-speaking advice to Sweden, Denmark *et al.*);
- the need for appropriate purchaser/ provider incentives and relationships to be complemented by a focus upon community health (unlike in most US HMOs) (Light, 1994);
- the need for unified clinical and financial information systems, to allow clinical evaluation, cost-effectiveness measurement and audit;
- the desirability of clear managerial accountability from providers to purchasers (a trend by no means apparent in the NHS reforms at present);
- meaningful choice of the primary provider, in the UK the general practitioner (whether fundholding or non-fundholding);
- appropriate political clarity and compatibility of different governmental and managerial aims (again by no means apparent in the current NHS situation!).

LESSONS FROM SWEDEN

The more interesting developments in purchasing in Sweden are naturally based on the County Council model, in that the County Council commissions health care in the decentralized Swedish system. Central government has more of a regulatory and 'intelligence' role. As in the UK, there was no purchaser/provider distinction in Sweden in a meaningful way until recently. The main lesson from Sweden is the creation of a **purchaser/provider functional distinction** rather than an **institutional purchaser/ provider split**. Although, under a continuing right-of-centre government, 'ideas from the NHS reforms' may be transplanted at least in part into Sweden, currently there are different models for increasing purchasing and commissioning (within the context of purchasing and provision still being the County Council's overall responsibility). In other words, Swedish providers are 'directly managed', to use the British language.

The money follows the patient more directly in the Swedish 'experimental models' than in the UK. This has been one of the biggest problems for British purchasing: input by patients and GPs (of the non-fundholding sort) has been limited by an inability of 'bureaucratic' purchasers to allow money to follow the patient. Indeed in some cases this situation has been significantly worsened by comparison with the pre-reform NHS.

Four prominent cases from Sweden come from the County Councils of Stockholm, Sormland, Bohus and Dalecarlia (Bergman, 1994). They vary in terms of the patient's right to choose, and in the type of contract used with the provider – although in most cases there are extra payments for extra work according to agreed principles. Saltman and von Otter (1992) have argued that the Swedish case is in effect a kind of 'public competition', where the patient chooses and the money follows, rather than the NHS reform case, which they call a 'mixed market' in that managers make choices and patients follow the contract, with a greater ideological desire to promote private provision in the UK than in Sweden (for the moment). In reality, the money following the patient is not a market at all, but a system of reimbursement of popular and efficient providers by agreed criteria.

The difference among the four models lies in the degree of centralization of purchasing (with some moving towards what would in the UK be known as more of a locality model) and also variation in terms of central regulation as to pricing; variation in terms of type of contract, ranging from block through 'sophisticated block' to in effect cost per volume; and so on. It will be important to monitor effects in Sweden from a British viewpoint.

LESSONS FROM THE NETHERLANDS

The primary lesson from the Netherlands is that opening up a purchaser/provider split may necessitate new mechanisms to allow significant choice for the patient and citizen. The British socialized system prior to the NHS reforms at least allowed the right of referral, without bureaucratic contracting to limit this. Other fee-for-service systems in Europe which incorporated the principle of National Health Insurance were also systems of free referral, with third-party reimbursement in this case being private (rather than public as in the UK pre-reform).

The common trend in the UK and other European countries, such as the Netherlands, is to limit free referral (whether to public providers in the UK or to private providers in the Netherlands), and to 'manage care' in the interests of cost control as well as quality. In some European systems, such a move is compatible with greater socialization – as indeed with the Clinton Reforms in the United States. The Netherlands in one sense is like the UK, in that, despite private (mostly non-profit) hospitals and the like, it was a largely publicly funded and publicly regulated system allowing free referral and free access.

In the interests of cost control, a market in provision is being sought, along with competition amongst purchasers. The Dutch reforms have been slower than the British reforms, reflecting the Dutch political system based on consensus and incremental reform.

The main lesson for the UK is that, if free patient/GP referral is to be limited, greater mechanisms for ensuring the accountability of purchasers to patients, consumers and citizens (not the same thing) must be sought. Again locality-based joint commissioning may be a way forward.

CONCLUSION

The main challenge for commissioning in the UK is to ensure that local needs assessment is rendered compatible with districts' (and regional, and central) resource allocation. It is very easy to conduct sophisticated and worthwhile, ethnographically based local needs assessment exercises, only to find that the money available to meet the required needs is not there. Furthermore such needs are likely to be for non-hospital services. The best means for 'assessing needs' for hospital services is probably to tap into the expertise which already exists and which always existed – although in an unsystematic way – at the level of the referring GP.

The challenge is to incorporate effective resource allocation from the centre through regional directorates to purchasers, in the future, into a system which also includes local sensitivities. While innovation is to be encouraged – witness the plethora of 'innovative schemes' in purchasing and commissioning which have grown up – the danger is that systematizing all the best practice locally – and all the need for regulation and resource allocation and market management, nationally and regionally – will lead to a very bureaucratic system indeed. In a worst case scenario, we will have the 'worst of both worlds' – the fragmentation of the market and the bureaucracy of an overplanned system. The challenge, therefore, is to unify budgets at the purchaser level, or find mechanisms whereby non-unified budgets can lead to effective joint commissioning nonetheless. The following literature provides many insights in that direction.

DISCUSSION

- Before considering the modern terms of 'purchasing' and 'commissioning', one should define the territory within which these concepts are intended to have operative meaning. Strategic planning refers to the identification of objectives and the mobilization of means to achieve these objectives. To that extent it is the broadest activity within which commissioning and purchasing (respectively) occur. Commissioning refers to the wider process of responding to needs identified in the planning process, and sometimes indeed refers to the wider planning process itself. More commonly, however, commissioning refers to the identification of services required and means of securing them. Purchasing in this context refers slightly more narrowly to the specific services, with a price tag attached, which are then 'contracted' from providers.

- Purchasing at its best is in fact a modern form of achieving the objectives identified in plans. Thus the public, GPs and other actors ought to 'feed into' the purchasing process, which should then be used to provide both capital and revenue to providers. In this sense, the term 'purchasing' is neutral as to whether 'the money follows the patient' or 'the patient follows the money'.

- A system whereby the money always follows the patient is simply a system of reimbursement – whether carried out in the private or public sectors (as discussed in earlier chapters of this book). A system

where the patient always follows the money is a system of managerially-based prioritization and even rationing, where clinical referral and patient choice are subordinate to 'the purchasing plan' quantified in terms of available resources.

- Confusion between the above two possibilities – and indeed the existence of both in practice – has led to confusion as to both the descriptive reality of purchasing in the post-reform NHS and indeed as to the prescriptive *desiderata* of 'purchasing'. Some agree with purchasing as a means of mobilizing resources to follow people's (and therefore patients') wishes. This is what is meant by purchasing in Sweden, by and large, although there are some purchasing mechanisms being developed by some Swedish county councils whereby contracts limit the availability of care. In the British sense of purchasing, however, contracts made by managers – which non-fundholding GPs and patients have to follow – are more common. This reflects the origin of the NHS reforms in the desire to control costs and 'do more with the existing money'. As a result, the financial origins of purchasing are dominant by comparison with the use of purchasing as a tool for either choices in health care made by the public or indeed by general practitioners or other experts.

ACKNOWLEDGEMENTS

I would like to thank the Audit Commission for commissioning me to submit a paper on purchasing that uses much of the material in this chapter (the Audit Commission is not of course responsible for my views). Thanks are also due to Kevin Hunt, who helped draft a section of the paper.

APPENDIX 1: CRITERIA FOR COMMISSIONING FOR HEALTH

The need to combine 'traditional expert' opinion and other sources of expertise: much of the medical profession is currently disaffected by the idea that 'managers are making contracts without consulting us'. At worst, this can lead to a bureaucratic system of purchasing and contracting which produces a worse result than the less bureaucratic system of referral to established services (and advice on new services, as in the old system).

The three main advantages of an overt purchaser/provider split are allegedly:

- an end to a professional dominance and 'provider capture';
- input into the purchasing system from public opinion;
- attention to cost-effectiveness in placing contracts.

It is important to ensure that an end to 'provider capture' is not simply the beginning of 'capture' by newer interests (such as the temporary priorities of temporary governments; local management priorities dressed up as science; or, for example, unsubstantiated claims about 'priority services'). The purchaser/provider split established to create a competitive market among providers may create 'purchaser power' in reducing 'production costs' and labour costs (if not transactions costs). But the purchasing process must of necessity involve decision by experts (based in providers) who could often make their input in a less bureaucratic way in the old system – whether as hospital clinicians or as GP referrers.

There is, therefore, a need to ensure non-bureaucratic and robust systems of commissioning which involve close collaboration between purchasers and both local and non-local providers.

The need to measure current health status and map a transition to desired health status: drawing on information drawn from mortality statistics, morbidity statistics, social statistics generally, surveys of the population, and so forth. Only after this is done can prioritization begin. Methodologies for making priorities – such as the quality adjusted life year –

have a role to play as servant but not master. Formal analysis of outcome and costs may be useful in showing within specialties (or even conditions-specifically) how different client groups can benefit differentially from different treatments, at different costs. Between specialties QALYs can also help, if one accepts the values behind the figures derived for 'utilities' for individuals and groups. But overall the QALY ought to be treated cautiously. Its best role may be in suggesting areas of minimal cost-effectiveness or areas of great cost-effectiveness in health care that may currently be receiving excessive or inadequate investment.

The need to recognize that purchasers 'have their hands tied' by national (governmental and managerial) priorities, and that very small sums of money (relatively speaking) are available for new local priorities in purchasing because of both this factor and the 'inevitable demand' factor of (primarily) acute care.

This is another argument for ensuring that the building of 'purchasing empires' under the guise of strong purchasing is not undertaken disproportionately to the benefit of so doing.

The problem, of course, is that under the internal market, autonomous providers can invest with greater freedom in rival information systems, or rival approaches to needs assessment generally, that force the purchasers to indulge in a policy of mutual deterrence! Just as providers need to invest large sums in order to compete with each other for contacts, purchasers need to invest in order to have information *vis-à-vis* providers. Again, there is something of a vicious circle here – which long-term stable relationships encouraged by Government policy ought to be geared to minimizing.

REFERENCES

Bergman, S. (1994) *Purchaser Provider Systems in Sweden: An Overview of Reforms in a Swedish Health Care Delivery System*, Spri, Stockholm.
Carruthers, I. (1992) *The Development of Purchasing*,

Dorset Health Commission, Ferndown, Dorset.

Centre for Health Planning and Management (1994) *A Primary/Secondary Care Interface Medical Audit Project*, Centre for Health Planning and Management, Keele/Staffordshire Medical Audit Advisory Group (FHSA), Keele.

Freemantle, N. et al. (1993) Talking shop. *Health Service Journal*, 17 Jun.

Glennerster, H., Matsaganis, M. and Owen, P. (1992) *A Foothold for Fundholding*, King's Fund Institute, London.

Ham, C. and Willis, A. (1994) Perspectives on purchasing: think globally, act locally. *Health Service Journal*, 15 Jan.

Hornby, M. and Wistow, G. (1994) Perspective on purchasing: ready, steady, go. *Health Service Journal*, 24 Feb.

King, N. and Newton, P. (unpublished) Patterns in practice. Department of Primary Care, Manchester University, Manchester.

Lane End Group (1992) *What is a Good Purchaser*, North West Thames Regional Health Authority, London.

Light, D. W. (1994) *Strategic Challenges in Joint Commissioning: Challenges and Strategic Issues in Comparative Perspective*, North West Thames Regional Health Authority, London.

Manning, S. and Dunning, M. (1994) Perspectives on purchasing: every day and every way. *Health Service Journal*, 10 Mar.

NHSME (1993) *Purchasing for Health – A Framework for Action*, Health Publications Unit, Heywood, Lancashire.

North West Thames Regional Health Authority (1992) *Developing Primary Care*, North West Thames Regional Health Authority, London.

Saltman, R. and von Otter, C. (1992) *Planning Markets and Public Competition: Strategic Reforms in Northern European Health Systems*, Open University Press, Bury St Edmunds, Suffolk.

FURTHER READING

GENERAL, BRITISH

Applegate, G. F. (1994) An investigation of purchaser/provider relationships and their importance for effective purchasing of health care. Unpublished MBA dissertation, Centre for Health Planning and Management, Keele University, Staffordshire.

Heginbotham, C. and Ham, C. (1992) *Purchasing Dilemmas*, King's Fund College and Southampton and South West Hampshire Health Authority, Southampton.

Hunter, D.J. and Harrison, S. (1994) *Effective Purchasing for Health Care: Proposals for the First Five Years*, (commissioned by the NHS Management Executive), Nuffield Institute for Health, London.

NAHAT and CASPE (1994) *Patterns of Priorities; A Study of Rationing in Health Authorities*, NAHAT Research Paper No. 7, London.

NHSME (1991) *Purchasing Intelligence*, NHSME, London.

HEALTH SERVICE JOURNAL AND ITS PURCHASING SERIES

Anonymous (1992) Smart moves (countdown to community care). *Health Service Journal*, **29 Oct.**

Layzell, A. (1994) Perspectives on purchasing: local and vocal. *Health Service Journal*, **20 Jan**.

Raftery, J. and Gibson, G. (1994) Perspectives on purchasing: banking on knowledge. *Health Service Journal*, **10 Feb**.

Raftery, J. *et al.* (1994) Perspectives on purchasing: band aid. *Health Service Journal*, **17 Feb**.

Reeves C (1994) Perspectives on purchasing: on cabbages and things. *Health Service Journal*, **3 Mar**.

Stockford, D. (1993) Perspectives on purchasing. *Health Service Journal*, **Dec.**

RESEARCH AND PROJECTS, BRITISH

Audit Commission District Reviews (plus Synthesis of DHA Recommendations).

Coulter, A. and Bradlow, J. (1993) Effective NHS reforms and general practitioner referral patterns. *British Medical Journal*, **306**, 433–437.

MORE GENERAL/BACKGROUND

Audit Commission (1993) *Practices Make Perfect: The Role of the FHSA*, HMSO, London.

Beecham, L. (1993) Clinicians must be involved in contracting. *British Medical Journal*, **306**, 935.

Bowling, A., Jacobson. B. and Southgate, L. (1993) Health service priorities: explorations in consultation of the public and health professions on priority setting in an Inner London health district. *Social Science and Medicine*, **37**, 851–857.

Bromley, N. (unpublished) Other modes of FHSA DHA integration in the NHS. South East Thames RHA, London.

Butland, G. (1993) Commissioning for quality. *British Medical Journal*, **306**, 251–252.

Department of Health (1993) *Managing the New NHS (The Langlands Report)*, HMSO, London.

Forsythe, M. (1993) Commissioning specialist services. *British Medical Journal*, **306**, 872–873.

Ham, C. (1992) *Locality Purchasing*, Health Services Management Centre, Birmingham.

Ham, C. (1993) *Partners in Purchasing: Models of DHA/FHSA Collaboration*, NAHAT Discussion Paper, NAHAT, Birmingham.

Huntington, J. (1993) From FPC to FSHA to... Health Commission? *British Medical Journal*, **306**, 33–35.

Huntington, J. (1993) Integrated commissioning for health. *Primary Care Management*, **3**, 2–4.

Joule, N. (1993) *Partners in Purchasing: Role of CHCs*, Greater London Association of CHCs, London.

King's Fund College (1993) *The Commissioning Experience: Learning the Art of Purchasing*, Paper 6, King's Fund, London.

National Association of Health Authorities and Trusts (1993) *Listening to Local Voices*, Research Paper No. 9, NAHAT, London.

NHSME (1992) *Purchasing for Health: The Views of Local People*, NHSME EL1, London.

Nuffield Institute for Health (1992) *Purchasing for Health Gain – The Public Health Role*, Nuffield Institute for Health, London.

Nuffield Institute for Health (1992) *Health Care Needs Assessment – The Public Health Role; Guidelines for Audit*, Nuffield Institute for Health, London.

Office for Public Management (1993) *Towards an Effective NHS*, HMSO, London.

Young Samuel Chambers Ltd (1993) *Effective Purchaser/Provider Relationships*, Young Samuel Chambers, London.

THE MANAGEMENT OF HUMAN RESOURCES AND INDUSTRIAL RELATIONS

8

INTRODUCTION: THE POLITICAL CONTEXT

Firstly, it is necessary to distinguish the two terms – 'industrial relations' and 'the management of human resources'. **Industrial relations** is a term heard less these days, outside academic Departments of Industrial Relations (increasingly renamed Departments of Human Resource Management, given the Conservative hostility to the concept of industrial relations and therefore to funding its study) and outside of trade unions. Industrial relations refers to the relations between different groups within industry – primarily employers and workers. In an age when trade unions were still 'respectable', even on the Right, this generally referred to the relationship between employers and trade unions, including a possible role for the state in joining or regulating such relationships. There is increasingly a trend on the right wing of politics to de-emphasize trade unions, through legislative and other social means, and to replace collective bargaining in industry and in state organizations with individual contracts for employment. Even where collective bargaining remains, it is now conducted more often on a local basis rather than a national basis. This does not, of course, negate the use of Industrial Relations as the discipline in which to **study** these changing relationships.

The management of human resources may be a value-neutral term that refers to how, in any political and industrial context, people are best managed. On the other hand, it may represent a prescriptive set of techniques for managing employees individually rather than through the collective process or the recognition of trade unions as the significant representatives of workers in terms of their rights, negotiation of terms and conditions and other aspects of employment. To the extent that it is the latter, the new discipline known as 'human resource management' (HRM) has an ideological content rather than simply being a general term to describe management of people by any means, in any political environment. In the NHS today, MHR often is the latter, posing as the former when necessary for political or propagandist reasons. Euphemistic or 'soft' language, to hide a 'hard' reality, is unfortunately the order of the day.

SETTING THE SCENE

The transformation in industrial relations in the National Health Service from the 1970s to the mid-1990s provides a fairly graphic illustration of a change – from a recognition of the different social and industrial interests employed in the health service to an assumption that labour is simply a factor of production to be managed (however this is dressed up in 'progressive' language). The different theoretical perspectives within industrial relations which interpret both the NHS and the public sector more generally, as well as the whole economy, are outlined below. Meanwhile a few illustrations of the changed climate will bring home the point early in this chapter. The questions of 'productivity' and 'skill mix' are now high on the agenda for very clear political and economic reasons.

It may be said that the following were the ruling assumptions of the Conservative government in the early to mid-1990s. Firstly, there is not much more money, if any, available for the National Health Service. Secondly, therefore, if quantities of patient care are to be increased, labour productivity must increase. If there is no more money available, national pay rises must either be avoided or, if granted, must be funded from local savings rather than from extra national money. In consequence, wage rises such as that granted in 1993 of 3% for certain key public sector workers (such as the nurses) means that, if 'efficiency savings' are unable to foot the bill, then either less patient care or fewer nurses employed or both would be a consequence at the local level. That is why Eric Caines and other right-wing supporters of the market strategy in health care argue that nationally mandated pay rises are unhelpful.

The argument is that pay rises should only occur locally in response to increased productivity (problems in measuring this will be discussed below). A 3% rise across the board, it would be argued, cannot be as a result of productivity – unless at a local level, when it is afforded by taking more business from a rival trust hospital or unit. (If it is not the result of higher productivity, it will mean less output as more of the budget is spent employing the same workers or the same budget is spent employing fewer workers with lower output.)

A 3% rise even with more productivity – say, in a trust – will mean cuts elsewhere in the system, if there is not more purchasing money in total.

The assumption that 'any rise must come from productivity', of course, denies the argument for higher wages from equity, or to cover inflation. That is, the fundamental and historic role of trade unions – the negotiation of higher wages in real terms – is denied. It was once memorably pointed out that 'socialism is about equality but trade unionism is about differentials'. Whatever the truth of this, trade unionism always used to engage with overall distribution of income between capital and labour, irrespective of intra-labour conflicts. That role is denied to them, on a minimalist reading of their role in the market philosophy now (re)emerging, especially under US tutelage.

A static sum of money for the health service means that, if units (trusts or directorates) become more productive – for example, treating more patients and therefore incurring more expenditure even if wages stay the same, by an earlier point in the financial year – then they run into financial problems. There is therefore a choice in terms of the labour force: to employ the same people for 9 months (say) rather than a full year, or to employ fewer people to do the same work over the financial year. The problem with the latter strategy is that the work is 'spaced out' rather than completed as efficiently as possible and yet a greater burden is put on those doing the work. It is hardly an efficient strategy. The problems with the former strategy are even more self-evident. Both strategies therefore create a bias to 'flexible' contracts, or part-time work, calling for more intensity of work (and, in practice, often reduced conditions and rights) (UNISON, 1994a).

One might ask: if the unit has done the work more quickly, cannot it find extra resources to do more work and keep its workers employed throughout the financial year? That is where the idea of the market in health care comes in. If there is no more money available in total in the national health system, yet units (trusts) are competing to take work from each other, then a unit can do exactly this. That is why the market and local pay flexibility, plus local searches for productivity, are part of a coherent strategy.

What this does mean, of course, is that higher pay as a result of productivity is only achieved at the expense of workers in other units or trusts. A 'beggar my neighbour' policy is the essence – indeed is part of the philosophical and ideological foundation of such a policy. People working in the NHS are expected to compete rather than cooperate – to change their behaviour in line with a new means of viewing the world of work.

In consequence, it is a matter of simple logic to see that, if the total money available for the National Health Service does not change and labour costs as a whole are not allowed to rise but are indeed encouraged to fall as part of the total expenditure on the health service, then more pay in total to some units (based only on productivity and not on ideas of equity) means less pay elsewhere. This can happen within or between professions. Some doctors can end up being paid more and others less. Or doctors as a whole can end up receiving less of the total pay bill while other professions get more, and so forth. It may be that everyone gets less under certain considerations. The political agenda to enforce such a policy is likely to be to 'divide and rule' – to prevent united opposition by the whole medical profession, nursing profession, etc. That is where 'HRM' and management responsibilities for doctors, nurses and others employ a useful political role.

The only way in which one can envisage a longer-term scenario of productivity rewarding more people than it punishes, within a static pay bill, is to re-establish the NHS labour force in the short-term in such a way that the total pay bill is significantly less. Hence the strategies for 'changes in skill mix', in the right-wing variant of that policy sometimes referred to as 'reprofiling the workforce'. Changing the skill-mix need not be a 'political' strategy in so blatant a sense. But recently, in the NHS, it has been.

This involves, for example, replacing doctors at a high level of expertise with less specialized workers at a lower remuneration. This is known as 'reprofiling upwards'. 'Reprofiling downwards' means getting professionals or workers generally to do more ancillary tasks associated with their job (for example serving meals to patients and so forth). One can in pure theory have the idea of a generic health-care worker doing as much as possible 'upwards' and 'downwards'. In practice the aim of re-profiling purely in order to cut costs (UNISON, 1994b) – or rather substantially in order to cuts costs – is to move as far as possible in the direction of cheaper employees doing as much as possible – which tends to mean reprofiling upwards in the case of the current National Health Service.

If the whole health-care workforce is 'reprofiled' (and Eric Caines, for example, sees massive scope for diminution and replacement of doctors and nurses as part of a generalized attack on professionalism) then the paybill could be reduced significantly and more work done – if one assumes that the same work is possible in terms of patient cure and care! – throughout the financial year. But this is somewhat in the realms of fantasy, as such a strategy has never been implemented, nor is it likely to be, on the grounds of its impracticality and lack of a research base. There is no evidence that such changes are possible without seriously affecting both the quantity and quality of patient care. And in this sense, it is important to ask what one means by productivity – does one mean simply economy and indeed even exploitation of workers, or does one mean looking in a broader sense at what one achieves in terms of patient cure and care (as well as prevention, in the longer term) through an integrated health-care strategy?

There is little evidence that labour can in aggregate be much cheaper without quality reductions (allowing the same money to produce more health care and therefore prevent hospital 'go-slows' throughout the financial year). Sacking health-care professionals in the name of productivity therefore leads one to the absurdity that – if the money saved is to be used for patient care – the sacked labour must be re-employed! Or – and here's the rub – part-time and 'contract' doctors and nurses replace the tenured, career-grade staff. This gives opportunities to private agencies and providers, but does potential harm to quality of care and also to the public service.

The debate about productivity dominates increasingly in a financially squeezed National Health Service, and what is known as the 'unitary' view of the organization has the capacity to drive out alternative ways to interpret the management of human resources, specifically, and industrial relations, more generally.

We now turn to the explanation of such theories, the bedrock of 'industrial relations' theory underlying attempts to explain trends in the 'management of human resources'.

PERSPECTIVES IN INDUSTRIAL RELATIONS

There are three major approaches to industrial relations, by which is meant three schools of thought by which the field can be interpreted:

- the unitary approach;
- the pluralist approach;
- the radical or Marxist approach.

THE UNITARY PERSPECTIVE

This perspective argues that work will involve inequality and hierarchy and that 'the right to manage is inevitable, legitimate and not negotiable'. It assumes that all employees accept the inequality and hierarchy and all are willing to work in these circumstances for the aims of the organization, with which they identify their own interests. The perspective therefore is resistant to fights for change in the system and hostile to collectivism (as expressed through trade unions), which is

seen as subversive to economic and industrial logic in the organization. This was very much the view of 'industrial relations' in the 1980s (if the term was used at all) and the Government's heroes of the time (such as Lord King and Sir Ian McGregor) embodied the virtue of the 'right to manage'.

The implications of this perspective are that, at one 'hard' extreme, the worker is seen as a resource for whom it is legitimate to make decisions and changes without consultation. The 'softer' version of unitarism sees the worker as someone whose needs can and will be met through the aims of the organization. As a result 'human resource management' is often a doctrine (quite prescriptive in most cases, rather than analytically based upon a universal truth) which argues that the aim in the management of human resources is to meet jointly the aims of the organization and the aims of the individual.

EFFECT ON MANAGEMENT OF HUMAN RESOURCES: LEADERSHIP

Thus a 'strategic' effort directed to 'positively managing' human resources could be either hard (explicitly excluding unions and being very dictatorial or at least prescriptive as regards individuals' rights) or soft. The latter approach would encourage withdrawal from the collective bargaining arena (certainly at national level), but perhaps through a traditionally strategy such as local bargaining by groups as a transitional device to reach the ideal system of 'personal contracts' with the firm.

In both the hard and soft version, leadership becomes a useful concept to managers, in that the values of the organization are expressed through various forms of leadership, which is then used to mobilize the workforce. There are of course different types of leadership.

Leadership may operate through charisma (Weber, in Pugh, Hinings and Hickson, 1986); it may operate through force; or it may operate through rational demonstration of 'necessary facts'. The fact that Hitler, Pol Pot, Margaret Thatcher and Fidel Castro have all been charismatic leaders in their way shows us that the content of leadership may be less important than its ability to mobilize. Leadership became a buzz-word in the National Health Service in the early 1990s – but unfortunately it was adopted for its propaganda value rather than for any scientific or consensual approach to analysing what leaders ought to be achieving. This reflected a rather uncritical call upon the business world for examples of 'charismatic' or effective leadership. The conclusion to this book, in Chapter 13, reflects upon the nature of power and leadership in the current NHS.

In the unitary perspective, personnel would be encouraged to share the same aims and values of the organization. Often the 'soft' version of unitarism will stress that core values ought to be negotiated, and that 'worker participation' ought to be encouraged – but through quality circles, 'total quality management' and other self-regulating devices rather than through trade union channels.

In other words, it is participation on the basis of **obligation**, not **rights**. There is a severe tension here, however: if such participation leads to a surreptitious change in what are seen as the necessary values of the organization, it is ethically illegitimate. Thus, for example, in the sphere of 'total quality management' there is stress upon participation through 'quality circles' and other devices, yet also a strict and often severe **quantitative** monitoring of workers' outputs. At the end of the day, such techniques are about replacing the policing of workers through self-policing – and where self-policing breaks down, conventional policing is usually not too long in re-emerging from the closet.

Enforcement of the 'necessary objectives' of the company can therefore either be through force and economic necessity; economic incentive to individuals or groups or the development of shared values. Achieving consensus through values which are genuinely shared throughout the organization is of course a laudable aim. A critical theorist, perhaps a Marxist, however, is best described as a thwarted unitarist – someone who would like society or the organization to reflect shared values but who thinks that, in a capitalist or similar form of society, such consensus is impossible unless workers are duped (through what Marx called 'false consciousness').

This raises an important distinction between **descriptive unitarism** and **prescriptive unitarism** – a distinction applicable to all three perspectives in industrial relations. Descriptive unitarism (or positive unitarism) argues that unitarism is a theory that reflects reality. Prescriptive unitarism suggests that unitarism is desirable – but may or may not be the prevailing reality. In other words, one might have to change society in order to achieve it. Or alternatively, one might have to use propagandist means to achieve a seeming unitarism.

THE PLURALIST PERSPECTIVE

This perspective also acknowledges that work will involve inequality and hierarchy, but that many parties within an organization have legitimate rights and demands to be considered – indeed, that it is important to recognize such rights and demands because of relative inequalities, to prevent unfairness and exploitation. But, on this view, inequality and hierarchy is not so steep, or determined in form, that it is impossible to represent different groups at the workplace. The pluralist perspective leads to a belief (in practice) that all parties can best obtain recognition of their rights and demands through negotiation and consultation. There is a 'right to manage', but this is negotiated through collective forums.

The pluralist perspective by and large

dominated industrial relations in both private and public sectors in the 1950s, 1960s and 1970s. Indeed, it could be argued that it was due to tensions within the pluralist perspective – and increasing failure to achieve consensus through existing pluralist channels – that there was a polarization into the 'new macho' unitarist perspective on the one hand and a more radical perspective, on the left wing of industry, on the other hand, by the end of the 1970s in the UK.

In political science, for example, it would be argued that pluralism is self-evidently truer than unitarism: dealing with all of society, there is no 'unitarist' view outside totalitarian or utopian theory, or only in a simplified Marxism which sees all conflict as class-based and therefore soluble through socialism. But industrial relations deals with industry or services and therefore unitarism within that sphere is at least theoretically more tenable. Nevertheless pluralism is a more plausible statement of reality.

The ethical implications of the pluralist perspective are that the worker is someone whose legitimate demands should be expressed in ways which include collective bargaining forums if the worker wishes. As far as the management of human resources is concerned, efforts will therefore be made to reconcile workers' demands within the scope and objectives of the organization. Where these cannot be met, means will be sought to alleviate unmet demands through other channels. These may consist in job redesign; 'humanistic' techniques within the management of human resources; and so forth. (Pugh, Hickson and Hinings, 1986)

Again, as with all three perspectives, there is a parallel between the perspective of industrial relations and the wider perspective concerning the whole of society, drawing on political science. Indeed, in this sense, industrial relations is political science applied to the specific sphere of industry within society. Political science distinguishes between pluralism and elitism – the latter not being a prescriptive, desired situation but a perspective used to describe a society in which power is monopolized by one or more stable elites. Equally, within industrial relations, elitism may be a better characterization of industry than pluralism: decisions are monopolized by a powerful elite, which uses its world view (e.g. of 'necessary company policy') to 'persuade' workers that 'there is no alternative' (i.e. unitarism!).

Within industrial relations theory, then, what is called pluralism probably incorporates the theory of elitism, and one may best distinguish between egalitarian pluralism and inegalitarian pluralism – the latter characterized by a situation whereby workers have significantly less rights and power, but where these are still allowed to be represented through collective means within the organization and where at least some autonomous power for these workers is circumscribed both by law and by industry practice.

THE RADICAL AND/OR MARXIST PERSPECTIVE

Marxism is of course a perspective to interpret the whole of society and the economy, at its most ambitious. It sees capitalist society, and the workplace within capitalist society, as characterized by structures of exploitation in line with the needs of 'the market' – which is in fact a device for extracting surplus value from those who own only their labour and for distributing profit to those who own capital. A Marxist perspective argues that the pluralist view trivializes what really goes on between employees and employers, and is a class-based theory. The implication of Marxism is that the worker is an exploited person who can never be satisfied as long as others control society (either capitalists in private industry or the state acting on behalf of the interests of private industry, in providing public services). There is no solution to this problem short of radical change, and the Marxist perspective on the management of human resources in capitalist society is therefore a cynical one: it argues that the management of human resources in whatever form is a device to maintain allegiance to the status quo; however gently, reluctantly or motivated by goodwill.

One can distinguish, again, between descriptive and prescriptive Marxism; the former characterizes the just-described situation as a scientific view of society. The latter type of Marxism argues for change to alleviate or transform such a situation. Technically therefore one can be an analytical 'Marxist' who does not care about what one perceives! More likely, however, is that the Marxist will see change as morally desirable. In original 19th-century Marxism, this tension was obscured by the fact that Marx saw the replacement of capitalist society as 'scientific' or 'inevitable'. In consequence, the descriptive (or positive) Marxist characterization of society led to the depiction of a situation which was inevitably to be changed in any case.

This is no longer plausible today, and the best approach for Marxists is to use Marxism as an analytical tool for describing society, industry and the public sector but to acknowledge that change is not inevitable. Values to inspire change, as well as strategies to achieve it, are therefore within the realm of political autonomy.

THEORIES AND PARADIGMS IN INDUSTRIAL RELATIONS: SOME CLARIFICATIONS AND SUGGESTIONS

We can therefore see that industrial relations (IR) has followed political science and other disciplines in social science by creating different theories – in the case of IR, to explain the coordination (or otherwise) of interests in private sector companies and public sector organizations. The best known theories, described above (unitarism, pluralism and the Marxist perspective) concern the interests of different groups within the productive process. They may be considered to include and interact with other perspectives which refer to structure and behaviour within organizations, such as social action theory and systems theory (Farnham and Pimlott, 1991).

It is fair to call these three main perspectives **theories** and not **paradigms**, in that they are seeking to present generalizations from facts which themselves are not contested between the three perspectives. That is, the three different theories are justified by conclusions from empirical research around the content of which there is at least consensus. For example, pluralists might seek to debate and test with Marxists of the radical perspective whether or not there were in fact 'two distinct sides' of industry, as opposed to merely plural groupings whose interests are not those of class interests in the Marxist sense.

There might be difficulty in defining an appropriate empirical test, but the challenge of doing so is generally accepted by both sides, unless abstract theoretical positions are taken up which themselves are mutually exclusive *vis-à-vis* empirical research implications.

It makes sense to reserve the word **paradigm** for the sense intended by Thomas Kuhn (1970). Otherwise 'paradigm' becomes merely a synonym for theory or, more confusingly still, an imprecise attempted synonym for value or perspective in the broadest sense. A paradigm in the Kuhnian sense is a new way of organizing reality and its perception, based on particular concepts used to describe reality, which generates a whole host of new theories. Paradigm change occurs when the old constellation of theories, which together are applied using concepts that themselves are about to be discarded, gives way to the new.

The above three perspectives might be considered to be competing paradigms if they each involved separate ways of 'looking at' reality, such that mediation between the different perspectives was not open to an ambiguous or 'static' empirical test. Instead, the paradigms would be seeking ascendancy *vis-à-vis* each other, in seeking to convert, by a process beyond that of merely empirical science, the 'critical mass' of experts in the field. Thus is 'normal science' established, according to Thomas Kuhn – when one paradigm gains ascendancy.

In teaching students of industrial relations, the three main perspectives are sometimes confusing, in that the descriptive and prescriptive elements are inadvertently combined. For example, the unitarist perspective may be observed in reality by someone who is prescriptively a radical and who wishes, as it were, that unitarism were not true. In other words, he wishes that staff or 'workers' were able to detect that they had interests separate from those of the management, and values separate from those of the 'core values' presented for the organization.

The implication, of course, is that there is a basis for deciding interests, whether 'scientifically' or normatively, separate from the subjective views of the worker. It is moreover an open question as to whether unitarism extends to workers as opposed to merely managerial staff – how democratic is it in the first place? Does it really argue that the cleaner shares interests with the chief executive – or rather, does it seek to impose such a view so that the 'weakest one-third' in society (and its industries) accept the logic of the market in determining their conditions? It is no coincidence that the NHS market is accompanied by an 'imposed unitarism' with myriads of management consultants advising on 'the organization and its needs'.

Similarly one can imagine a descriptive 'Marxist' who is prescriptively a conservative, i.e. someone who sees conflict but wishes to ignore it. If Marxism is a science as presented by Marx and is not what Karl Popper termed 'vulgar Marxism', whereby values are dressed up as an amalgam of science and a prescription for activism, then the above phenomenon should not be surprising.

The Marxist perspective observes conflict in capitalist industrial relations, but might envisage a future in which a unitary organization is possible because the contradiction preventing it in capitalist society has been resolved. This, of course, is a classical Marxist perspective.

Further refinement concerns the Marxist who sees an essential or 'objective' basis for conflict in the organization, yet who sees behaviour patterns effected or created to prevent this conflict being expressed. What Lenin called 'opportunism' might in modern parlance be considered to be the provision of incentives for groups (within what used to be called the working class) to hold allegiance to the dominant or core values of the organization. Thus conflict 'in essence' becomes unitarism of a particular sort in practice. Put bluntly, workers can be bought off by a policy of divide and rule.

A radical view need not be Marxist. An elitist perspective may argue that pluralism fails to understand the systematic nature, or particular form, of 'interest group activity', but that economic bases for workplace equity are only capable of providing a partial explanation. Classical elite theory includes Vilfredo Pareto's *The Mind in Society* (treatise of general sociology), Gaetano Mosca's *The Ruling Class* and Robert Michels's *Political Parties*. It is possible to add to these Burnham's *The Managerial Revolution* and C. Wright-Mills's *The Power Elite* (see Parry, 1969 for a discussion of these views).

A THEORETICAL FRAMEWORK FROM WHICH TO UNDERSTAND MANAGEMENT STRATEGIES IN TODAY'S PUBLIC SECTOR

Based on the above and related considerations, I propose the following categories:

1a. **'ideal' unitarism,** where all members and groups within the organization subscribe as free and autonomous individuals to the goals of the organization as consonant with their interests, whether egoistically or altruistically interpreted;

1b. **'authoritarian' and/or 'utilitarian' unitarism**, whereby direct sanctions or material incentives are applied to forge a unitarism (or at least a majoritarian) subscription to the values and practices of the organization as currently managed (in the majoritarian version, the 'worst-off third' may simply be coerced, in line with society's overall distribution of power as mirrored in the particular industry or service in question);

1c. **'totalitarian' unitarism**, whereby ideological or propagandist means are used to persuade people that their interests lie in a particular direction; this is akin to Steven Lukes's 'third dimension' of power (Lukes, 1974);

2a. **descriptive pluralism**, which describes the behavioural reality that there are many groups operating with different claims within an organization, but which passes little judgement on either the distribution of power or the ethics of such a situation;

2b. **micro-pluralism**, which points to the existence of a large number of groups, which cannot be 'controlled' by a unitarist strategy;

2c. **corporatist pluralism**, which argues that there is a tendency to centralize negotiation (on the corporatist model of the national economy involving representatives of the state and 'both sides' of industry – employers and employed) in order to make pluralism manageable;

3a. **descriptive Marxism** (as discussed above), which stresses the existence of conflict on the basis of economic class without passing judgement as to the morality of its resolution one way or another;

3b. **non-Marxist radicalism**, in which 'two sides of industry', in opposition, are perceived – but the explanation for inequality is not only related to economic class;

3c. **prescriptive or critical radicalism**, which argues for acknowledging and promoting separate interests, in order to sponsor the interests of the repressed.

It should be pointed out that the above perspectives are not mutually exclusive. One may subscribe to behavioural 'micro-pluralism' as a 'common-sense' depiction of reality, while being a Marxist in perceiving 'deeper' power; and so forth. Experience in teaching the management of human resources on the MBA (Health Executive) Programme at Keele University, and in researching within the National Health Service, reveals that some, but not many, senior managers subscribe to unitarism as the best descriptive theory of the organization, while also, of course, favouring it normatively. The radical perspective, interestingly, has more adherents, as 'things get tougher' in the NHS of the 1990s, even among managers who have no choice but to cooperate with the system. The more worldly-wise but conservative in the professions and management tend to the pluralist perspective. When pressed further, many subscribe to the perspective of 1b above – that of a unitarism manufactured rather than natural, created through the provision of incentives to the 'pivotal' groups amongst the professions and the labour force generally.

'Creating unitarism where it does not or cannot exist' is a pithy means of describing the job of the 'Director of Human Resources' in an NHS trust today!

As in society generally, what might be called conservative coalitions can be manufactured, such that there is a 'contented two-thirds and discontented one-third'.

The NHS has some particular features, of course. Whether it is interpreted as a socialist island within a capitalist economy, or as a mirror image of capitalist organization (albeit in a public sector context), or something in between, there may be greater change in it (and other public sector organizations which are having to change their ethos rapidly) than in the sphere of private business. If interpreted as the proverbial 'socialist island', the

NHS may be capable even in the eyes of prescriptive Marxists of benevolent unitarism.

Paradoxically, the more the NHS is encouraged to mirror private sector techniques (extraction of value from its employees through private sector techniques), the more the perspective (1a) of 'ideal' unitarism is unrealistic, but equally the more important to the Government is the task of manufacturing unitarism (1b. or 1c. above).

On this perspective, the National Health Service (although not hitherto providing as many opportunities for private investment as elsewhere – a state of affairs itself altered by the Conservative government) creates class and group relations analogous to those in the private sector.

This characterization is all the truer if the public sector 'exploits' workers to provide a 'cheap' subsidiary product or support service (health care, education) of use for the production of greater profit in the capitalist economy. If, for example, the NHS serves industry's needs for a fit workforce, the analogy may be extended. And if such services are produced in quasi-capitalist institutions such as trusts, then more conventional exploitation may occur.

THE ENVIRONMENT WITHIN WHICH INDUSTRIAL RELATIONS OPERATE

The most central issues in analysing industrial relations concern the following components of the economy and polity: capital; the state; management; and labour.

Capital may best be defined as both the means of production and the source of profit, thereby embracing property as well as the resources for production. In a capitalist economy, profit maximization (or profit generation) is the rationale for production. It might be argued that this has little relevance to the NHS, and perhaps in the past the NHS didn't have much of a tendency for capital to have an effect on its 'human aspect'. The NHS was seen as a paternal employer, albeit offering through a centralized policy low wages to many categories of staff. As public expenditure on the NHS was however restricted throughout the 1980s, both for party-political reasons and also because of the UK's relatively shrinking income, it was perceived that there was a greater need to work within tighter and tighter budgetary controls, producing maximum throughput and 'output' in the NHS. This led to a drive towards mass production and to 'reprofiling' the workforce to 'produce more for less'.

Management is the coordinator of such an activity, on behalf of the state. Management controls resources on behalf of the state – whether at purchaser or provider level (a trivial distinction at this level of analysis). Management therefore has the function of controlling the workforce to achieve the maximum output from such resources, if the NHS is to mirror the industrial sector of the economy and indeed provide 'a healthy workforce' to it.

It was fashionable in the middle part of the 20th century to argue, mostly with a private sector focus, that there was a growing distinction between the owners of capital and the managers of firms or companies. This argument has recently been revived, in 'post-modern' accounts of society. Organizational and behavioural theories of the firm, in economics, replaced simpler microeconomic approaches to profit maximization. It was argued that often 'satisficing' (or simply doing well enough) was a new perspective on the motives driving the firm, and that the interests of managers were not necessarily the same as the interests of shareholders, or indeed direct owners. At the organizational and behavioural level, this no doubt contained some truth.

It can be argued, however, that this reflected the relative 'plenty' of the time. But the more internationally competitive the environment, the more the need for profit maximization and the subjugation of management to the aims of the generation of surplus becomes more crucial. That is because profit margins are lower for most companies and profit maximization therefore implies the search for **any** profit. Profit maximization is necessary, except for stable international and national oligopolies. Even there, the international hunt for greater profit becomes competitive, between rival giant multinationals.

Thus, although large organizations have characteristics of their own and can be treated at the behavioural level as 'organisms' worthy of study, rather than simply profit-maximizing machines, a number of characteristics of the modern economy have developed to suggest that downplaying the 'capital/labour' divide is mistaken. Profit maximization, both from necessity (in the domestic economy) and from 'the new greed' (in the international economy), is re-established, if it were ever disestablished. One should not confuse the instrumental goals of managers (not just economic) with the overall functioning of the economy.

Firstly, free movement of capital means that capital will seek to produce where labour is most productive. Capital is now much more multinational. This does not *necessarily* mean cheap labour, but, given an equivalent output (productivity), capital will seek to relocate to where labour is cheapest. This is the phenomenon through which all the countries of the industrialized West are 'losing out' in certain sectors of the economy to the newly industrialized economies such as Malaysia, South Korea and Thailand.

Internationalized capital is seeking internationally competitive labour – whether to produce 'locally' for local consumers or whether to generate a hierarchy of consumers spread around a world increasingly colonized by scarce international capital. The idea of the local, or national, firm – and of 'exports' themselves – has less meaning over time. This is why 'international Thatcherism' is destroying middle-class stability as well as working-class stability in the hitherto 'advanced' countries.

Capital will either move to more productive or cheaper labour, or seek to have labour move – depending upon whether trade is free enough to allow overseas-produced goods to be 'imported' for home sales, and related factors. Additionally, where labour and capital are cheap or scarce *vis-à-vis* each other, different techniques of production (what economists call 'production function') may apply. Labour-intensive production will occur when labour is cheap. For the NHS, therefore, if labour is seen to be expensive – by the state, acting in concert with capital – attempts will be made either to cheapen it or to find less labour – intensive ways of 'producing' services. This is because the NHS – on such a scenario – must produce a cheaper service in a more stretched inegalitarian economy.

International regulation may of course prevent competition by labour to attract capital within the international grouping, or between the grouping's labour and that of the rest of the world, (such as is attempted by the Social Chapter of the European Community). If so, then either such an international grouping will lose out as a whole to the rest of the world or capital will remain within it where, for a given wage, the workforce is more skilled and developed (and where, for example, the EC has a comparative advantage, despite its higher costs). Nevertheless, protectionism – or restriction of capital flows to 'cheap' countries – may be necessary. That is why the 'new protectionism' embraces elements of both right and left, and often includes suggestions for 'free trade' within protectionist blocks of countries. The problem then, of course, concerns equity for the excluded in the international economy.

The key question is, how scarce is capital *vis-à-vis* labour? The international generalization is, very – if, by scarce, we mean only available for high-profit, low-wage investment and employment, due to increased internationalization of capital in what is euphemistically called 'the global economy'. There is thus a problem for international equity. Where there are restrictions, legal or practical, on the international location of scarce capital, the migration of labour may of course occur, as from Mexico to the United States, from the south to north generally, and so forth. Or, within a country, labour may migrate to where the jobs are. Or, within the NHS, labour may migrate to where trusts are flourishing, not closing! Alternatively, trusts that 'win in the marketplace' may re-employ the labour of their 'losing' competitors by takeover and merger, without relocation of services.

All in all, labour power is in inverse proportion to the scarcity of capital and to labour's relative plenty.

While Marxism may – at the behavioural level – have less explanatory power within advanced Western economies as labour forces become differentiated, as an international phenomenon it nevertheless has significant power in explaining the competition by capital to produce profit. Labour is in surplus, yet the capacity to produce profit (partly because of limited international purchasing power) is restricted. This may not be the earlier form of 'free market' competition within particular countries, but may lead to competition of large multinational conglomerates to dominate the market and extract profit both through international production and international sales.

In earlier times, high unemployment meant slump, as capitalists required mass production and mass consumption to prosper. Now, however, technology means that 'islands of the rich' can be ever more 'productive' and wealthy alongside swathes of the poor (in both the developing and the developed worlds).

Such a perspective has a particular explanatory value not so much in depicting tensions between capital and labour in one country **but in analysing the imbalance of power between capital and labour globally**. The consequence of this is that, in all countries, labour's bargaining power is reduced.

Inequalities Marx could not have dreamed of are the reality in 'the global economy'!

This occurs differentially, of course – and there is much that governments can do to alleviate such a trend. Nevertheless, a labour-dictated agenda in either production or the provision of public services is less possible in the absence of widespread international planning of trade: rendering a country less competitive by international criteria may simply be the consequence. As a result, calls for cuts or restricted public services arise, as a seemingly more 'logical' alternative to higher and fairer taxes, higher expenditure and **planned** participation in the world economy.

THE PUBLIC SECTOR AND THE NHS

In consequence, management within the public sector has tended to mirror management within the private sector, and such an effect has been exacerbated by political phenomena such as 'Thatcherism' in the UK. Management in the National Health Service is therefore increasingly charged with delivering 'more for less'. The NHS traditionally was seen as a 'model' employer, using Whitley council frameworks to explore concepts of equity. Yet the NHS reforms are bringing a market ideology into both the management of patient care and the management of the NHS workforce. The development of trusts, in particular, institutionalizes a competitive situation whereby even constant income for the organization is only achieved on a 'beggar my neighbour' basis. In consequence, there is an attempt to produce what was described above as an 'enforced unitarist' situation, which has a kind of ironic logic – the 'real enemy' is, after all, elsewhere!

In this situation, there may be a specific conflict between the needs of the organization on the one hand and traditional and worthwhile notions such as clinical decision-making based on the clinical needs of the patient on the other hand. Let us consider one example.

A trust, whether large or small, is facing a financial deficit and possible closure or merger. It can mobilize extra money only by reducing labour costs or by winning extra contracts. The district contract has already been 'exhausted' and doctors are being urged not to admit patients under the district contract, i.e. referred by non-fundholding general practitioners. (This will produce extra workload without extra money.) Doctors are asked instead to admit patients from GP fundholders, where such business can be 'drummed up'. This leads to an admissions policy on the basis not of clinical need but of the financial requirements of the organization. The doctor is, however, faced with a dilemma. If he ignores such an instruction, the financial position of the trust may worsen, and the upshot may be no local hospital (rather than differential admission, not on the basis of need, to the local hospital). It may lead to denial of local care to all local patients rather than simply to some!

The doctor is therefore faced with a choice: does his obligation to the individual patient at the present time override his calculation as to the best means of proceeding for the future? Will it be better simply to admit patients on the new 'corporate' basis and rely on public pressure to change policy? Should tactics be in line with the strategy of 'shaming the powers-that-be' or of maintaining the trust's finances? One can understand a pessimistic approach to such a situation: it may well be the case that no such public pressure would be either forthcoming or effective. In consequence, going along with the 'unitarist' needs of the organization may be seen as the lesser of the two evils.

And this is indeed the intention of provider competition within the public service: to enforce 'labour compliance' (including doctors) with a finance-led agenda. There is a trade-off between equity in patient care and maximum productivity, given the institutions used by the NHS reforms (trusts on the one hand, and GP

fundholding on the other) as a stimulus to greater 'provider efficiency/exploitation'.

Thus a self-governing trust in a competitive environment both enables and necessitates the 'freedom' to:

- reprofile the workforce;
- derecognize trade unions;
- develop individualized contracts;
- divide the labour force into core and periphery, whereby the latter have their 'expensive' rights (pensions and various other forms of protection) removed;
- remove centralized pay bargaining.

In order to implement such policies, National Health Service management is in fact an agent of the state. 'Management' in the public sector is the Government's tool, especially when governments have a tight and clear agenda. If the Government's aim is ideologically and practically pro-capitalist, public sector management is likewise. Witness how 'top management' in the NHS organizes its agenda (and conference agenda!) around the buzzwords of the day ('private partnerships'; 'mergers'; 'private capital'; 'productivity').

THE EVOLUTION OF INDUSTRIAL RELATIONS – FROM STABILITY TO INEQUITY

One can depict three phases in the history of industrial relations within the National Health Service. The first phase, from 1948 to the beginning of the 1970s, was represented by commitment to full employment; commitment to the development of the welfare state; a belief in the mixed economy, including the nationalized industries sitting alongside the private sector; and a Keynesian approach to economics to embrace all the above.

As regards industrial bargaining, this was increasingly collectivized and centralized, and principles of equity such as comparability and stable pay were institutionalized through devices such as arbitration. There was a tacit understanding that if central government, and public sector managers operating on its behalf, were good or model employers, then trade unions and employers would avoid conflict and the widespread commitment to the notion of the public service would also help to do so.

The second phase is best represented by the mid to late 1970s, and was a time when inflation and public expenditure problems began to dominate the agenda of the whole economy. Incomes policies were seen as inadequate to restrict an increasing fragmentation and 'interest group jostling' in politics, which led to less stability within trade unions themselves and less consensus between the various segments of society as a whole.

Within trade unions, there was growing divergence between the strategies of leadership and activists; and greater left-wing presence in leaderships of trade unions also led to less manageable 'corporatism', the system whereby the state, employers and employees (as represented by trade unions) were intended to reconcile industrial needs and worker demands. The TUC does not control individual unions and unions could not easily control their members, or local shop stewards. As a result, planning the economy was difficult. This process culminated in what is now popularly known as 'the Winter of Discontent' of 1978/1979.

The series of disputes in the mid-1970s initially concerned attempts by lower-paid workers to secure greater equity within the Government's 'incomes policy' (after a wage freeze) and was not an attack by 'privileged workers' upon the Government's right to govern. But some higher-paid workers sought to maintain differentials in a manner which led eventually to many groups of workers fighting the Government's pay policy. Denis Healey's memoirs (1989) reveal that the policy nearly succeeded. It failed because the Government could not in the end offer enough to the lower-paid workers (such as those in NUPE) because it perceived that such a decision would lead to more demands

on the public purse from **all** workers than could be afforded. There was a concealed split between, on the one hand, national TUC leaders and activists of the unions representing the poorer workers (such as NUPE) and, on the other hand, leaders and activists of unions representing richer workers – who wished to maintain differentials.

Ironically, a maintenance of the 'flat rate' increase of the earlier part of the pay policy (£6 per week for all, which naturally was a higher percentage for the lower-paid) might have maintained greater equity and affordability than the new, less 'redistributive' policy of 5%. But the key union leaders could not deliver a 5% pay policy (for different reasons). And so the Winter of Discontent; and the return of the Conservatives after the Labour government was defeated in the Commons on a devolution bill.

The third phase is represented by the attempt to diminish the salience of trade unions altogether, by Conservative governments in the 1980s. Conservative governments believed that 'incomes policies' and consensus had not worked. Ironically the Heath government of 1970–1974 had sought incomes policies, as part of a strategy to control both prices and incomes, but also to maintain industrial consent. Unfortunately, political conflict over the content of the incomes policies – and the greater strength of the trade union movement at the time, resisting Conservative governments often as a matter of principle and Labour governments when necessary or practical – led to a perception that incomes policies were a source of overt industrial conflict. It was also believed in the Conservative Party, with some truth at the time, that the Labour Party – if likely to form the next government – would always be able to 'outbid' Conservative governments as regards trade union rights and therefore undermine Conservative policies.

It was therefore resolved by the new Conservative leadership, after Margaret Thatcher's election early in 1975, that, instead of controlling labour through overt discussions and disputes over incomes policies, a more brutal strategy would be adopted. This would consist in using economic policy (monetarism, in its broadest political rather than simply technical economic sense) and unemployment to discipline labour and also legislation to limit and remove key trade union rights. (Trade union rights in the UK generally consisted in immunities from an individually based law, rather than positively established collective rights.) In the early years of the Thatcher governments, the trade unions still had some strengths and the Conservative government pursued a series of strategies which involved 'picking the right fight at the right time'. The miners, for example, were not 'taken on' until there was a surplus of fuel for generating power: the dispute of 1980 was settled quickly but the battle lines were drawn up for later, 1984/1985.

Ironically enough, the unwillingness of the Heath government to remove trade union rights on the scale of the later Thatcher governments led to visible conflict (based on a search for consensus!) yet the more brutal policy of the Thatcher governments led to a gradual economic and industrial defeat of the trade unions – and overt conflict became less evident.

This might be described as an 'enforced unitarism', in the whole of society: 'there was no alternative' to compliance with the dominant industrial and managerial approach. Within the NHS, the impact of cash limits and the Government's response to strikes (the demise of arbitration; the increasing economic costs of strikes to unions; legal attacks such as sequestration of funds and the removal of immunities) led to the diminution of effective collective bargaining.

A variety of tactics were used – pay review machinery was set up (but selectively ignored) for nurses and others, while the rhetoric of decentralization and 'flexibility' for the generally more unskilled workers in the health services was increasingly mooted. The diminished power of the NHS labour force reflects the diminished power of the labour force in the economy as a whole.

One may ask here whether there is a distinction between public and private sectors. At the broadest level of generalization the trend has been in the same direction for both. In the private sector, temporary areas of boom in certain sectors of the economy have temporarily led to sudden demand for certain forms of skilled worker (not least because of the UK's failure to maintain a skilled labour force). Elsewhere, however, the picture has been one of industrial restructuring, involving lower pay and fewer social and environmental rights as well as fewer individual rights for the worker. The rhetoric has been of flexibility, but genuine flexibility linked to workers' rights has not been forthcoming. Part-time jobs, for example, should be part of a strategy involving acceptable income and choice of type of job, not a brutal necessity whereby part-time jobs with few rights replace full-time jobs as a aggregate trend.

TYPES OF BARGAINING

One can construct a typology of systems of bargaining as follows, in order to combine the various theoretical possibilities with some practical observations.

'National planning' of wages, terms and conditions

Whether we are talking about an industrial work force, public sector workers or all cadres (including professionals and managers), the rationale for such an approach is to decide what is affordable and (ideally) equitable, and to pay each cadre appropriately. It is a 'national plan' because such decisions are made centrally. Although decisions may be made separately for each cadre, naturally there is a logic (whether based on power or equity) relating the different decisions – or at least there should be! In the past, elements of this system have been used in the UK, although institutions such as pay review bodies for different cadres – and coordination between them – have been imperfectly developed and used.

National bargaining on a unified spine

It is unlikely that in any country one would see full national bargaining on a unified spine for an industry (or enterprise, or organization such as the National Health Service). This is because it is unlikely that there would be political or managerial agreement to allow a unified spine comprising 'top management', the professionals and the 'workers' to fit into such a system. The idea is, however, there: there are moves towards establishing unified spines both for national and local bargaining – and for a combination of both (supported by management and pragmatically accepted by trade unions such as UNISON, as well as having been proposed for the higher education sector. Note one of the differences from the first system, above: we are talking of bargaining and not simply 'centralist planning': there is therefore scope for disagreement between, on the one hand, Government and its agents, the managers, in the public sector (or an amalgam of Government and private sector managers, in the private sector) and, on the other hand, 'the workers', whether or not these include the managers. In consequence systems for resolving bargaining disputes, without recourse to industrial action, have to be devised – and again in the UK we are familiar with systems such as arbitration, the services of ACAS and schemes such as pendulum arbitration which 'decide one way or the other' without compromise or finding a third way.

National bargaining, group by group

This is bargaining conducted at the national level, but cadre by cadre, without a unified workforce subscribing to a spine or agreed set of differentials (whether changing or not). In an era of national bargaining, diminished somewhat in the UK by the early and mid 1990s, this is quite a familiar system – bargaining conducted (especially in the public sector) nationally but group by group. Thus, for example, doctors, dentists and nurses might negotiate (or have their review bodies in a 'central planning' system) but this would be conducted separately from the bargaining exercises conducted on behalf of other workers by different trade unions.

These trade unions may have evolved as 'craft/skilled' trade unions or as general unions (such as the Transport and General Workers Union) representing in an *ad hoc* manner groups of workers from different industries and occupations.

There is a move now towards industrial unions or 'organization'-based unions – such as UNISON, which seeks to unify the representation of workers in the National Health Service (and indeed moving beyond that to local government, being a merger of the former NALGO, the National Association of Local Government Officers; NUPE, the National Union of Public Employees; and COHSE, the Confederation of Health Service Employees).

Local bargaining on a unified spine

The principle of the unified spine has already been defined. If bargaining is conducted locally, the idea is that differences in the labour market from region to region or locality to locality will – and should – affect the bargaining power of both employers and employees (whether the employer is the Government acting through a surrogate, such as the health service purchaser or provider). The primary theoretical reason for implementing local bargaining is to 'clear labour markets,' according to free market microeconomic theory – such that where workers are 'oversupplied' their wage will fall and where 'undersupplied' their wages will rise; and so forth. In other words a shortage will bid up wages; a surplus will bid down wages.

In the health service in the 1990s, local bargaining is promoted under the guise of efficiency – and even, on the wilder shores of fancy, under the guise of equity. The latter claim is made where it is pointed out that, where prices are higher locally or lower locally, wages should be likewise in the interests of equity. What is not pointed out in this claim, however, is that regional differences are therefore solidified rather than diminished by such a policy.

Moreover the political agenda behind local bargaining is to move away from 'Government's responsibility' for remuneration (yet to maintain Government as the Wizard of Oz pulling the levers). It is widely expected that local bargaining will lower the cost of the wage bill. Where this might not be the case, it is rigidly controlled by the Government. Recent moves to 'performance-related pay' for doctors (paid according to the success of their trust) are centrally mandated and regulated.

Local bargaining in a unified spine has the advantage of greater simplicity, in that local bargaining can be a very cumbersome exercise despite the accompanying rhetoric of freedom and flexibility. It can be cumbersome in the private sector, let alone in a public sector organization such as the NHS where Government will always keep its 'hands on' in one guise or another.

A negative side of local bargaining on a unified spine is that – within the spine – some workers may be in shortage while others are not. Thus, for example, computer staff may be in shortage in the NHS while cleaners are not – yet the unified spine may have been compiled either nationally or regionally without reference to the local situation. Thus, for example, local bargaining around a unified spine dominated by the need to recruit professional workers who are in shortage may set workers who are not in shortage (lower down the spine) at wages higher than necessary. This may distort the labour market elsewhere, in that workers will be attracted to

move – if one believes in the assumption of such free market theory that mobility is relatively easy or 'perfect'.

In reality, differential introduction of local bargaining, accompanied by only the rhetoric of a 'single table bargaining' for all a hospital's workers, is the means of proceeding. Thus 'care assistants' (the weakest of the nursing labour force) have in 1994 commonly been the first group 'allowed' local pay determination!

An even greater downside might be that, where local bargaining 'bids' the overall remuneration of the whole spine downwards because of a surplus of the 'dominant' or salient workers upon which the bargainers choose to concentrate, workers in shortage in the spine may not be remunerated adequately to attract them. This gives an impetus to the next system.

Local bargaining group by group

This is the 'free market' approach to recruiting cadres of workers, although of course it is not decentralized to the level of the individual which is done in the next system.

Individual contracts for all workers in all localities

This is the opposite extreme from the first system, a national plan for the whole workforce. Instead we have here a market-oriented contract for the individual. Often dressed up in the 'human resource management' language of meeting the needs of the individual and the enterprise together, where cost constraints or cost reductions are paramount as the main political objective, this progressive language normally hides the reality of a market approach.

There is a fundamental conflict between 'free bargaining', whether collective or individual, and 'socialist' planning. This conflict bedevilled trade union and Labour Party debates of the 1970s, when 'free collective bargaining' was often seen as a rallying cry of the left ('in a capitalist economy, at least') yet in practice aided the strong and weakened the weak. Arguably it was a precursor to Thatcherism, when it was of course shorn of its 'socialist', or rather syndicalist, veneer (with such a veneer based on the Government's willingness to maintain high employment levels and a range of workers' rights and benefits as the backdrop). Without these, it easily degenerates into the politics of the pig-trough.

DISCUSSION

It is constructive to revisit arguments for and against various types of bargaining. The political imperative of cost control, in a publicly funded social service such as the National Health Service, ought not to be underestimated. Thus, if the aim is to control and reduce costs, using the market to bid down the wages of unskilled workers will be paramount.

Exercises in 'contracting out' occurred in the early 1980s for domestic services, and for other services later on – and then came the internal market itself as a result of the NHS 'reforms'. The cumulative effect has been that, rather than moving to an NHS of **higher pay albeit with lower numbers of workers** we have – for many cadres – moved to a system of **fewer workers with lower pay**. This reflects the poor bargaining power of unskilled workers. It gives the lie to the rhetoric that 'Whitley has failed lower-paid workers and local freedom is better'. It also reflects a strategy of deskilling in order to pay people little – rather than producing more skilled workers who can be paid more (even on market principles). This is a strategy which has many disadvantages, some of which are pointed out below.

Meanwhile, it can be noted that the system of contracting, purchaser to provider, for overall health services, and then subcontracting, provider to worker, has disadvantages even for the Government's employment and pay objectives. Scarce workers may actually 'bid up' providers' costs to purchasers in such a system. In the absence of a highly educated and properly trained workforce, shortages produce bottlenecks (or high pay) at times of demand, and then workers are simply discarded at times of slump. There is nothing necessarily party-political about a properly maintained, planned workforce.

The only cadre to be paid significantly more in fact is the management cadre responsible for implementing the NHS reforms, which have witnessed higher pay and higher numbers of plentiful managers! Such defiance of economic logic causes me to look for another explanation: such managers are the political agents of the Government. In fact political embarrassment from such a tactic has been such that ministers in 1994 were seeking to reverse (at a superficial level) the bonanza in bureaucracy and the pay of the bureaucracy that has occurred as a result of the NHS reforms.

For the professions, however, it is different. Even where cadres are in short supply, such as nurses and in some cases the medical profession (whatever one thinks of consultants or junior doctors), there is often a politically motivated attempt to argue that there is an effective oversupply of key professionals. This then enables reprofiling exercises to point to a 'surplus', real or imaginary, and then the market can be used to bid down salaries or wages and conditions. There is thus an amalgam of political imperative and market logic, to produce the desired result of the same or more services at lower cost.

BUT WHAT IS THE MARKET?

A complicating factor in considering the NHS market, and its effect upon the bargaining power of workers and bargaining systems, is the fact that it is what might termed a two-stage market. Accepting the purchaser/provider split, there is a market process between purchasers and providers but also a market process between providers and their suppliers, especially the workforce. This produces sometimes unanticipated sources of bargaining power.

Starting from conventional economic theory, one can consider in a market whether the buyer or seller has the 'bargaining power' in terms of relative supply and demand – perhaps translated into the scarcity of one or other (buyer or seller). To put it simply, if there is one purchaser and many competing providers, the buyer (purchaser) has the power. Such economic factors may of course be constrained or enhanced by the structure of the market: if purchasing is fragmented and uncoordinated (for political or bureaucratic reasons), its economic bargaining power may be diminished.

Alternatively, what appears to be fragmentation may simply be a complicated means of organization. In other words (as with GP fundholding in some respects) the 'fragmentation' of purchasing – an intrapurchaser split between districts and GP fundholders – may in fact enhance the power of purchasing, especially in the context of a surplus of competitive providers. This is because the separate purchasers have different rather than competitive roles *vis-à-vis* each other in the purchasing process: for example, GP fundholders often 'soften up' providers, which other purchasers can then use to their advantage (albeit short-term).

Nevertheless the basic economic model of demand and supply and relative scarcity, is important. A two-stage market is, however, characterized by three actors – in an NHS context, these are: (1) the purchaser; (2) the provider; and (3) (for our purposes here) the labour force, from consultant to cleaner. A market operates between purchaser and provider. A market also operates between provider and subcontractor, i.e. the workforce. Other two-stage markets, providing an analogy, are: firstly the oil industry, composed of (1) consumers, (2) oil companies and (3) primary providers such as the OPEC

States; and secondly the newly commercialized rail industry in the UK, which in its privatized form will have (in theory) companies competing for access to the track, yet also competing for labour and resources to employ. This is an even more complicated market, involving a continuum from the consumer (the traveller), through the rail company in question (whether organized regionally or competitively), to Railtrack and the various workforces (e.g. of the rail companies and of Railtrack).

It could be argued that the two-stage market is a truism, in that all markets involving companies as provider involve three actors – the consumer, the company and the contracted resources 'working for' the company, primarily labour and capital. Nevertheless, the concept is useful in particular circumstances in which the provider has to acquire subcontracted resources in order to make a tender to a purchaser. In the British NHS, the purchaser is a buyer separate from the consumer (the patient). In the oil example, the bulk consumption of oil from the oil company (the provider) is a separate process from consumption of petrol at the pumps. In the rail example, the companies have to acquire their resources, including the workforce, and then secure contracts with Railtrack.

Some two-stage markets involve a process whereby, instead of simply selling themselves to the purchaser (whatever relationship that purchaser has with the consumer), the provider has to secure access to the purchaser or consumer by making a bid (as with the rail companies' bids to Railtrack). Whether the tendering process between purchaser and provider involves payment for access to the market by the provider (as with the rail example) or simply an offer to supply a service at a given cost (as with hospital trusts tendering to purchasers), it is worth considering the relative power in the two-stage market (or a supplier of natural resources, such as the oil States in the oil example); of the company providing the service (such as the hospital trust); and of the purchaser. The oil example can indeed be considered a three-stage market, as there are the basic supplier of oil, the oil company, the bulk buyer and the consumer at the pumps. In the NHS, it is analytically more straightforward in that providers contract with labour and other resources in order to sell themselves to purchasers. There is no subsequent financial relationship between the purchaser and the consumer/patient – the purchaser is a surrogate consumer. In the rail example, again there is greater complexity in that one of the key factors of production (the track) is owned and managed by a regulatory body which in effect determines conditions for the consumer.

It might be argued that none of these arrangements alters the basic economic logic. For example, if labour is scarce, companies will have to pay more to employ it, which will affect the price they can offer to the purchaser. If companies are paying for access to a market (as in the rail example) then the price to the eventual consumer (the traveller) will be all the higher if – additional to recompensing scarce and therefore expensive labour – the companies also have to pay a large access fee to Railtrack.

In the health example, providers will be 'squeezed' in the sense that they will be seen to attract scarce labour, therefore outbidding each other to offer labour terms but also seeking to make contracts with purchasers by cutting their costs. In the rail example, the companies will have the same relationship with labour and will be seeking to minimize the amount they have to pay to Railtrack. This is because the rail companies then sell their services direct to the public. Health providers are seeking to minimize their costs for provision and maximize their income from purchasers, so that they can then supply health care to the public, who are free to 'walk through the door' in a hospital service that is free at the point of use. So there are

analogies but also differences. The 'market logic' is nevertheless clear: suppliers seek to minimize their costs and maximize their income (or ability to meet their obligations as in the case of hospitals). If access to the market is regulated (as with Railtrack, contracting with companies) and furthermore access to the market guarantees good income and profit, then suppliers will be willing to pay for the privilege of entering the market. A more direct example is provided by the famous case of waiters in expensive Riviera restaurants paying for the privilege of having their job, rather than being paid for the job, in the expectation that they can make a significant income from tips. An analogy in health care, I suppose, could be found if doctors were willing to pay for the privilege of operating from lucrative private hospitals.

All of this, of course, assumes that a market works as the textbook would imply. This is far from the case. In the rail example, it is most unlikely that companies will be competing on free market principles for access to track. Instead, the privatization is simply based on a desire to create private companies that distribute dividends to shareholders, for political reasons as well as economic reasons. In health care, it is reasonably well known which cadres within the labour market are relatively scarce and relatively plentiful. How the market is likely to work in practice should be analysed.

Consider the following. Where labour is plentiful rather than scarce (or where there are attempts to make it plentiful, by changing skill-mixes – see below), competing employers such as hospital trusts may lower the price of labour even more than a monopsonistic employer (a single or monopoly buyer of labour). This is because, in a context of plentiful labour, one hospital sets a trend in cutting wages and they all then compete to do the same in order to appeal to purchasers. Paradoxically, plentiful labour may actually have more bargaining power under the conditions of a monopsonistic employer (as in the old health service, when trusts were not competing). This is because that monopsonistic employer – what would have simply been called the hospital service, in the old days – has more power *vis-à-vis* its purchaser, as a monopoly supplier. (In the pre-reform NHS there was not even a divide into formal purchaser and formal provider, and it was a political decision as to how to reward labour and therefore cost services in the NHS.)

Where labour is scarce, it might be thought that their employers – the hospitals/ providers – would be better to be unified, to buy that labour on a monopsonistic basis (as monopoly purchasers of labour). Nevertheless competing hospital/providers may be forced into a less powerful relationship with their purchasers (the health authorities) and may therefore tender to the health authority on the basis of an assumed price for labour. The provider that wins the tender may then be the only source of access for the labour into the health service market, and may therefore be able to limit the power of what is otherwise a scarce and powerful resource.

In other words one has to look at the **dynamics** as well as the **statics** of the market place. In this connection, how regulation and Government policy (indeed politics) affects the operation of the market is crucial. To put it another way, scarcity, and relative supply and demand, may not always lead to foreseen results. In the example just provided, labour may retain its bargaining power and competitive providers may be forced to seek economies in other ways in order to please purchasers. This would presumably be a desirable way of operating the market. An important question therefore concerns the means by which the tendering process operates. If providers win and lose tenders with purchasers before employing their subcontractors (the labour), the power of even scarce labour is reduced. If prices are agreed with labour on the basis of a labour marker characterized by scarcity, on the other hand, then

prices in general are raised for the purchaser – and the purchaser seeking to cut costs under Government instructions may have difficulty in doing so. This is where political decision can again enter the process: how much is labour really left to offer itself in a free marketplace, in the reformed NHS, and how much is labour 'directed'? This will be discussed below.

Meanwhile, it can be pointed out that, in a two-stage market, how coalitions are formed between the three actors is important. If purchasers and providers form a coalition, in whatever form, then the bargaining power of the subcontractor (labour) may be reduced. If, however, providers and the subcontractor (labour) form a coalition, then the bargaining power of purchasers may be reduced. It is crucial that desired objectives in labour policy in the management of human resources in particular are rendered compatible with other objectives in operating such a system, otherwise unforeseen results may ensue. If purchasers and providers make alliances to reduce labour power rather than improve services, regulation will be necessary in the interests of equity.

Perfect competition, monopoly, state ownership and industrial relations

How does the existence of competition (however 'free') or its opposite, private monopoly, affect industrial relations and therefore human resources policy? The pure model of perfect competition assumes that companies compete freely, with no problem in access to markets, and that therefore profits are bid down to zero through competition. Therefore profit maximization under conditions of theoretical perfect competition involves zero profit as the best one can hope for! Add to this an assumption that there is perfect competition by these competing companies for labour, and one ends with the assumption that labour is paid its 'marginal product': in other words, labour's own 'profit maximization' is reduced to zero and that they are therefore paid in relation to what they produce without a 'profit margin'.

All markets in practice involve a degree of monopoly: the question is, how much, rather than whether monopoly exists. There is not perfect competition between companies; equally there is not perfect competition between labour. If labour is scarce it may be able to extract higher wages or 'profit' in neoclassical terms; or if it is plentiful, it may well be exploited, in that it will be paid less than its productive value. The free market assumption that this situation will be rectified by an exodus of labour to other industry is of course belied by the existence of unemployment – whether local, national or international. Already therefore one can see the political utility of unemployment to cost-cutting governments.

Companies which have power due to selling their services in monopolistic markets or oligopolistic situations (domination of the market by a few providers) may have more power *vis-à-vis* their purchaser of their services. They may also have therefore more ability – if they are so inclined – to give workers better conditions and insist that the purchasers agree to that as part of the overall agreement of the contract. Equally, they may 'take the purchaser's side' and use their power to weaken labour, especially if it is plentiful. Again therefore 'politics and policy' in a heavily managed service such as the NHS (whether market-oriented or not) are arguably even more crucial than economics. The generalization nevertheless remains that, if unemployment exists on a significant scale (or as threatened as a political tactic, as with threats to the medical and nursing professions to use them more selectively through skill-mix changes), then 'perfect competition' is a myth in the employment of labour. Labour's conditions will depend on attitudes to redistributing 'profit' from monopoly providers: that is, labour has less bargaining power within the company but the company may nevertheless have more profit redistributive wishes.

In the case of the National Health Service today, the Government may seek to diminish the power of providers who are not operating in free markets (who would therefore otherwise be fairly monopolistic or oligopolistic) by threatening to use purchasing health authorities and direct regulation to reorient health care away altogether from traditional providers. This is part of the political motivation behind the rhetoric of the policy concerning 'primary care' and closure of the secondary sector, i.e. the hospital sector.

It is then an open question as to whether a combination of monopoly and semi-monopoly, plus political objectives, is best addressed by state ownership rather than by regulation of 'the market'.

DISCUSSION: TOWARDS A LIBERAL VIEW OF PRODUCTIVITY

It is both a truism and a matter for controversy that productivity has become the buzz-word for the new NHS. It is a truism because nobody can really be against productivity, in at least some sense of that term. It is, however, also a matter for controversy because the demand for 'productivity' is being used to force the economics of the sweat shop on the NHS. What is the reason for this and what can be done about it – both in theory and in practice?

In economic matters generally, the present Government has taken the view that the UK can best compete by providing a low-wage alternative to the rest of advanced Europe. In other words, we are competing at the low end of the market. The belief that it is either desirable or necessary to do this is closely associated with another belief – namely, that the economy will only be productive if taxes and therefore public spending are low. Low public spending means lack of investment in both training and public capital, and so workers can only be 'productive' by being paid low wages. A more enlightened approach would invest in workers and therefore combine productivity and high wages.

The corollary for the NHS is that times are inevitably going to be hard, if the Conservative view is accepted. As a result, if legitimate demands for patient care are to be met, the maximum must be squeezed out of the workforce. A traditional Marxist view would have seen this as clear exploitation – with the NHS providing a support service to the private economy, where the state acts as financier and provider of health care on behalf of that economy. Although workers are not exploited directly by private employers, they are exploited by the state on behalf of these employers. The extent to which profitability in the rest of the economy is boosted by a 'cheap' NHS is the measure of such exploitation.

The NHS need not be like this. But ironically it seems that the Conservative government is determined to revitalize (analytical) Marxism! If it is true that 'there is no more money', then any wage increases – on this argument – have to be financed from 'productivity gains'. This argues against national pay norms, as they mandate increases that have to be paid for locally. Ironically it is correct to point out that **unfunded** national pay rises are bad news for the service, as they mean either less employment or the maintenance of employment only through generalized, extra, local productivity which secures extra funding from contracts.

As discussed here in the market NHS, however, with no additional purchasing money, even productivity gains may not allow extra remuneration. Consider the position of a trust, competing for markets. If its workers become more productive – and, say, complete what was traditionally a year's work in less than a year – it is only if extra purchasing money is forthcoming through new contracts that the workers can 'get more by working harder'.

A trust can only reward its workers for greater productivity in a sensible manner if it receives extra money, which means at the expense of other trusts – given the basic assumption 'that there is no more money for the NHS'. Thus 'more pay' requires harder work – and a 'beggar-my-neighbour' policy.

This depressing situation can only be avoided – in the absence of more money – if a radical 'reprofiling' of the workforce takes place, such that there is a once-and-for-all diminution in the numbers of doctors and nurses and indeed a diminution of their basic pay wherever possible. (This is rendered easier if doctors and nurses are alleged to be in surplus and therefore less in demand.) Once such a once-and-for-all saving on the total wage bill for professionals and workers in the NHS has been achieved, incremental increases in later years could presumably be countenanced. It is only by resort to such tortuous logic that one can give the benefit of the doubt to the rhetoric that says that people can earn increases (albeit at other people's expense).

Before the beggar-my-neighbour policy of the internal market (which has clearly been proposed as a means of forcing the workforce to come to heel), national pay bargaining allowed the state to act as the arbiter, acting of course through intermediary bodies such as the pay review bodies. This represented reality – in that it was rightly seen as the state's responsibility to balance the appropriate provision of health care with appropriate financing and appropriate terms and conditions for those employed to provide that health care or the support services for that health care. Now, however, this reality is disguised and workers are forced into an obedience to the dictates of their local trust, with the alternative being unemployment or worse conditions.

A more liberal approach to skill-mix would look at job satisfaction, and would therefore 'manage the human resource' without this simply being finance-driven. For example, both cleaners and patients used to get considerable job satisfaction and comfort respectively from conversations on the occasion of meals being served. With the privatization of ancillary services, however, cleaners experience intensified labour (with lower pay) and bureaucratized jobs that prevent them doing this; a 'reprofiling downwards' of part of the nursing workforce is in effect the situation.

A more liberal approach to productivity would undoubtedly involve some 'reprofiling upwards' but would not use this as an excuse simply to get rid of specialist doctors, instead employing them differently, **using adequate finance to do so**. Where nurses can legitimately undertake roles currently performed by doctors, such a policy should be not simply a means of firing doctors or making savings. Currently exercises in 'needs assessment' by both purchasers and providers are often driven by defensive mechanisms such that real debates about what outcomes are sought and who is best placed to provide the services to meet these outcomes are less possible. Doctors are defensive about maintaining their contribution; so are nurses – whether we are talking about a hospital service or a school health service. Where there is a mood abroad (with a lot of truth behind it) that 'they are out to get you', frank sharing of information as to more appropriate means of providing more appropriate services is less likely.

Any meaningful exercise in considering skill-mix will look at desired outcomes and then consider the services required to provide these outcomes, and then consider the most appropriate workers and professionals generally to provide that service under conditions of fair employment. An obsession with productivity in a narrow sense – which has a narrow view of output, has little view at all of outcome and translates efficiency into mere economy – tends to ignore the need for comprehensive health care in a number of specialties. For example, advice provided on the hospital ward to patients by nurses, in

informal settings and in perhaps conversation, may be quite significant in preventing readmission or later morbidity.

Alternatively, consider a situation in which a patient requires care in the community after a hospital stay – either care at home or care from community services generally. A narrow view of productivity would not necessarily invest in appropriate 'seamless care', despite the prevailing rhetoric – and indeed, there is an incentive for hospital trusts to 'cost-shift' and 'patient-shift' to community trusts and *vice versa*! That is, there is an incentive to complete episodes rather than complete care.

Research on productivity should link broader definitions of outcome to appropriate services, which are then in turn linked to appropriate skills. No one is arguing simply for a 'producer-driven' service which doesn't take account of the needs of the user (the patient). What some of us are, however, arguing for is a research agenda on skill-mix, productivity and remuneration that prevents the adverse consequences of the market for industrial relations and service conditions, on the one hand, and liberalizes rather than rejects the skill-mix agenda.

PERFORMANCE MANAGEMENT – THE EVOLVING AGENDA

The following pages briefly set out some trends in 'performance management' in the NHS in the first half of the 1990s, with significant implications for the intensification of 'labour'.

On what actual criteria will hospitals and individual directorates be judged, whether or not they choose these criteria? The Government, acting through the NHS executive, has recently assembled a number of key indices of efficiency. It is fair to say that technical efficiency has come to dominate other criteria in recent years as to the indication of performance. The aspiration is naturally to include quality as a central concern in the contracting process. The reality, however, is that, unless cost improvement and quality improvement are luckily going in the same direction (as they sometimes but not very often are), then the name of the game is cost advantage.

The efficiency index is a mechanism for institutionalizing 'efficiency gains' into the NHS (for example in the 1993 budget the Government decreed that NHS efficiency gains of at least 2.25% must be made, and that any pay rises must be funded by such efficiency savings) and for judging local providers. What is the efficiency index? It aims to develop a single number for each purchasing district and provider unit, to measure each unit's efficiency gains. Efficiency is measured in a simplistic way and is defined as the change in activity (the numerator) divided by the change in (real) spending, the denominator.

Activity is a weighted average of different types of health service activity, known as the **cost-weighted activity index** (CWAI). The measures of activity used are finished consultant episodes for ordinary admission in day cases; outpatient, accident and emergency and day case attendances; community contracts; and ambulance journeys. These are weighted according to their share of health spending so that, for example, a consultant episode is given more weight than an ambulance journey (UNISON, 1994c). The efficiency index is, however, flawed, as it only measures some types of health activity – most notably, those that can be measured! It therefore may give a boost to things that can be quantified rather than, for example, community and preventive health services. The accuracy of the data is generally poor, as it relies heavily on the finished consultant episode (FCE) as an activity measure. However this data is assembled in ways which do not necessarily correlate the number of FCEs with the number of patients actually treated. There is great arbitrariness in how to measure consultant involvement in patient care, let alone the appropriateness of measuring effec-

tive patient care by such a means. To deal with the objection that the measure fails to address the question of quality, the Department of Health is introducing the idea of 'quality offsets'. Such offsets will amount for 1994 to £54 million, equivalent to 0.3% of regions' total allocations (UNISON, 1994c) Perhaps more fundamentally, which spending to include and which to exclude from the efficiency index is not clear.

The efficiency index is in fact used constantly by ministers to claim that the NHS reforms have worked. This is, however, dubious. How do we account for the fact that the efficiency index has introduced a new means of measuring efficiency, contemporary with the introduction of reforms? Secondly, how do we disentangle the effects of the reforms from other initiatives, such as: centralized initiatives on waiting lists; Patient's Charter action and central monies related to it; inputs of cash connected with political priorities such as winning the 1992 general election; and so forth? In the longer term, developments in medical practice and changing treatment regimes which are completely divorced from existing health policy, let alone the NHS reforms, may be responsible for changes in the measures which make up the efficiency index.

It might be considered more sensible to take less aggregated measures and apply them more sensitively and more locally. There are political and other problems with so doing, of course. Indeed a **productivity index** based on 'unit labour costs' (derived from FCEs as output and the number and pay of staff) was devised specifically to measure workforce productivity, but was – sensibly – abandoned by central policy-makers as too analytically blunt yet politically sensitive. The danger with all such measures, in any case, is that they measure a simple relation of inputs to outputs, and therefore can lead to a conclusion that improvement is down to efficiency, whereas it may simply be down to economy or exploitation of labour.

A significant element of performance management is the new system of league tables that has been introduced for hospitals, based on a 'star system', hotel-style, for hospitals, which can be rated highly or otherwise.

Star ratings are given depending upon a hospital's performance (and the system is for community providers as well as hospitals). The better the performance against the standard, the more stars, on a range from one to five. There are five indicators on which providers are judged. These are:

- percentage of patients having their operation within 12 months;
- percentage of patients having their operation within 3 months;
- percentage of patients seen in outpatients within 30 minutes; within accident and emergency within 5 minutes; and operations cancelled;
- Ambulance services meeting rural and non-rural targets concerning percentage of ambulances arriving within an agreed number of minutes;
- percentage of patients having their procedures through day-case surgery rather than overnight stay.

In 1995, time of wait for outpatients appointments was added.

The first point to make is that the public certainly has a right to know about hospitals' quality. The second point concerns the audience for such a star system. Will regions use such a system – or even manipulate such a system – to ensure that the hospitals that they wish to favour for the future (through capital policy as discussed above, and through other means) emerge well from the system? Thirdly, are the relevant measures being used? For example, although the amount of time the patient has to wait on the day of an outpatient appointment is included, the amount of time one has to wait **for** an outpatient appointment is not included – a major omission. Fourthly, since managers and to some extent GP fundholders decide where to

place contracts, is it the point of informing the public that 'consumers' will then bring pressure to bear upon their purchasers? If so, how will this square with other policies, notably cost control and managed reductions in the size of the hospital sector? Next, is the data accurate? The Audit Commission in fact failed to authorize use of the star system for one in six providers, based on suspect data. Next, the data is based on small samples and may not be meaningful for comparison. Moreover, the data may be used illegitimately. For example, it may not be a measure of quality that one hospital has more day-case surgery than any other. Whereas **appropriate** day case surgery is generally a good thing, day-case surgery for patients who do not have adequate support at home, or to travel home, to give just a couple of examples, may be a bad thing.

In other words, as one would expect with any performance indicator, there is a whole range of criticisms that can be made. These should not be made merely negatively – for example, the indicators could be extended. There are, however, difficulties here also: should, for example, hospital mortality rates or individual consultant waiting times and waiting lists be added to the list, as some advise? Firstly, a hospital's mortality rate may not be an indicator of its quality. The best hospitals may attract the sickest patients. Furthermore, and more frighteningly, a hospital can discharge early to the community in order to reduce its mortality rate. Individual consultants' waiting times and waiting lists, which naturally affect the hospital's performance, may increase in relation to the consultant's quality. Solving the hospital's problem by bringing in extra clinical staff may bring in part-time clinical staff of (sometimes, not always) lower quality. As a result, waiting times may be reduced in relation to a reduction in quality.

Even when the measures are used for individual specialties, they may produce inappropriate management decisions. For example seeing more patients within 30 minutes in outpatients may diminish the effective use of a clinician's time. It may lead to the doctor waiting rather than the patient waiting – which may be appropriate if there is unlimited money but which is highly inappropriate in a system whose primary objective is to deliver the maximum care at agreed levels of quality within strictly limited resources.

More fundamentally, such a system of performance indication creates a centralist bias that prevents the local hospital tackling local problems and making its 'business plan' in line with local purchaser objectives. All in all, it is likely to be used as a mechanism for regional leverage on local providers, in line with broader policy objectives such as hospital closures, mergers and redirection of care.

WAITING-LIST INITIATIVES

Not exactly unrelated to the league table system is the increasing reliance upon 'waiting-list initiatives'. This again shows greater continuity with the pre-reform NHS than is widely believed to be the case. In the pre-reform NHS, waiting-list initiatives were geared to addressing waiting-list problems and were allocated to districts on the basis of bids made to the region, using regional and central monies. The new system is essentially the same, except that providers, working with their host districts, make the bids. A lot of energy goes into preparing the bid, agreeing the bid entirely within the hospital and negotiating over price – often a political process based on the available money. Such a system naturally gives regions – and the centre – power over which hospitals do well in the future and which do not. It is interesting to note that the internal hospital politics of managing a waiting-list bid and implementing it are a time-consuming and expensive process and lead to much fraught activity unrelated to effective patient care. It would be more sensible to allocate purchasing resources in relation to need and then allow purchasers and providers to work sensibly together to address such issues.

Most significantly of all, waiting-list initiatives are manipulated by politicians – either to 'win elections' or to provide a short-term solution to a long-term problem. for example, the 1994 regionally based waiting-list initiative, which some regions are implementing more enthusiastically than others, is geared to reducing waiting times in order to 'soften up' the public for bed closures, which are part of the Government's plans. This is not a conspiracy theory, in the light of the Secretary of State's desire to close 40% of acute beds within 8 years. In such a context, both waiting-list initiatives and league tables allegedly geared to the public are likely to become PR measures to aid a centrally driven planning process. The need to translate this into market language through the business plan causes clinical directors, business managers and hospital boards endless sleepless nights.

More centrally, such initiatives are being used to 'force' a shift to (improperly funded) greater GP responsibility for acute patients. This is allied to political agendas of claiming the reforms have worked not only in efficiency terms but in tipping the balance to primary care! In reality, however, the 'market' is *Diktat*, accompanied by competitive tenders by providers and directorates, to survive!

INTER-PROVIDER RELATIONSHIPS

Another complication affecting the measurement and management of performance is the rapidly changing relationship between providers. Firstly, the hospital sector is being 'right-sized' (i.e. downsized, i.e. cut) in order allegedly to put more money into primary and community care. In practice this means secondary care in a community setting. Secondly, a 'lead provider' model is developing, whereby hospitals take contracts for total patient care in particular specialties and subcontract community services (e.g. for cases where patients require both hospital and community services). Alternatively, community units can be the 'lead provider' and can subcontract to hospitals. As well as this, we see the 'hub and spoke' policy developing whereby trusts that have the infrastructure subcontract consultants to units in the community. Again, this may or may not be good practice locally and should not be a general policy. The hub and spoke principle may produce a situation whereby community units can offer services more cheaply because they employ consultants at marginal cost but do not cover the infrastructure and overall costs of the hospital. The hospital may therefore be undermined financially, yet the community service depends on the hospital for its very 'efficiency'! Safeguards are necessary in this area.

Thirdly, the fate of specialized services is often adversely affected in such an environment. Where local purchasing decisions affect which specialized services are purchased, the protection of services which all wish to maintain yet which local purchasers do not wish to maintain individually without ensuring that other local purchasers pay their share, may be adversely affected. Regional protection and management of such services is crucial.

Another mechanism affecting inter-provider relationships is the possibility of cost-shifting, for which read patient-dumping, from one provider to another. Regulation is necessary, where hospital and community trusts are separate, to ensure this does not occur – especially under block contracts, where both community and hospital services are squeezed to provide the relevant quantum of care. Pressures for early discharge based on the need for economy may increase the desire to 'dump' patients on another facility and thereby to save one's own budget. Again tight regulation is necessary to prevent this.

It is within this environment that new initiatives such as 'patient-focused care' and 'business process re-engineering' are being developed. In reality, there is always a need to evaluate conflicts as well as convergences between quality for the patient and cost control. 'Business process re-engineering' is in fact a hospital-wide system for using resources more efficiently and, if linked to patient-focused care, it is related to attempts to 'reprofile' staff and staff mixes in order to meet patient-defined objectives. As a neutral process, it may simply be a worthwhile means of relating input to desired output and outcomes. On the other hand, there is a need to ensure that it is not a mechanism for cost-driven standardization, in other words the opposite of its claim to be 'patient-focused'. Where a cost agenda is forcing hospital workload on to GPs to shorten length of hospital stay, 're-engineering' is being used also to introduce managed care. In this, protocols are used to try to ensure GPs only 'deliver' patients to hospital on the basis of an agreed care plan and that the hospital only discharges patients when their 'GP and home' circumstances have been agreed. In principle, it is an open matter as to whether this is a good thing or not. The patient does not always want 'discharge as early as possible'. But, again, finance is the name of the game. As with community care generally, such a policy might not, however, be cheaper if the necessary investment is made in primary and community services!

Regarding patient-focused care, practical examples are found in the initiatives known as 'one-stop clinics', 'near patient testing' and the just mentioned 'hub and spoke' principle whereby services are devolved from the hub to spokes such as GP fundholding surgeries and other community units. Identifying the costs and benefits of alternative strategies and making decisions accordingly is an important challenge. These policies run the danger of becoming all things to all men.

For example, the hub and spoke principle – the latest jargon – may fundamentally involve relationships between the hospital and community units. On the other hand, it is now being invoked in the context of takeovers of one hospital service by another – which may be justified either economically or otherwise but is different from the hub and spoke principle. Equally, it is important to ensure that cost and benefits are measured separately from any prevailing political agenda. For example the one-stop clinic may indeed be useful to the patient – who can have an outpatient consultation, have a test commissioned and get the test results all in one go. However, it may be a means of ensuring that consultants' time is used less productively and therefore that less is available for other priorities. All in all rigorous evaluation is required of what – somewhat inevitably in a frenetically managed NHS – become fads and badges of virtue at a superficial level.

The implications for the management of human resources of all these, and other, initiatives in performance management are great. This chapter has already considered the issues of 'reprofiling upwards' and 'reprofiling downwards'. Alongside initiatives to intensify productivity such as those just described, we find changes in the mix of medical manpower mandated by separate initiatives such as the New Deal for junior doctors' hours and conditions; the Calman Report on the future of medical education and training; and the changing nature of – and differentiations within – the nursing profession.

The question of reducing junior doctors' hours (which are still at extremely high levels by international standards) means that, without additional resources, junior doctors will work slightly fewer hours more intensively. Consultants may be encouraged, asked or expected to do more 'on call' work, to replace junior doctors. Nurses are often expected to 'reprofile themselves upwards' in order to take on duties formerly undertaken by medical staff. There are, however, complaints from various nursing bodies that such extensions of the nursing role are not being promoted as part of a holistic approach to nursing but simply by 'tacking on' tasks to

certain categories of nurse.

Inevitably there will be a clash between short-term needs of reconciling these various initiatives in the absence of adequate resources and longer-term attempts to provide more effective medical education, more humane medical training and more satisfying professional careers generally. At present, the agenda is one of squeezing more widgets off the production line – and the squeeze is causing significant problems of morale, specifically in the professions but also in the management cadre.

KEY TERMS AND CONCEPTS IN THE MANAGEMENT OF HUMAN RESOURCES

SCIENTIFIC MANAGEMENT

This is the approach to management that uses specific techniques of measurement and control to achieve specific objectives. It was seen as 'scientific' in that previous approaches to management (both historically and conceptually speaking) were less quantitatively based and relied on old-fashioned notions of 'obedience to orders' and on hierarchical relationships without aims, objectives and outputs being clarified. Such a philosophy of management derived naturally from the industrial and commercial sectors, and the relevance of such concepts of management to the delivery of services can be debated.

The relevance to the management of human resources, and the worker's role and relative power in the production or service-delivery process, is that scientific management became increasingly criticized for compartmentalizing the worker's contribution. Related to this, the lack of a 'human' aspect of the philosophy has also been criticized, although in its day scientific management was seen in some contexts as progressive.

HUMAN RESOURCE MANAGEMENT (HRM)

The school of 'human resource management'

is (in most of its manifestations) an attempt to give **descriptive** content to what is a **prescriptive** aim – the maximization of the individual's potential and satisfaction (and potential for satisfaction), jointly – or compatibly with – the best contribution to the organization's objectives. It is within this context that one therefore comes across conceptual approaches from psychology such as Maslow's 'hierarchy of needs'. There is a vast literature on human resource management, which deals with the organization, the individual's role in it (stressing the manager's role but also focusing on the motivation of the 'worker'), leadership, organizational development and so forth.

HRM seeks a 'humanistic' approach to management, whereby the individual is responsible for understanding the contribution of his job to both the organization's overall output and the culture of the organization. The extent to which the individual's objectives can be rendered compatible with the organization's objectives is of course a moot point: often propaganda rather than the achievement of direct consensus may play a role in persuading the individual that 'his interests are being maximized'.

In this sense, the perspectives of industrial relations are relevant: the pure unitarist view, for example, argues that all individuals can pool their interests without conflict in order to meet the organization's objectives. Whether or not an individual's interests are described in terms of the collective welfare of society and the content of the pay packet, as well as the 'intrinsic' job satisfaction possible in theory is of course a different question. It would be idealistic to assume that conflicts do not arise between the individual's objectives and the organization's objectives. Tom Peters – a leading US 'management guru', for example, used to be fond of an anecdote about the need to 'train, retrain and then train again' – but he made the argument that, often, it was less functionally necessary for the organization than good for the morale of the individual and was therefore **indirectly** beneficial to the organization. For example, companies that subsidize extracurricular activities and hobbies for workers are claimed to be on the right lines: the sausage factory that trains its workers in drama is not doing so because of the correlation between dramatic art and sausage stuffing but for other reasons!

The literature on human resource management is relatively recent but vast, and some key texts are listed at the end of the chapter, under 'Further reading'.

JOB EVALUATION

Job evaluation is an approach to measuring (at best) the content, intensity and qualitative nature of a job – for the purposes of remuneration, principally, but also for the purposes of more appropriate job design and redesign, within the context of the whole organization. Market forces may be used to determine – or allow – particular wage structures, for groups or for individuals, but job evaluation is concerned, at least indirectly, with equity rather than simply market forces, in that it seeks to measure the worth of a job. This worth has some 'intrinsic' content, irrespective of local market conditions, although this may be a contentious point with some.

One way of 'squaring the circle' between approaches based on job evaluation and market bases for reimbursing workers is to argue that the market will determine the overall wage structure, but that individuals' jobs can be enhanced and therefore rewarded through training and other programmes of development. In this sense, it could be argued that job evaluation is a means of measuring but also enhancing the productivity of the job (with productivity being used in a wide sense to cover all the dimensions of the job) such that the appropriate market reimbursement can be better devised and even improved. Thus it can be a form of 'action research'. Those who reject the market, unfettered or otherwise, as the basis for reimbursement would rely on a more radical version of job evaluation to feed into a process of either bargaining or wage determination.

One difficulty is that it is sometimes not clear if one is talking about 'the shop floor' or the management cadre, or both, for such purposes. In principle the term can be applied across the board – 'a job is a job' and its specific content can be analysed, at whatever level within the organization the job is based. Recently, a lot of NHS money has been spent on gaining management consultants' advice – superficially as to job evaluation but more fundamentally for the purposes of legitimizing contentious change.

PERFORMANCE MEASUREMENT AND PERFORMANCE RELATED PAY

Especially in the context of local rather than national pay bargaining, assessing what a job is worth takes on a new and sharper meaning. Generic systems of evaluation may overlook the particular skills and contribution of particular professions. What is more, the high costs of assessing both a job in itself and the performance of the worker in it are not to be underestimated. In practical terms, there is often a debate as to whether job evaluation should be conducted 'in house' by an employer (favoured generally by the trade unions, where they have accepted local pay bargaining and job evaluation as a political reality) or by outside consultants and 'experts'.

More specifically, performance-related pay is one of the most controversial areas currently in human resource management. Some argue that it is an arbitrary process and only worth implementing if performance can be measured accurately and with the consensus of the majority of those in the organization.

It can have a damaging effect on morale in an organization such as the National Health Service where, if there is not additional money forthcoming, one's performance is being evaluated in effect to avoid redundancy or a pay cut rather than to achieve an extra increment of income or other form of remuneration. There is an emerging research literature now on whether or not performance- related pay is correlated with effectiveness or improved performance in particular organizations, both private and public (Storey, 1992).

More theoretically, how can one assess an individual's contribution to a team effort or judge an individual's professional skill when the organization's objectives are financial? Recent decisions to abandon controversial plans to pay NHS doctors 'by performance' and replace them with plans to reward the organization as a team for improved performance (e.g. the hospital trust) perhaps take account of the first point but not the second.

INDIVIDUAL PERFORMANCE REVIEW AND LOCAL AGREEMENTS

These two may be different, in that individual performance review is naturally concerned with the specific evaluation of the individual, whereas local agreements may be conducted on a group or trade union basis. It has been pointed out that, irrespective of the political complexion of the ruling party, many Western countries are moving towards more devolved management structures within large organizations and enterprises, whether public or private. It is therefore argued that wages and remuneration generally, and also training and management development strategies, ought to be localized as well.

However this is not a logical so much as a psychological link. It is possible to have decentralized management (with autonomous units operating within companies, for example) yet centralized strategies for pay, training and development. There is no 'hard' research on this topic, perhaps not surprisingly, although it is increasingly being suggested that an organization which has the capacity to raise its own revenue as a direct result of production can reward local initiative and local productivity more effectively than a centralized public sector organization.

The National Health Service, despite recent discussions about devolution of operational responsibilities, still has a centrally planned purchasing budget, and there are therefore constraints upon rewarding local initiative – for financial reasons rather than for reasons of preference. Again the costs and benefits of such an approach have to be taken into account. It is interesting to note that moves to decentralization in the private sector have often been partially **reversed**, for the reason that employers think they have more bargaining power when dealing in unified negotiations with the whole workforce! (Railtrack might reflect ruefully on this, following the 1994 strike by the signalmen.) This may be a question of psychology or a question of economics. If industrial relations are left to local markets within a company's field of operations, prices (wage costs, etc). may be bid up by a market bargaining process, especially where workers are in scarce supply. If one considers, in the case of the Health Service, the situation of the purchaser (health authority) dealing with the provider (hospital and other units), one can consider local pay bargaining as a form of subcontracting by the provider unit (i.e. employing its staff, as discussed above). Doing this through market means at a local level (rather than through a hierarchical system involving more centralized negotiation and stipulation of pay and conditions) may actually bid up wages rather than the reverse. On the grounds of both economy and reducing bureaucratic costs (what economists call transactions costs) the argument for local bargaining is far from won – before one even reaches the political realm of national comparabilities, equity or the question of trade union rights.

DISCUSSION

- The fundamental distinction within the territory of 'human resource management' and 'industrial relations' is between, on the one hand, the 'scientific' analysis of industrial relations and human behaviour in organizations and, on the other hand, the advocacy of prescriptive techniques to 'manage the human resource' according to prevailing norms (such as producing more output with less costly input; the resulting changes in skill-mix to achieve this and so forth).

- Concerning the former, the main disputes in the academic study of industrial relations are between the schools of unitarism, pluralism and Marxism or radicalism. These different schools – in their descriptive rather than prescriptive sense – take different perspectives as to whether interests within the organization are unified, plurally differentiated or differentiated on a class basis.

- The question of productivity in today's NHS stems from two characteristics of the present-day service – the absence of extra finance and the need to do more with the available money. If labour were still to be rewarded through national agreements, this would mean that it would have to be made explicit that people were doing more for the same money. Local pay bargaining therefore has two functions – as well as allowing local productivity to be rewarded (if it can be measured and dealt with appropriately), local pay bargaining also allows the political fact that work is being intensified to be obscured. The rhetoric of 'rewarding the productive' can be adopted.

  People can earn more money by doing more, but only at the cost of less money elsewhere in the system – either in their own hospital, or rather trust, or by reducing income for other providers. If everyone is more productive or if every trust is more productive, there is not enough money to pay for this.

The question then arises, what about increases merely to cover inflation, let alone increases based on a desire to give more money to the lower paid for their existing amount of work? The answer in the current system is that this is only possible through 'efficiency savings' – which ironically means in practice unemployment or lower wages for other workers, i.e. economy rather than efficiency.

- Local pay bargaining is a means for allowing successful trusts to take work from others and thereby to pay their employees more (for more work). In the long run, as rival providers are put out of business, there is less of a competitive market – and it is then a question for policy-makers as to whether regulation is used to seek to restimulate a market or simply to regulate the income of the new monopolies. Either way, central regulation is necessary alongside local action, as recognized in the NHS Executive document *Local Freedoms, National Responsibilities*, published in December 1994 (NHSE, 1994).

- This combination of localism and centralism is reflected in the approach to performance-related pay. Local pay bargaining is not the same as performance-related pay – one can have local pay for trusts but central bargaining within these trusts. If one moves further towards performance-related pay, either for groups of workers or for individual workers (doctors; nurses; cleaners; everyone), then it is likely that local market forces will only be part of the story. Using performance-related pay to control the workforce will have to be part of a national strategy to minimize costs (especially labour costs) and maximize output.

- There is therefore a problem in distinguishing the different purposes of performance-related pay: is it to regulate (and control) the workforce; to motivate the workforce in a positive manner; or for recruitment purposes? These, of course, may overlap in practice, but the problem with performance-related pay in a service with increasing productivity demands yet static income (in aggregate, for the whole National Health Service) is that it is likely to be a stick rather than a carrot. And this is where the 'reprofiling of the workforce' comes in: substituting cheaper workers for expensive ones allows some to be rewarded (albeit for more intensive work) while others are dispensed with altogether.

ACKNOWLEDGEMENTS

I would like to thank the editor and publishers of *Nursing Management* for permission to draw on a short article, 'A Liberal Dose', from the June 1994 issue, which was used in the final pages of this chapter.

REFERENCES

Farnham, D. and Pimlott, J. (1991) *Understanding Industrial Relations*, Cassell, London.

Healey, D. (1989) *The Time of my Life*, Michael Joseph, London, pp 388–408, 461–464.

Kuhn, T. (1970) *The Structure of Scientific Revolutions*, 2nd edn, University of Chicago Press, Chicago, ILL.

Lukes, S. (1974) *Power – A Radical View*, Macmillan, London.

NHSE (1994) *Local Freedoms, National Responsibilities*, Department of Health, London.

Parry, G. (1969) *Political Elites*, George Allen & Unwin, London.

Pugh, D. S., Hinings, C. R. and Hickson, D. J. (eds) (1986) *Organizations: Readings*, Penguin, Harmondsworth.

Storey, J. (1992) *Developments in the Management of Human Resources*, Blackwell, Oxford

Storey, J. (1992) *New Perspectives on Human Resource Management*, Routledge, London.

UNISON (1994b) *Skill-mix*, UNISON, London.

UNISON (1994a) *The Market Menace*, UNISON, London.

UNISON (1994c) *The NHS Efficiency Index: A Briefing*, UNISON, London.

FURTHER READING

MANAGEMENT OF HUMAN RESOURCES AND INDUSTRIAL RELATIONS: PERSPECTIVES AND ANALYSIS

Burchill, F. and Seifert, R. (1993) Professional Unions in the NHS: Membership Trends and Issues, Paper at Annual Conference, Employment Research Unit, Cardiff University, Cardiff.

Fox, A. (1985) *Man Mismanagement*, 2nd edn, Hutchinson, London.

Lloyd, C. *et al.* (1993) Why trusts need unions. *Health Service Journal*, **28 Jan**, 31-32.

Salamon, M. (1992) *Industrial Relations, Theory and Practice*, Prentice Hall, Englewood Cliffs, NJ.

Seifert, R. (1992) *Industrial Relations in the NHS*, Chapman & Hall, London.

Sisson, K. (ed.) (1989) *Personnel Management in the UK*, Blackwell, Oxford.

Storey, J. (1992) HRM in action: the truth's out at last. *Personnel Management*, **April**, 28–31.

Towers, B. (1992) Choosing bargaining levels: UK experience and implications, in *Issues in People Management 2*, Institute of Personnel Management, London.

MODELS OF MANAGING HUMAN RESOURCES: PRINCIPLES AND PRACTICE

Bishop, G. and Lewin, R. (1993) Shortcutting old bargaining machinery. *Personnel Management*, **Feb**, 28–32.

Cohen, P. (1994) Just rewards [on the costs of local bargaining], *Health Service Journal*, **17 Mar**.

Geary, J. F. (1992) Pay control and commitment: linking appraisal and reward. *Human Resource Management Journal*, **2**, 36–54.

Griffin, R. P. (1992) Why doesn't performance pay work? *Health Manpower Management*, **18**, 31–33.

Handy, C.B. (1986) *Understanding Organizations*, Penguin, Harmondsworth.

Kessler, I. and Purcell, J. (1992) Performance related pay: objectives and applications. *Human Resource Management Journal*, **2**, 36–54.

Pugh, D.S., (1991) *Organisational Theory*, 3rd edn, Penguin, Harmondsworth.

LEADERSHIP THEORY

Bryman, A. (1986) *Leadership and Organisations*, Routledge & Kegan Paul, London.

Bryman, A. (1992) *Charisma and Leadership*, Sage Publications, London.

Kotter, J. P. (1990) *A Force For Change: How Leadership Differs from Management*, Collier Macmillan, London.

Harvey-Jones, J. (1989) *Making It Happen*, Fontana, London.

Stewart, R. (1989) *Leading in the NHS: A Practical Guide*, Macmillan, London.

EDUCATION AND TRAINING

National Audit Office(1986) *NHS: Control over Professional and Technical Manpower*, HMSO, London.

NHS Management Executive (1989) *Working For Patients: Working Paper 10 – Professional Education and Training*, HMSO, London.

MANAGEMENT DEVELOPMENT

Garratt, B. (1987) *The Learning Organisation and the Need for Directors Who Think*, Fontana/Collins, London.

Harrison, S. (1988) *Managing the NHS: Shifting the Frontier?*, Chapman & Hall, London.

Handy, C. (1989) *The Age of Unreason*, Business Books, London.

Morgan, G. (1986) *Images of Organisations*, Sage Publications, London.

NHS Management Executive (England) (1991) *A National Development Strategy for the NHS*, NHSME, London.

NHS Training Authority (1986) *Better Management, Better Health*, NHS Training Authority, Bristol.

Pedlar, M. *et al.* (1991) *The Learning Company: A Strategy for Sustainable Development*, McGraw-Hill, New York.

REPROFILING AND SKILL-MIX

Advisory Conciliation and Arbitration Service (1988) *Labour Flexibility in the UK: The 1987 ACAS Survey*, ACAS, London.

Atkinson, J. (1984) Flexible employment strategies. *Industrial Relations Review*, **Report No. 325**, 13–16.

Atkinson, J. (1984) *Manning For Uncertainty – Some Emerging UK Work Patterns*, Institute of Manpower Studies, Brighton.

Atkinson, J. (1986) Is flexibility just a flash in the pan? *Personnel Management*, **Sep**, 26–29.

Audit Commission (1991) *The Virtue of Patients: Making Best Use of Ward Nursing Resources*,

Department of Health, London.

Bevan, S., Stock, J. and Waite, R. K. (1990) *Choosing an Approach to Reprofiling and Skill Mix*, Institute of Manpower Studies, Brighton.

Dyson, R. and Naylor, A. (1991) *Skills Mix Issues and Choices in Hospital Theatres*, Department of Health, London.

IMS (1991) *Choosing an Approach to Reprofiling and Skill Mix*, University of Sussex, Department of Health, Brighton.

Income Data Services (1992) *Skill Based Pay, Study 500*, IDS, London.

Patton, M. (1987) *How to Use Qualitative Methods in Evaluation*, Sage Publications, London.

Tigou, F. (1991) Just rewards. *Human Resources*, **Autumn**, 147–150.

GENERAL AND INTERNATIONAL HRM

Anderson, G. (1993) *Managing Performance Appraisal Systems: Design Implementation and Monitoring for Effective Appraisal*, Blackwell, Oxford.

Bamber, G., Snape, E. and Redman, T. (1993) *Managing Managers: Strategies and Techniques for Human Resource Managers*, Blackwell, Oxford.

Beaumont, P. B. (1993) *Human Resource Management: Key Concepts and Skills*, Sage Publications, London.

Brewster, C. (ed.) (1993) *European Developments in Human Resource Management*, Kogan Page, London.

Bridgford, J. and Stirling, J. (1993) *Employee Relations in Europe*, Blackwell, Oxford.

Kakabadse, A. and Tyson, S. (1993) *Cases in European Human Resource Management: Teacher's Manual*, Routledge, London.

Oliver, N. (1992) *The Japanization of British Industry: New Developments in the 1990s*, Blackwell, Oxford.

Teague, P. (1989) *The European Community: The Social Dimension: Labour Market Policies for 1992*, Kogan Page, London.

Williams, A. (1993) *Human Resource Management and Labour Market Flexibility: Some Current Theories and Controversies*, Avebury, Aldershot.

PERFORMANCE

Appleby, J. (1994) Evaluating NHS Reforms *Health Service Journal* 10 March p32

Appleby, J. and Little, V. (1993) Health and efficiency, *Health Service Journal*, **6 May**, 20–24.

Audit Commission (1991) *A Shortcut to Better Services: Day Surgery in England and Wales*, HMSO, London.

Audit Commission (1991) *Measuring Quality: The Patient's View of Day Surgery* (NHS occasional papers), HMSO, London.

Audit Commission (1992) *All In A Days Work: An Audit of Day Surgery in England and Wales*, HMSO, London.

Audit Commission (1994) *Trusting in the Future: Towards an Audit Agenda for NHS Providers*, HMSO, London.

BAM, BMA, RCM, IHSM (1993) *Managing Clinical Services: A Consensus Statement of Principles for Effective Clinical Management*, IHSM, London.

Beech, R. and Morgan, M. (1992) Constraints on innovatory practice: the case of day surgery in the NHS. *International Journal of Health Planning and Management*, **7**.

Berwick, D. (1989) Continuous improvement as an ideal in health care. *New England Journal of Medicine*, **320**, 53–56.

Berwick, D. (1900) Appraising appraisal, in *Quality Connection*, a publication of the Institute for Health Care Improvement, Brookline, MA.

Dixon, M. (1993) Board games [on unitary and non-unitary boards]. *Health Service Journal*, **29 Jul**.

Editorial (1994) Is anybody up there? *Health Summary*, **May**.

Grainger, C. and Griffiths, R. (1993) Over the obstacles: management issues for running day surgery. *Health Service Journal*, **22 Apr**, 24–25.

Harper, J. (1991, updated 1992/93) *Unit Labour Costs: A Guide*, NHSME, London.

National Association of Health Authorities and Trusts (NAHAT) (1983) *Health Boards*, NAHAT, London.

NHS Management Executive (1994) *Managing the New NHS: Detailed Analysis of Functions*, Progress Report, NHSME, London.

NHSME (1994) *Code of Accountability for NHS Boards*, NHMSE, London.

NHSME (1994) *Code of Conduct for NHS Boards*, NHMSE, London.

Petchey, R. (1991) NHS Internal Market 1991–2: towards a balance sheet. *British Medical Journal*, **306**, 699–701.

Slater, G. and Del, K. (1994) Capital planning: investing in excellence. *Health Services Management*, **Apr**.

Health Business Summary *The Economics of Day Care Surgery* (edited version), available from Zeneca Pharma.

Yates, J. (1994) A league of their own [on league tables]. *Health Director*, **Jun**, 8–9.

SELECTED PRESS VIEWS

Anonymous (1993) The new proletariat [on how soon most British employees will be women but with low pay and poor conditions]. News item. *The Independent on Sunday*, 16 May, 19.

Anonymous (1994) Britain adopting 'Victorian' type of employee relations. News item. *The Times*, **15 Feb**, 2.

Anonymous (1994) After the performance begins [on the BMAs opposition to changed pay and terms and performance related pay]. *Guardian, Section 2*, **17 Aug**.

Anonymous (1994) Performance pay plan for NHS ditched. News item. *Guardian*, **17 Aug**.

Hutton, W. (1993) A country of casuals [on part-time work involving less pay and fewer rights]. *Guardian*, **30 Mar**, 20.

Hutton, W. (1993) The latest cut is the deepest [on pay freezes and public sector workers]. *Guardian*, **15 Sep**, 16.

For a defence of performance-related pay, changes in skill-mix and reprofiling, see regular articles by Professor Eric Caines in *The Health Services* and *The Times*.

MEDICAL AND CLINICAL AUDIT: TOWARDS QUALITY?

9

*Calum Paton and Anne McBride**

INTRODUCTION

Audit of clinical care has become a central concern in many health-care systems. The reasons are many, and a section of this chapter outlines the origin of the policy of medical audit in the UK. The broader reasons for the importance of audit are substantial.

Firstly, guaranteeing effective care to the individual patient where possible is the primary purpose of audit. Secondly, where overall resources are constrained, it may be important to ensure that resources within particular clinical specialties are put to the most appropriate use – which includes audit as a means of reconciling cost control with quality control. This is not to deny there will often be awkward trade-offs between 'quantity and quality' so much as to assert that, where effective audit can prevent the need for 'readmission or repair', it will be a useful accompaniment to effective management of resources.

The policy of medical audit predates the NHS reforms, although *Working Paper No. 6*, accompanying the launch of the White Paper *Working for Patients* (the blueprint for the NHS reforms), concerned medical audit (Department of Health, 1989a, b). In providing medical services, the pursuit of quality has been an assumed norm and although subject to certain forms of external regulation, there has been a traditional reliance on self-regulation. Thus many doctors viewed the introduction of medical audit with suspicion, seeing it as a device by managers to control their behaviour or their resources, or both. There is reason for this suspicion, in that – by the mid-1990s – the policy of medical audit has been superseded or rather absorbed into a more general concern with control of the 'clinical product'. To this extent, it may be an integral part of the managerialist agenda which has been reinforced by the NHS reforms. Nevertheless, medical audit in itself is obviously a worthy activity – it is a means for doctors to agree on appropriate standards in delivering effective outcomes and appropriate standards for the processes involved or associated with such outcomes.

With these considerations in mind, it can be seen that, in principle, medical audit may be a **voluntary** activity, internal to the medical profession; a **semi-mandatory** activity commissioned by the funders of health care but not prescribed in detail by such funders (for example, as to which particular conditions have to be 'audited'); or a **mandatory** part of the 'business process' – whether it is prescribed by the provider, or purchaser, or both acting together. The appropriateness of medical audit being applied within any one of these frameworks is an important question – and one which this chapter addresses.

This chapter begins by outlining the nature and impact of traditional methods of health-care quality assessment and comparing this with more recent developments in the

* Formerly, Research Fellow, Centre for Health Planning and Management, Keele University.

management of health-care quality. The chapter reviews the key components of the new framework for managing health-care quality in the NHS and argues that the introduction of medical audit within such an environment could have a radical impact on improving health-care quality. However, the lack of scientific evidence underpinning many clinical interventions necessitates the pursuance of a large research agenda before the implementation of medical audit proper. Three studies are reviewed to illustrate the continuum of research activity, which runs from clinical research to audit proper. In addition, each study raises questions concerning the basis upon which clinicians should change their clinical practice. The concluding sections describe how these issues are further complicated by the introduction of medical audit within a framework of cost-containment.

TRADITIONAL METHODS IN THE MANAGEMENT OF HEALTH-CARE QUALITY

Prior to the introduction of medical audit in April 1991, the quality of clinical practice was mainly assessed on an informal and voluntary basis by the medical profession itself. This 'freedom' to regulate oneself is often justified on the grounds that only clinicians have the requisite expertise required for determining and monitoring their own standards of practice. As noted by Shaw (1989), it also reflects the high degree of clinical autonomy which clinicians in the UK have compared to those countries such as North America and Australia where standards of practice are monitored by external bodies.

Within this self-regulatory framework, the method of quality assessment used most frequently was that of **peer review**. Peer review is the evaluation or review of one's work by one's equals. In the medical profession, this takes a variety of forms ranging from an informal peer group discussion of case note presentations by colleagues through

to the more systematic and formal review which exists in the confidential enquiries into maternal deaths and perioperative deaths (Buck, Devlin and Lunn, 1987; Department of Health, 1991). However, the status of peer review as a voluntary exercise may well have led to its usage being haphazard and less than comprehensive. The confidential enquiry into perioperative deaths (CEPOD) noted that many surgeons and anaesthetists did not hold regular reviews of their operation results (traditionally known as mortality and morbidity meetings) (Buck, Devlin and Lunn, 1987).

IMPACT UPON CLINICAL CARE

If participation in peer review is only conducted on a voluntary basis, then changing one's practice as a result of this review tends also to be only of a voluntary nature. Although clinicians may participate in peer review, the review group has no means of ensuring that evaluative expressions by colleagues are acknowledged or appreciated, or that recommendations for a change in clinical practice are effected. The CEPOD report mentioned above illustrates this point: although the cases reviewed in CEPOD were not self-selected – encompassing all deaths within 30 days of an operation – and they revealed a number of practices which were not considered to be of an appropriate standard, participation in the enquiry was only voluntary and the report itself was only able to make recommendations as to appropriate changes in practice. It was not able to effect any change. Confirmation of its ineffective nature is found in the latest report of the National Confidential Enquiry into Perioperative Deaths (Campling *et al.*, 1992), which reports similar findings to those reported in 1987. Although the prevailing standards of surgery and anaesthesia are reported to be excellent and improving, the report highlights a number of deficiencies in medical practice.

In addition to the limitations of peer review caused by its voluntary nature, McColl notes that within 'informal audit', consistency and clarity are often lacking in the formulation of standards and their comparison with practice (McColl, 1979). Irvine argues that if practice is compared with a standard based on a subjective opinion at the time of comparison, these standards are unlikely to be greatly consistent amongst a group of subjective opinions – and even less reliable (Irvine, 1990). Furthermore, a typical mortality and morbidity meeting will concentrate on the discussion of unexpected deaths and exotic cases and as such there can be no conclusions drawn on the standard of routine practice and treatment. Not surprisingly, peer review has tended to have little significant impact upon patterns of clinical care (Van't Hoff, 1986).

DEVELOPMENTS IN MANAGING HEALTH-CARE QUALITY

To limit the subjective nature of peer review, Lembcke and his fellow pioneers in America concluded, from a number of studies, that using explicit criteria and standards enabled a more objective, systematic and repeatable assessment of the quality of health care (Brook and Appel, 1973; Lembcke, 1967).

Criteria are aspects of medical care which, when measured, give us an indication of quality. Standards are those measurement levels which it has been agreed represent appropriate levels of quality. An illustration of this two-pronged quantification of quality is given by Black, who suggests that a criterion for the care of patients with acute abdominal pain could be 'that appendectomies should be performed only when appendicitis is present'. The standard to be set would be an acceptable number of inflamed appendices which were removed in relation to the total appendectomies (e.g. 75%). Thus the removal of appendices of which only 65% were inflamed would indi-

cate a need to improve the care of patients with acute abdominal pain – which in this case might require an improvement of the diagnostic practice of the clinicians (Black, 1990).

From their respective studies, Rosenfeld determined that the method of measurement should be sensitive; objective; valid; applicable; practical (Rosenfeld, 1957), and Lembcke laid down six 'cardinal points applicable to all criteria': objectivity, verifiability, uniformity, specificity, pertinence and acceptability (Lembcke, 1967). Thus evolved a more measured approach to assessing health-care quality, through which the examination of practice and comparison with standards was much more organized and systematic, often involving the collection of statistical data and the development of clearly defined standards. This process became known as 'medical audit' and was the first step in systematically identifying specific deficiencies in the quality of care which required correction.

CRITERION-BASED AUDIT

Donabedian usefully categorizes the development of quality standards into two sources: **empirical** standards, which are derived from actual practice (but which may not reflect current medical knowledge), and **normative** standards, which derive from bodies of 'legitimate knowledge' (but which may not reflect actual practice). Attempts to combine the characteristics of both types led to the development of normative criteria and empirically based standards (Lembcke, 1967), which were designed to 'take account of the contingencies not foreseen in the standards themselves' (Donabedian, 1966). This process – and its derivatives – has become known as **criterion-based audit** (Shaw, 1990).

The attraction of this categorization of quality standards lies in its potential for merging the advantages of both 'bottom up' and 'top-down' approaches to quality assessment and addressing the tension which exists between groups setting their own standards and gaining 'ownership' of the data, and ensuring achievement nationally of a minimum level of service (Black, 1990).

OUTCOME, PROCESS AND STRUCTURE

The quality of a product or service is usually assessed in its final form and the extent to which it meets the needs for which it was obtained. Although it was this concept of 'final form' which underlined the work of the much earlier pioneers of health-care quality assessment (such as Dr Codman – Lembcke, 1967 – and Florence Nightingale – Maxwell, 1984), it can prove difficult to relate final outcome to antecedent care – and thus to accurately identify the appropriate remedial action to be taken, if needs are not satisfied.

Donabedian attempts to counteract this difficulty by suggesting that medical care can be assessed by three approaches: the assessment of outcome, process and/or structure. **Outcome** is still considered the ultimate validator of the quality of health care since it refers to the results of a medical intervention – in terms of the changes in the patient's current and future health status – which can be attributed to health care at the GP surgery, at the hospital or both. Since outcome can be difficult to measure with a degree of accuracy, process and structure can be used as a proxy for outcome, when the relationships between outcome, process and structure are known. **Process** relates to the interaction between practitioner and patient and includes clinical interventions and the use of treatments and investigations. **Structure** relates to the settings in which these interventions take place and the related processes that support and direct the provision of care (Donabedian, 1966).

Donabedian himself notes that this three-way division is a somewhat arbitrary abstraction from the provision of medical care, but suggests that it is a way of organizing one's thinking and enables the generation and classification of specific indicators of quality (Donabedian, 1980). It also ensures that the whole spectrum of medical care is taken into account when its quality is assessed: an important factor, when recognizing the multi-dimensional nature of medical care.

DIFFERENT PERSPECTIVES

The World Health Organization Working Group on Quality (WHO Working Group, 1989) suggests that quality must reflect at least four concerns:

- performance (technical quality);
- resource use (economic efficiency);
- risk management (identification and avoidance of injury, harm or illness associated with the service provided;
- patient (or client satisfaction).

Notwithstanding that these four concerns may – in some instances – conflict with each other, the heterogeneity of priorities and expectations of, and between, health service professionals, managers and clients will generate further diversity and conflict to be reconciled within this particular framework of quality.

A number of commentators have attempted to provide the definitive framework for determining quality, but no one criteria set encapsulates the totality of quality that could be assessed. Nonetheless, these debates serve a useful purpose in illustrating the dynamic nature and diversity of competing interests, expectations and priorities of health service professionals, managers and clients, and highlight the manner in which these perceptions influence the criteria by which each 'player' believes a quality health service system should be judged (see Cochrane, 1972; Donabedian, 1966, 1980; Holland, 1983; Hopkins, 1990; Jennett, 1988; Maxwell, 1984; Mooney and Ryan, 1991; Ovretveit, 1992; Pfeffer and Coote, 1991; Steffen, 1988; Williamson, 1992 for a range of frameworks within which to highlight and prioritize the quality of health care).

CHANGING CLINICAL PRACTICE

As noted above, the process of quantifying and measuring health-care quality facilitates the identification of specific deficiencies in the quality of care which require correction. In order to improve the quality of health care in these identified instances, it is likely that one, or more, individuals will be required to change their particular way of doing things. As individuals, we all react differently to changing circumstances, and take up new innovations at different rates (Rogers, 1983). Clinicians are perceived as particularly resistant to change (Eisenberg, 1986), a feature variously attributed to their position as 'dominant-interest-holders' with 'familiar patterns of work; old skills; comfortable assumptions; institutionalized support or sanction; established relationships and patterns of communication with each other' (Williamson, 1992: p. 17); and the unrealistic expectation that unaided practitioners will be able to effectively synthesize the large amount of complex information which characterizes modern medicine (Eddy, 1990a).

Eisenberg acknowledges the variety of influences which exist within the individual clinical decision-making process and suggests that no one approach to changing practice can be expected to be comprehensively effective (Eisenberg, 1986). His research leads him to identify six major ways of altering practice which he suggests be used in an orchestrated combination rather than one by one. These are reviewed below, together with the findings of other commentators in the field.

Education

Eisenberg defines education as the imparting of new knowledge and a number of commentators note the limited success of education in changing practice (Eisenberg, 1986; Standing Committee on Postgraduate Medical Education, 1989). Eisenberg highlights the importance of professional leadership in education, and the existence of a perceived need for education within the physician, to the success of educational activities.

Feedback

A number of studies have been conducted into the effect which feeding back information on current practice has on changing future practice. A review of such studies by Mitchell and Fowkes (1985) concluded that the passive feeding back of information on performance had almost no impact on changing clinical behaviour, while feedback combined with other educational measures appeared to have some success – termed 'active feedback'. In addition, a number of commentators argue that the effectiveness of feedback is determined by traits of 'maturity, honesty and selfless commitment to the goal of improving clinical skills' possessed by the recipient of feedback (Ende, 1983); the individualization of data; comparison among peers; delivery of feedback by a physician in a position of clinical leadership (Eisenberg, 1986); and the proximity of feedback to the clinical decision-making process (Mugford, Banfield and O'Hanlon, 1991).

Participation

Eisenberg notes that the value of physician involvement in efforts to change their own practice is one of the most important lessons of the literature about quality assurance, with there being general agreement that clinicians need to feel invested in the programme of change in order to respond to the benefit of medical practice. This reflects the earlier findings by Nelson: that physicians who did not participate in the development of peer review criteria challenged the validity of the criteria when the data suggested an unacceptable level of compliance with the criteria (Nelson,1976); and has been more recently supported by Mugford, Banfield and O'Hanlon's review of practice (1991).

Administrative rules

These refer to the development of guidelines, protocols, checklists and algorithms which clinicians can use in their assessment and treatment of patients. There is some evidence to suggest that the use of such 'tools' promotes desired changes in clinical behaviour (Fowkes, 1982; Schoenbaum and Gottlieb, 1990; Packer *et al.*, 1991).

Incentives and penalties

Studies by Rice (1983) and Krasnick *et al.* (1990) illustrate the potential impact of incentives on changing clinical behaviour (see also Beech and Morgan, 1992).

Theory of continuous improvement

Another approach to managing changes in clinical practice is outlined by Berwick (1989) (see also Berwick, Enthoven and Bunker, 1992), and refers to the theory of continuous improvement which Deming (1982, 1986) and Juran (1964; Juran, Gryna and Bingham, 1979) developed from their non-health-care studies in the 1930s. They discovered that problems of quality usually emanated from 'poor job design, failure of leadership, or unclear purpose', and concluded that opportunities to improve quality were more likely to emanate from the study of complex production processes than the motivation of the people involved in the processes. Berwick translates the operation of these principles into the arena of health-care management and argues that leadership; investment in education and study; re-establishment of respect for the health-care worker; maintenance of open dialogue between customers and suppliers of health care; the use of analytical tools; and the placing of quality improvement on a par with finance within the organization, are all steps towards continuous improvement in the quality of health care (Berwick, 1989).

AUDIT AS PART OF THE REFORMS

In America, where the concept of medical audit was initially developed, it has evolved into a quality assurance programme whereby action is required to be taken regarding any deficiencies of quality, and procedures are established to ensure that these deficiencies are unlikely to occur in a similar way in the future (Black, 1990). Given the methodology of medical audit and its introduction within an environment which encourages its regular usage, its potential to make a significant impact on the quality of medical care delivered in the NHS is quite substantial. The following section considers the extent of its potential for improving health-care quality, highlighting the key determinants of its success.

From April 1991, every doctor has been required to participate in a regular and systematic review of the quality of medical care (known as medical audit). Although not given legal force in the NHS and Community Care Act 1990, the Government's prescriptions for audit contrast significantly with the Government's previous requirements for the quality assessment of medical care. For example, *Working Paper No. 6* indicates that medical audit is to be:

- undertaken by every doctor;
- regular and systematic;
- central to quality programmes;
- conducted within a clearly defined organizational framework;
- agreed locally between the profession and management;
- the responsibility of local medical audit committees;

and is to include reference to

- the patient's perspective;
- the use of resources (Department of Health, 1989b).

It is argued that the introduction of a competitive element in the NHS will ensure that purchasers will be establishing progressively more advanced quality standards and outcome measures in the health-care contracts they agree between themselves and the service providers – forcing providers to demonstrate the existence of formalized quality assurance programmes and meet jointly agreed standards (Bowden and Walshe, 1991).

AUDIT AND QUALITY – THE LINKS

The introduction of medical audit could mean that voluntary and sporadic quality assessment which rarely resulted in significant alterations in patterns of care, could be replaced by systematic and informed discussions that enable the development and assurance of agreed standards of care on a regular basis. It might be useful at this stage to provide examples of how these standards can be used in the audit process. An audit of the hospital care of acute asthma was able to set its standards of care in accordance with the standards recognized by the British Thoracic Society (Bell, Layton and Gabbey, 1991). Similarly, an audit concerning the care of diabetes in general practice took as its standards the eight clinical interventions identified by the British Diabetic Association as being critical to the effective care of diabetes in the community (Hill, 1991). Using nationally recognized guidelines as the basis for their explicit criteria enabled both audit groups to compare their current local practice with national standards and determine where they were not being met. Having previously agreed that achievement of the guidelines was an appropriate objective, in the absence of this achievement, both groups were in a stronger position to take remedial action.

In the new environment where purchasing organizations are able to purchase health care from any provider organization, the purchaser is arguably able to determine what services are required both in terms of quantity and quality, and require provider organi-

zations to compete for these services. If the Royal Colleges and the medical professional generally are reaching consensus about national standards of practice to be achieved, then these too could inform the content of health-care contracts.

So, for example, a purchaser could conceivably require its provider to provide respiratory medicine for the treatment of asthma in accordance with the British Thoracic Society guidelines (British Thoracic Society, 1990). If the contract for these services were placed on that basis, the respiratory physicians in the provider unit would be obliged to work in accordance with these guidelines with the possible added incentives that (1) the purchasing authority might require evidence from time to time that these guidelines were being adhered to; and (2) if the purchaser were not satisfied that the guidelines were being adopted on a regular basis, the contract could be placed elsewhere the following year.

RESEARCH AGENDA FOR CRITERION-BASED MEDICAL AUDIT

Notwithstanding the perceived intention of medical audit to have an impact on the quality of medical care, the Government's definition of medical audit did not refer to requirements to change practice as a result of medical audit – although subsequent Directives and policy have attempted to address this aspect. Instead, it has been the proponents of the process who have incorporated this aspect of change into their conceptualization of medical audit, arguing that to be effective, medical audit needs to follow a 'cycle', 'spiral' or 'staircase' of continual clinical development, which involves the determination of appropriate standards of care, the measurement and comparison of practice and a commitment to change (Shaw, 1980; Mitchell and Fowkes, 1985; Standing Committee on Postgraduate Medical Education, 1989; Irvine, 1990; Baker and Presley, 1990; Brice, 1989). This interpretation of medical audit addresses the tension – in part – that exists between medical audit being perceived on the one hand as an educational activity and on the other as a regulatory device (Berwick, 1989). It may also reflect a desire to rely on the new internal market to provide the necessary incentives for the promotion of change (McBride, 1992).

The use of criterion-based audit is not widespread as yet in the UK and only represents one technique used at present. Criterion-based audit requires a sophisticated knowledge of the relationships that exist between structure, process and outcome or – at the very least – the generation of criteria which are rigorously tested to validate their usage (Lembcke 1967; Brook *et al.*, 1973; Eddy 1990a). In particular, Eddy argues that it is 'dangerous to call something a standard unless the outcomes are truly known, the preferences are truly known, and the preferences are truly virtually unanimous'. Anything less is most likely to lead to the generation of practice guidelines which have an 'optional' status, and are entirely arbitrary in use (Eddy, 1990a).

The lack of scientific evidence to underpin effective clinical practice has long been the subject of discourse (Cochrane, 1972; Eddy, 1990a–l; Maynard, 1992), and it is only relatively recently that central monies have been invested to address this issue. In the absence of 'hard' standards, since the formal introduction of medical audit, 'softer' data has been collected by audit groups across the UK in non-criterion-based audits which have led to the identification of: potential criteria and standards for future validation; issues which can be addressed in the absence of 'harder data'; and additional information which could provide a sounder basis for clinical decision-making. That is, one can consider a continuum of questions underpinning clinical research through audit research to audit.

Medical research is used to decide how best to treat patients – whether using surgical techniques, drugs, or other means – by measuring and adjudicating the effect of clinical process on the patient. It is intended to answer the question 'what should we do?' at the broadest level and entails systematic investigation to explore cause and effect in the world of clinical science.

Audit research is a phrase coined here to describe the collection of local data to support an adjudication between alternative processes of care, when the basic clinical research has already been done. It is a grey area as to where clinical research stops and audit research starts: both are concerned with seeking better outcomes. Audit research is more limited in its overall pretensions, dealing with smaller populations, and local treatment regimes, rather than challenging basic clinical knowledge. The distinction between medical research and audit research is illustrated in the case studies detailed below.

The need for audit research is greatest in the absence of both **empirical** standards (which are derived from actual practice), and **normative** standards (derived from legitimate knowledge), with which the peer group agrees. It seeks to address the questions 'what are we doing?', 'what impact is it having?' and, given that knowledge, 'what should we do/change?'. Thus, if standards are to be set on the basis of an improvement of prevailing quality rather than the adoption of an ideal standard – for example from the relevant Royal College – it will be necessary to appraise current practice. The absence of agreement on either empirical or normative standards creates an initial difficulty in deciding which data should be collected as part of this appraisal, but if we hypothesize that certain criteria in care are related to better outcomes, we can call these **candidate criteria** and collect information in relation to them. Once collected, the data is available for peer group discussion and analysis. Tests can be performed to determine whether different processes or care regimes produce better outcomes, and substantive criteria and standards can be agreed by the local peer group.

Finally, once both clinical research and audit research have determined appropriate means of treating patients and appropriate treatment regimes within those means, it should be possible to develop standards and guidelines for future practice. Medical audit itself ensures that the appropriate procedures are carried out, and addresses the question 'are we doing what we are supposed to be doing?'. If the answer were in the negative, information collected within this stage could well provide the answer to the question 'why are we not doing what we should be doing?'

STUDY NO. 1: THE AUDIT OF DAY-CASE SURGERY

DAY-CASE SURGERY – THE NATIONAL PICTURE

In its report on day surgery, the Audit Commission highlighted the uneven distribution of day-case surgery in England and Wales (Audit Commission, 1990). Their analysis indicated that the extent to which some common appropriate procedures were treated as day cases varied from 0% to 100% between district health authorities. The Commission indicated that if all district health authorities performed day surgery consistently at readily achievable levels for 20 common procedures, an additional 186 000 patients could be treated each year without increased expenditure. The Commission noted the support for increased day-case surgery by the Royal College of Surgeons but also noted various obstacles that stood in its way:

- the difficulty in assessing and monitoring current and potential performance;
- poor management and organization of day-case facilities;
- clinician preference for more traditional approaches.

In its report, the Audit Commission recommended that these obstacles could be overcome and day-case surgery could be expanded, if the following were undertaken:

- a robust method of assessing performance, recording and monitoring progress;
- measures to improve the use made of day-case units, drawing on best practice in this country and elsewhere.

Subsequent to this Audit Commission report, the NHS Management Executive have selected four day-case surgical procedures for inclusion as performance indicators in the Patient's Charter comparative 'league' tables (Department of Health, 1994). The tables allegedly indicate how hospitals perform on 'allowing patients to go home on the same day as their operation' (p. 4), but there is an absence of discussion regarding the ambiguity of this seemingly benevolent action. For example, a hospital performing these procedures as day cases for 100% of its patients will receive the maximum of a five-star rating ('the more stars the better the performance'). However, this rating (based on throughput) will not be taking account of the condition of the patient at the time of discharge; the rate of subsequent recovery or the possibility of readmission. In addition, by stating that 'more' equals 'better', critical assumptions are being made in aggregate about the postoperative recovery rates of patients undergoing such operations and the home environment of such patients.

DAY-CASE SURGERY – THE LOCAL PICTURE

In common with all hospitals, day-case surgery in the case study hospital was reviewed in accordance with the Audit Commission methodology, to determine the amount of day surgery that was being undertaken in comparison with national statistics and to determine if there was any scope for the improvement of the efficiency and effectiveness of facilities for day surgery. The review indicated that, for a number of surgical procedures, the case study hospital had day surgery levels that fell below the national average. Two factors appeared to produce this effect: first, the team noted that existing information systems were poor, leading to day-case activity levels being inaccurately recorded. Secondly, a number of consultants expressed reservations about performing certain procedures as day cases, objecting on medical grounds to the suitability of some of the basket procedures for day-case surgery and raising concerns that the quality of patient care might suffer an increase in day-case throughput.

In response to the findings of the local Audit Team report, the clinical directorate for surgery wished to increase day-case surgery where appropriate. To support this increase they wished to do the following:

- improve the accuracy of data collection on day-case surgical activity;
- obtain information about the quality of day-case surgery being undertaken at present;
- increase the level of day-case surgical activity;
- audit the quality of day-case surgery on a regular basis to ensure that increasing activity is not having a detrimental effect on the quality of service provided.

The Audit Commission has identified 20 surgical procedures which can be appropriately undertaken as day-case procedures. In this case study hospital, these day-case procedures are performed in two different settings: (1) the Adult Day-Case Unit and (2) a ward in the main hospital. Furthermore, depending on the location, timing and outcome of the operation, it is possible that the patient could be discharged the same day or required to stay overnight. Thus, the audit of day-case surgical procedures needed to include day-case procedures performed in all three categories of care:

- **Category 1**: Day-case procedure performed in adult day-case unit with patient discharged the same day;
- **Category 2**: Day-case procedure performed in hospital ward setting with patient discharged the same day;

- **Category 3**: Day-case procedure performed in hospital ward setting with overnight stay by patient.

PROJECT METHODOLOGY

- Which individuals are being selected for the different categories of care?
- What is the standard of care being provided **within each category of care**?
- Is there a difference in the standard of care being provided between the alternative categories of care and if so, is this a significant difference?

From the Audit Commission's 'basket' of 20 surgical procedures deemed appropriately undertaken as day-case procedures, the project team selected 10 surgical procedures for audit in this project. A major factor in this decision was the desire to involve as many surgeons as possible in the exercise:

- hernia repair;
- nasal fracture reduction;
- circumcision;
- extraction of teeth;
- cystoscopy;
- laparoscopy;
- sterilization (by laparoscopy);
- breast lump biopsy;
- dilation and curettage (D&C);
- cataract.

Information was collected along five dimensions (the items that make up these dimensions are contained in Appendix 1).

- patient characteristics (e.g. age, gender, medical characteristics, living arrangements);
- measures of structure (e.g. grade of surgeon or anaesthetist);
- measures of process (e.g. anaesthetic, tests, explanations);
- measures of postoperative outcome at 1–4 hours, 24 hours and 7 days (e.g. need for painkillers, complications, use of services);

- measures of patient satisfaction/perception (e.g. worries, aspects of hospital).

This information was collected through a series of questionnaires:

- four questionnaires completed by the patient (one preoperative and three postoperative);
- two questionnaires completed by the nurse (one preoperative and, for those patients discharged the same day, one postoperative);
- one questionnaire completed by the anaesthetist/theatre staff (postoperative).

OPERATIONAL ISSUES

The audit was able to elicit a considerable amount of information about the patient experience of those individuals undergoing a day-case procedure. However the distribution of questionnaires, collection and subsequent analysis of this information was very labour-intensive. This observation is borne out by Black in his discussion of the development of a national comparative audit service for day surgery (Black *et al.*, 1993), in which he notes

that: 'clinicians and managers locally must appreciate the need to commit realistic resources to the exercise. Without these resources the survey will at best be a waste of time and at worst produce misleading results which might lead to erroneous management decisions'.

It is worth noting too that the audit required considerable input and cooperation from anaesthetists, nurses, theatre staff and ward clerks, and ironically the surgeons (who commissioned the audit) were the least affected by it.

INPATIENT OR DAY CASE?

As noted above, consultants were concerned about performing day-case surgery. Using a Chi-square test on the collected data, the researchers tested the null hypothesis that there would be no difference in questionnaire response between those patients treated as inpatients and those treated in the Adult Day-Case Unit (ADC). The findings of this exercise are contained in Table 9.1.

This small project provided a guarded conclusion that, with careful monitoring and

Table 9.1 A comparison of day-case and inpatient care

Dimension of care	Expectations	Findings
Characteristics of the patients	Differences	Very few differences
Outcome of care	Differences	Very few differences
Structure supporting the treatment	Differences	Differences noted
Process of care supporting the treatment	No differences	Difficult to substantiate, but evident that some differences
Patient satisfaction/perception	Mixed as to whether any differences	The only significant difference between inpatients and ADC patients was that, of those expressing a preference (85% of respondents), patients were more likely to recommend the care that they themselves had received!

patient selection, there is scope to increase day-case surgery in selected areas. However, it obviously cannot guide any decisions where day-case surgery is not systematically used at present. Patient selection in any increase is crucial. Patients without appropriate transport or home facilities or environment may not continue to be 'satisfied' with day care. As a result, re-audit **after a significant increase in ADC for selected conditions** is crucial, and should involve patient satisfaction on a surveys on a comprehensive basis as well as clinical and medical audit by 'experts'. Such (re-)audit should pay attention to whether, within ADC, and inpatient care, satisfaction is maintained. Audit research of this nature provides a framework for cautiously changing local case management and a basis for continuing audit under new arrangements. But it should be noted that limited conclusions from small samples cannot provide a glib source of dramatic policy and management change. (Black *et al.* (1993) notes the difficulties of comparative audit using small numbers.)

Before dramatic increases in day-case unit throughput, attention should be paid to social, class and other characteristics to ensure that patient care is both adequate and equitable. Given the national drive towards day-case surgery, it is important that the policy is not adopted irresponsibly and later discredited.

STATUS OF DATA

The collection of a considerable amount of 'new' data in this project illustrated the need to set clear objectives as to the purpose of this data collection. As noted above, the surgeons were particularly interested to interrogate this data for any associations between particular outcomes and care settings, which could arguably be construed as 'poor man's research'. However, it is important to note that this data collection also represented the only systematic collection of information on the patient experience. For the first time

surgeons were able to discover how patients fared after discharge (something that a retrospective audit of process cannot do). Notwithstanding this, the survey did not look at the detail of surgical techniques used. Nor was any attempt made to set standards **before** the audit, thereby ensuring that the baseline of 'quality' (before the increase in day-case surgery) was taken as that which was prevailing at the time of the survey.

STUDY NO. 2: THE AUDIT OF POSTOPERATIVE PAIN RELIEF

INTRODUCTION

Concern over low standards of postoperative pain relief has been expressed nationally in the joint report by the Colleges of Surgeons and Anaesthetists (1990). The local Anaesthetic Department wished to audit postoperative pain relief in relation to all surgery which is conducted. Postoperative pain relief obtained by patients undergoing intermediate and minor surgery has been the subject of the first audit. In determining the 'quality' of postoperative pain relief, two themes were of particular interest to the Department: (1) the incidence and impact of preoperative discussions and (2) the nature of the drugs used preoperatively, in theatre and postoperatively, and their impact.

PROJECT METHODOLOGY

Hernia and varicose vein operations were selected to represent intermediate and minor surgery. The process and outcome of the anaesthetic process associated with these two surgical procedures were audited through the use of two surveys:

- one questionnaire to be completed by the patient (postoperatively);
- one review form to be completed by the audit assistant (postoperatively), using information from the case notes.

The lack of commonly agreed standards within the Department meant that information was to be collected and reviewed for itself, as opposed to being collected for comparison with predetermined standards. Information collected about the patient was categorized along four dimensions (the questions that comprise these dimensions are contained in Appendix 2):

- patient characteristics (e.g. age and gender);
- measures of process (e.g. preoperative discussions, drugs, postoperative advice);
- measures of patient satisfaction (e.g. satisfaction with postoperative pain relief);
- measures of outcome (e.g. experience of pain, requests for painkillers).

The incidence of postoperative pain was measured using a visual analogue scale, on which patients were asked to mark the pain they experienced (in the recovery area and on the ward). The scale was 10 cm long, with no divisions. One end of the scale was marked 'none', the other 'worst pain imaginable'. In all, 100 patients were surveyed in this particular project (50 patients per procedure).

THE INCIDENCE AND IMPACT OF PREOPERATIVE DISCUSSIONS

Kuhn *et al.* (1990) refer to a number of studies that indicate that information given either orally or in writing to the patient can reduce postoperative pain and anxiety. The data from this survey indicated the number of patients with whom postoperative pain and its control was discussed, and the extent to which patients had found it helpful with regard to postoperative pain and reducing anxiety. It is sometimes argued that collecting data about the patient process from the patient is a more reliable form of data collection than self-reporting by health-care professionals. However, the fact that 13% of patients said that they did not know whether or not postoperative pain and its control had been discussed illustrates the extent to which collecting data from both sources might be more appropriate.

FORMS OF DRUG USAGE

By collecting information from the case notes, it was possible to provide a summary of the complete anaesthetic/analgesic route taken by each patient in the sample. This summary graphically illustrated the range of clinical practice in this particular field. Including the analgesics prescribed postoperatively, a number of drug combinations were used for this sample population and it was anticipated that this variation in drug combination would be of considerable interest to the practitioners. The presence of different combinations in the administration of drugs to this group of 100 patients meant that it was not possible to statistically test the strength of association between each combination and its outcome. However, this did not preclude the sighting of apparent associations and a careful analysis of the data generated two hypotheses for discussion and/or later testing:

- a particular intra-operative drug is associated with reducing postoperative pain;
- a particular postoperative drug is associated with a high incidence of nausea and vomiting.

POLICY AND CONCLUSIONS

This 'audit' (which could almost be considered a pre-'audit research' audit) raised a number of issues for future policy on clinical standards in this area.

It has been suggested that patients have a low expectation of postoperative pain relief (or a high expectation of postoperative pain). Although 97% of the patients surveyed within this project said they were satisfied with their pain relief, the appropriateness of this as a valid measure of 'quality' needs to be discussed in the light of levels of pain actually experienced and the number of patients for whom pain was not relieved.

On what basis should a policy on future practice be agreed by the peer group? For example, given that there appears to be considerable variation in the combination of drugs administered to these patients, would it be possible (or desirable) for clinicians to agree to the use of a specific regime(s) only? Furthermore, what evidence do clinicians require before they are willing to agree to the use of specific regime(s)? Is the medical literature sufficient? Would a controlled trial be necessary?

Which criteria should be used for measuring quality? If it is desirable to measure process, with what levels of process are we comfortable (e.g. the specification of particular drugs, or overall regimes)? If it is desirable to measure outcome, do we wish to specify standards on an individual basis or do we wish to specify standards for the whole department? What do we think are 'acceptable' levels of pain to be experienced after an operation?

Who should be the constituents of the 'peer group'? Is it more appropriate to include nurses and surgeons, and thereby become 'clinical audit'?

STUDY NO. 3: PRIMARY–SECONDARY CARE INTERFACE AUDIT

MANAGING HEALTH-CARE QUALITY AT THE PRIMARY–SECONDARY CARE INTERFACE

Although comparative data illustrates that countries providing health care through a primary–secondary 'gateway' achieve a more efficient use of resources than those allowing free access to secondary care (Cartwright and Windsor, 1992; Frankel and West, 1993), a number of empirical studies of the primary–secondary care interface suggest that this might not be the case at a micro- or individual patient level. In particular, much research and discussion has focused on the variation in GP referral rates, the incidence of inappropriate repeat outpatient attendances and the lengthy waiting lists that exist for certain specialties.

Where there is inappropriate referral, inappropriate repeat outpatient attendances and

inappropriate waiting, some patients are suffering dissatisfaction, unmet need, unnecessary waiting, and a needless loss of their time and money. If hospital resources and time are expended on unnecessary consultations, citizens are also potential losers, since their future needs may remain unmet because of a wastage of finite resources and the 'blocking' of clinics by inappropriately booked outpatients.

Although the introduction of contracts for health care and a requirement to participate in medical audit may provide a powerful impetus for improving quality at the primary–secondary interface in the future, this potential is worth examining in more detail. Previous endeavours to address these instances of inappropriate patient care have focused on fostering closer collaboration between the two sectors – albeit on a voluntary basis only. Ironically, this important principle may be lost in the move towards encouraging and compelling change within a competitive environment. A more detailed examination of these new initiatives highlights that, without joint collaboration, some of the mechanisms will be insufficient to assure the quality of care for patients at the primary–secondary interface.

Medical audit has the potential to encourage more appropriate referrals and repeat outpatient attendances. However, while participation in medical audit within each sector might encourage individual improvements in the quality of primary and secondary care, the distinction between the providers of care in each sector may diminish the contribution which medical audit could make to the **complete** referral and discharge process. It is worth remembering that, in many cases, members from both sides of the purchaser/provider split contribute to patient care; the successful outcome of a surgical intervention, for example, might be dependent on the diagnostic skills of the referring general practitioner. Without specialist knowledge from secondary care, doctors in the primary sector might be under- or over-estimating their role in the management of certain conditions. Without reference to a patient's subsequent re-adjustment to life out of a hospital, a specialist may not realize the full implications of a particular process. In this way, the quality being defined and assessed within each sector may reflect only a partial 'truth' about the total needs of the patient. This is illustrated by looking at studies that have attempted to assess the appropriateness of referrals (see Sanders, Coulter and McPherson, 1989 for a comprehensive review of the literature).

Of these studies, only a few use standards derived from the medical literature to assess the appropriateness of referrals. In the vast majority of studies, appropriateness is judged by the hospital consultants. Coulter notes that, since clinical uncertainty and differences in opinion exist in hospital specialties as well as in the primary sector, looking to specialist opinion for a standard against which to judge the appropriateness of referrals may be misleading (Coulter, 1990). Just as important to note is that a specialist opinion often does not take account of the patient perspective. Over 80% of patients in the study of orthopaedic outpatient referrals in Doncaster reported that they were helped by seeing the consultant, despite consultants judging that almost half of the referrals were probably, or definitely, inappropriate (Roland *et al.*, 1991).

Although we have seen the introduction of GP contracts, the ability of patients to move their registration from one general practice to another, the introduction of Patient's Charter standards into the primary sector and an increase in GP accountability to the FHSAs, there is little in the primary care sector equivalent to the secondary care 'quality process'. Thus, through a re-alignment of roles, the patient is potentially being drawn outside the contract specifications and quality assurance programmes that purchasers are beginning to demand in the secondary sector. Although GPs are required to participate in regular

medical audit, the section above outlines the limitations of assessing care from one interface perspective only, and highlights the need for joint collaboration in this field.

DEVELOPMENT OF JOINT MEDICAL AUDIT

By encouraging joint collaboration and feedback of relevant information across the interface, joint medical audit, could provide an appropriate vehicle for improving the management of patients both within and between, the primary and secondary care sectors. This potential has not gone unnoticed by a number of commentators (Marinker, Wilkin and Metcalfe, 1988; Light, 1990; Cartwright and Windsor, 1992; Frankel and West, 1993).

The development of medical audit is underpinned by the continued development of explicit criteria and standards. Participation in joint medical audit by both general practitioners and hospital doctors would encourage the recognition and reconciliation of a number of different perspectives within joint standard-setting exercises. It could also lead to a wider focus on the structure, process and outcome of health care. Hitherto, each element has been defined – and assessed – within the confines of each care setting. Within joint medical audit, the structure, process and outcome of health care could be defined along a continuum of care that commences in the community, travels through secondary care and terminates in the community once the patient has been discharged from all medical care (rather like the 'end result' that Codman first envisaged (Lembcke, 1967).

Participation in joint medical audit could also play an important role in improving communications between general practitioners and hospital doctors. A number of studies of the referral process highlight the lack of clear communication that occurs at the interface. Jones, Lloyd and Kwartz (1990) highlighted the lack of information contained in 500 referral letters, and Kentish, Jenkins and Lask (1987) noted that insufficient information was contained in psychiatric reports to GPs for them to fully appreciate their role in relation to the child and family while treatment was carried out. Likewise, Williams and Fitton (1990) noted that a lack of information conveyed to the GP was a contributory factor in unplanned readmission to hospital (within 28 days of discharge) in 49 out of 133 cases. Inevitably, such events have a knock-on effect with regard to overall waiting times for outpatient and inpatient consultations. As noted above, this lack of clarity in intention and decision can also have an impact on the number of repeat referrals and repeat attendances which the insufficiently informed GP, or hospital doctor, may be making.

In recognition of their operational differences, the Department of Health made a distinction between the organizational structures, responsibilities and funding required for the development of medical audit within the primary and secondary care sectors. Thus, although there is a degree of interaction between the two organizational structures at a local level (the medical audit advisory groups in the primary sector and the local medical audit committees in the secondary sector), members of both groups have been more heavily involved in developing medical audit within their own discrete spheres of work than in sharing their endeavours at the interface.

RESEARCH AGENDA FOR JOINT MEDICAL AUDIT

An integral part of medical audit is the determination of appropriate standards by which to assess quality. Determining such standards at the interface requires considerable thought and skill, particularly if they are to reflect the views of all the participants in the referral process. Within the new environment of the NHS, managers may also need to express their opinion as to appropriate standards –

since their responsibility is to the population, as opposed to the individual.

In addressing the reconciliation of different perspectives, Irvine argues that doctors and managers have to attempt to develop a comprehensive blend of components that will reflect a 'reasonable consensus' across all the groups concerned and thus minimize the risk of misunderstanding the term 'quality' (Irvine, 1990). In addressing the same issue, Ovretveit argues that the way to proceed is to explicitly recognize these differences and accept that whilst – on occasion – quality can be improved from all perspectives, in other cases trade-offs will be necessary (Ovretveit, 1992).

The evaluation of one's work by one's peers is a delicate process and requires trust, respect and understanding among the peers. Within joint medical audit, these characteristics need to exist between members of the medical profession who do not work in the same settings, may never meet each other, do not work under the same conditions and do not necessarily share the same clinical expectations. Moreover, placing GPs and hospital doctors within a competitive environment could provide further barriers to the cultivation of a cooperative environment between such peers.

Reference has already been made to the range of mechanisms required to bring about a change in clinical practice. Encouraging a commitment to change in current practice, where appropriate, is a challenge in any environment. This challenge is intensified at the interface due to the diverse nature of the peer group involved and the different functions each clinician performs. A number of studies have attempted to address the issues of interface quality. Unfortunately, however, well defined and well argued their case for change might have been, the majority suffered from the absence of any mechanism to ensure that their recommendations were translated into positive action. Exploring the feasibility and appropriateness of joint medical audit in improving quality at the interface raises a number of questions to be addressed.

- Is it possible to determine jointly, appropriate standards of care and measure and compare practice, and what are the determinants of its success?
- Is it possible to develop a joint commitment to change and what are the determinants of its success?

PROJECT METHODOLOGY

It was the intention of the project team to address the research agenda of both criterion-based medical audit and joint medical audit, through a series of developmental audit projects with local GPs and hospital doctors. The project team conducted a series of exploratory interviews with a number of general practitioners and hospital doctors. A common theme running through these interviews was a perceived need for greater communication, collaboration, interaction and coordination between the primary and secondary sectors.

Particular concern was expressed about the structure, process and/or outcome of the following primary-secondary care characteristics:

- waiting times for first outpatient appointments;
- referral and postconsultation letters;
- the alignment of roles and responsibilities between the two sectors.

Each characteristic and its impact on the quality of patient care is capable of being perceived in different ways by the medical profession – particularly differently by GPs and hospital doctors, who do not work under the same conditions and do not necessary share the same clinical expectations. Thus, in order to obtain a more stable conceptualization of these characteristics and their relationship to quality health care, the project team conducted a literature review in each of the three areas, while at the same time targeting the second study on particular specialties (ENT, ophthalmology, dermatology) and the third study on a specific condition (upper GI discomfort). The literature reviews provided a frame of reference within which the project team was able to pursue the same basic methodology to different stages of fruition (Table 9.2).

Table 9.2 Project methodology

- Is there a variation in process?
- Is there a variation in outcome?
- Are some outcomes preferable to others?
- Is there joint agreement on this?
- Which processes are likely to lead to the better outcomes?
- Is there joint agreement on this?
- Do the preferred processes lead to better outcomes?
- What action is required to promote a joint move towards better outcomes?

OBSERVATIONS AND CONCLUSIONS

In the process of working towards the development of sets of criteria for a range of primary–secondary interactions, the project team was able to observe: the dynamic mechanism of developing audit criteria and standards; the changing relationship between the primary and secondary care sector; the potential contribution of joint medical audit; and the interaction between the market, internal quality management systems and professional collaboration. A summary of the project findings is contained in Table 9.3.

Table 9.3   Summary of project findings

Project methodology	Study No. 1 (Outpatient waiting time)	Study No. 2 (Referral and postconsulation letters)	Study No. 3 Upper GI endoscopy)
Is there a variation in process?	There is variation in the methods of calculating outpatient waiting time	There is variation in the content of letters and the extent to which the senders and recipients of referral and postconsultation letters share a mutual understanding of the appropriate patient-based information to include in the letter	There is variation in access, and follow-up, to upper GI endoscopy for patients being referred with upper GI discomfort. There is also variation in GP management of upper GI discomfort
Is there a variation in output/outcome?	The variance in formulae for calculating outpatient waiting times results in different answers being obtained to the same question. The information obtained does not enable valid comparisons to be made across districts, between units and between clinics	There is variation in the effectiveness with which the recipient can address the needs of the patient	The variation in clinical outcome was not tested. However, there is variation in the secondary care experience for the patient: at one end, the patient may need to travel to the hospital for a consultation on at least three separate occasions at the other, the patient only need visit the hospital once
Are some outputs/ outcomes preferable to others?	Outpatient waiting times that are comparable, accurate, validated, widely -available, regularly updated, case-specific and fit for a given purpose	Putting the recipient in the position of being able to meet the needs of the patient as effectively as possible	GPs and hospital specialists agreed that the desired outcome of the upper GI endoscopy itself was a timely notification of an accurate diagnosis, coupled with high patient satisfaction and low patient morbidity. The endoscopy was seen as one part of a sequence of events that led to subsequent investigations or the reassurance of the patient (in the case of a negative pathology), or timely management action (in the case of a positive pathology)
Is there joint agreement on this?	Yes	Yes	Opinion differed as to the cohort of patients/ population to which this sequence of events should apply
Which processes are likely to lead to the better outputs/ outcomes?	The calculation of outpatient waiting times from a distribution of prospective or retrospective waiting times	The joint determination of essential information to be included in referral and post-consulation letters	There was no agreement among GPs and hospital specialists as to which set of processes was more likely to lead to the desired outcomes

Table 9.3   (cont'd)

Project methodology	Study No. 1 (Outpatient waiting time)	Study No. 2 (Referral and postconsulation letters)	Study No. 3 Upper GI endoscopy)
Is there joint agreement on this?	Yes	There was joint agreement to the principle, but opinions differed as to whether it could be operationalized	Opinions differed as to the most effective means of selecting patients, reaching an accurate diagnosis, reassurance and organizing timely follow-up treatment
Do they?	Yes: as tested by East Anglian Regional Health Authority	Yes and no: it is possible to identify generic letter contents which senders and recipients believe would (on occasion) produce more effective letters. However, it is not possible for these contents to reflect the required specificity and sensitivity of each situation. It is possible, however, to use the generic letter contents as a base from which the primary and secondary care clinicians can reach mutual understanding as to which information the recipient requires in specific situations	This was untested in this study. There has been little localized research to illustrate which processes are likely to lead to the better outcomes. Each clinician has put forward what his/her clinical preference would be based on his/her own own individual experiences personal code of medical ethics
What action is required to promote a joint move towards better outputs/ outcomes?	The specification in health-care contracts that out-patient waiting times should be calculated from a distribution of prospective or retrospective waiting times (or an equivalent method that will allow outpatient waiting times to be comparable, accurate, validated and fit for the given purpose)	The establishment of joint peer review of referral and postconsultation letters on a regular basis	The conduct of local audit research, i.e. systematic study to discover the best care processes and which processes are leading to better outcomes

More specifically, the project has seen the following developments:

- a model for ensuring that outpatient waiting times are comparable, accurate, validated, case specific and fit for a given purpose (McBride *et al.*, 1993a);
- a model for the joint primary and secondary care peer review of letters (including the examples of desired letter contents developed in the specialties of ENT, ophthalmology and dermatology) (McBride *et al.*, 1993b);
- a model for determining an appropriate alignment of roles and responsibilities for patients with upper GI discomfort (McBride *et al.*, 1993c).

The project team believe that if the quality of information and the mutual understanding of that information were improved along the lines suggested within each study report, it would contribute significantly to improving quality at the primary–secondary interface.

It was argued above that secondary care health-care contracts and individual primary or secondary care medical audit were insufficient in themselves to ensure overall quality care for the patient. The findings of the three studies have confirmed this view. Without defining the responsibilities of GPs in the primary sector, contracts and audit will not be able to ensure the quality of care for the individual **who has not been referred**. Likewise, although GPs will be able to assure the quality of their community-based practice, through regular and systematic medical audit, they may not necessarily be able to assure the quality of their referral practice without the specialist knowledge of the secondary care sector.

However, despite the need for symmetry between the two professions, the studies highlighted the differences that exist between members within each care sector, as well as between the care sectors. This is not necessarily surprising. Within each care sector it can be a reflection of the different stages of education and experience which each physician possesses. Between the care sectors it can be a reflection of the respective roles of the primary and secondary physician and the different cohorts of patients that they see. The interviews with GPs highlighted the responsibility they held for individuals on their practice list, and interviews with hospital specialists highlighted the responsibility they held for individuals who were referred to their specialty (or who were likely to be referred to their particular specialty).

What is important to discuss is the extent to which these differences remain unresolved with reference to the total care of the patient. This is illustrated most starkly in Study No. 3, where there are a number of different ways in which physicians **believe** patients with upper GI discomfort are best managed – with no overall attempt to discover what is the best for the resident population.

VARIANTS OF AUDIT: SOME HARD QUESTIONS

Reference has been made above to the number of research questions that underpin the continuum from medical research to medical audit. The case studies have also illustrated the variants of these questions in clinical practice. As well as the policy question 'who commissions the audit, or in whose interests, or on whose agenda is it carried out?' there is the fundamental question 'what is being audited?'

One type of audit sees doctors looking at the internal quality of how they do things. That is, they do not question the practices in which they are engaged (i.e. what they are doing) nor do they question their use of different techniques. Instead they are merely checking that they are performing their chosen techniques properly.

A higher level of audit would question whether the most appropriate techniques or processes are being used to achieve desired outcomes. This might lead to conflict between doctors within a specialty who disagree on the most appropriate techniques or processes.

The highest level of audit questions outcomes and might therefore lead to radical questions as to whether activities themselves are worthwhile, and deserve continued funding. So, for example, an audit of dilation and curettage (D&C) operations could indicate that they are being performed to the highest standard. However, there is much disagreement about the effectiveness of this womb operation, some clinicians arguing that it is inaccurate and ineffective and its usage should be reassessed.

Naturally, if one moves to the more radical agenda, it can be seen that audit is merely one part of an integral management concern

– with effectiveness of care; with use of resources; and therefore arguably with health policy itself. In other words, audit can help answer questions concerned with the utility as well as the cost of medical interventions – and can be part of an economist's concerns as well as a doctor's concerns.

It is not surprising that, with the whole arena of audit embracing such a grey area, doctors have rightly often been suspicious of the agenda. If behind exhortations to medical audit is a health economist with a bee in his/her bonnet, or a manager with a budget axe to wield – or a politician with a combination of both – then it is as well to be clear about what audit is and is not!

The above discussion also shows that medical audit may easily become clinical audit: that is, it may be a concern for the whole health-care team and not simply the concern of the clinician. Equally, audit (whether medical or clinical) may become concerned with overall priorities and 'the business' of the hospital department concerned. That is, it may therefore (by default or otherwise), become the concern of the whole hospital – or indeed the whole community outside the hospital. Thus does medical audit become an integral part of quality management overall. Nevertheless, it is necessary to illustrate some of the complexities involved in what might seem a simple activity of simply assuring adequate quality:

- Consider the case of two different treatment regimes for the same diagnostic condition or disease. It is not simply a case of one being better than the other. Considered for their effect over different patients and the whole population, Treatment Regime 1 produces a higher percentage of excellent outcomes but equally a higher percentage of poor or even dangerous outcomes, including death. In other words, it may be a more risky treatment. Treatment Regime 2 produces less bad outcomes but less excel-

lent outcomes and (if we want to make our example even more interesting) a less good average across all patients. This assumes that outcomes can be ranked as 'utilities' for patients and averaged (itself a contentious assumption but one often used in economic studies of benefit and outcome).

There is no managerial or 'scientific' means of simply categorizing either Treatment Regime 1 or Treatment Regime 2 as 'the better one'. **Value judgements** have to be brought into play – does the patient, the doctor, the clinical director, the trust managers or the purchasing health authority prefer a riskier treatment with a better average outcome (or chance of excellent outcome for the individual patient) or a less risky procedure?

In such cases, it might be thought that the clinician should decide, (in conjunction with the patient or not, depending upon one's views of patient consent) which procedure to follow. In this circumstance, medical audit would simply mean that – whichever procedure was followed – the best processes were used, against a backdrop of the best resources available (the 'structure' of medical care), to seek the best outcome given the treatment regime adopted. But, in making this decision, consider the following.

- Although there is no better treatment regime by agreed criteria (i.e. values must come into play to decide which is to be used), the treatment regimes do not have the same **cost**. Furthermore, in a clinical directorate within a trust, the budget is naturally limited – not just for this particular diagnosis or disease but for the whole range of treatments available for the patients that present within the specialty. (It should be noted further that budgets have to be allocated not only within specialties, but between specialties.)

Even though doctors – and their patients – within the clinical directorate may have different values, they have to make decisions based on their share of pooled and limited resources. Some means must be found of deciding what to do if money is not available to fund all clinicians' preferences for treatment of patients with this diagnosis. A number of options arise.

Firstly, decisions can be taken on the basis of individual patients presenting, and the 'first call on the resources' through the financial year decides how they are spent. This may be the best way to proceed, even though it is not within the spirit of overt prioritization, or 'overt purchasing' after the NHS reforms. It may, however, be the best way for the reason that alternative means may be excessively bureaucratic without producing commensurate benefit to compensate for such bureaucratic costs.

Secondly, a means for mediating between values and getting the clinicians to agree on the procedure may be sought – taking into account the different costs but not necessarily in a decision-making process wholly dominated by cost. In this circumstance, audit is used as a means of making clinical choices, or at least of resolving clinical differences in a managerial context. One means of proceeding (untried as far as we know) may be as follows: the doctors with the different values, using the different treatment regimes (neither of which 'dominates' the other, either morally or practically), may rate the expected utility to the patients of using the regime, measure this against cost and then provide a cost–utility ranking for either the clinical director or the management of the hospital. (You can see already how we are into uncharted waters in transferring clinical decisions away from doctors.)

In this circumstance, however, clinicians will quite naturally wish to boost their own procedure by attributing high utility to it. It can therefore be seen that

the attribution of utility (in the economist's sense) is a somewhat arbitrary and value-laden process in itself. All measurements – such as the quality adjusted life year – are in fact translating values into numbers – it is a question of **whose** values (those of the doctors, patients, hospital or society in general).

• Such a situation is likely to lead to a search for further information. Which patients are those who – using the 'more exciting but riskier' procedure – are most likely to suffer? Can further research show which would benefit from Treatment Regime 1 as opposed to Treatment Regime 2 with greater degrees of certainty? The doctor might then be able to make a more unequivocal clinical choice in the long term.

This is how (what we have called) audit research can complement basic clinical research: in other words, audit in this circumstance consists in a means for adjudicating between procedures by deriving further information.

Even if this is possible (and it is unlikely to be productive of unequivocal results or a clear prescription for action, certainly in the short term), there is still the thorny problem of attributing different utilities to different patients from different treatment regimes, with different costs, in order to create a practical framework for decisions.

Again, it may be better simply to proceed informally than to systematize on the basis of imperfect information and producing an intimidating and bureaucratic means for regulating clinical behaviour.

• Further complexities are added by remembering that provider budgets are allocated **between** specialties and clinical directorates as well as within them. Is there to be a scientific attribution of expected cost utility in order to allocate resources to such directorates, or is historical data on funding to be used along with a respect for individual clinicians' preferences? Now we are at the level of board decisions within the hospital – individual directorates cannot decide other directorates' priorities!

But wait – we are not just in the domain of decision-making within the hospital. We are talking about the **purchaser's** wishes also. And whom does the purchaser represent? The purchaser represents the Government, which (in an ideal world!) represents social preference.

It may be argued that this is a hypothetical example – or rather that the argument follows from a hypothetical example, based on different treatment regimes – which will not apply in the real world. Mercifully such conundrums do not always apply. But they apply more often than the sceptic might acknowledge. Many pioneering medical techniques will be of this nature – they will produce better results in some cases and more dangerous or worse results in others – certainly in the short term until greater knowledge and greater skill is derived.

Furthermore, controlling for dangerous outcomes may produce success in small-scale research or small-scale audit settings – for example, in specialized units dedicated to such purposes. Yet, generalizing to the health service as a whole may prevent such effectiveness from being generalized (this is in fact the difference between **efficacy**, achieved under conditions of research, or pilot projects, and **effectiveness**, achieved generally throughout the system.

More commonly, different treatment regimes will over time be seen to be better or worse under different conditions. They will, of course, have different costs attached. A scientific approach to choosing priorities would therefore do some sort of a cost/utility calculation – based on the principle (from health economics) that procedures that generate a high utility per fixed cost ought to be adopted before others. In practice, however – especially in specialties where the NHS is

unequivocally expected to care for the patient – such scientific procedures will lie in the realm either of Utopia or Nightmare.

The danger is that standardization of clinical practice may occur through overt purchasing (i.e. interventionist choice by a budget-holding purchaser), where 'managed care' is chosen by the purchaser on the basis of cost considerations. This is the kind of grey area where management *Diktat* or management persuasion may seek to influence clinical decision-making. Clinical freedom is a valuable concept when properly used and ought not to be abandoned lightly. Standardization of medical or clinical process, in the name of quality, may produce quite the reverse for certain patients. It is important that fads allegedly adopted in pursuit of quality (such as 'process engineering' and all the other pieces of jargon adopted, in order to persuade professionals and workers of the alleged scientific basis of management), are adopted only as a result of an intellectual, indeed humanist, discussion and on the basis of consensus between managers and clinicians.

On the other hand, there is no doubt that, given constrained resources, it is not simply a matter for clinicians to decide what to do – there must be agreement between clinicians, whole clinical directorates, providers as a whole and purchasers as to how money is to be spent – even if there is flexibility in allocating resources and flexibility in spending it.

The danger of the new arrangements in the NHS, following the NHS reforms, is that standardization through the contracting process may lead to the adoption of 'cheaper and worse procedures', justified by an audit process. Such a process would not be medical or clinical audit, but management or 'resource management' audit. Clinical audit would be at its most useful when it could identify procedures that are both worse **and** more expensive.

There is no doubt that different outcomes with different costs attached are a matter for adjudication through the audit process. Indeed it is desirable, according to the Government, that audit ought to include questions of resources – and that therefore medical audit and 'resource management' ought to be linked to processes. Unfortunately, medical audit was 'sold' to the medical profession as something less threatening – in order to get a toehold for such a process within a sceptical profession, and to move audit (which has a lengthy pedigree) into the domain of resources.

DISCUSSION

- Medical audit originated as a limited policy to encourage doctors to audit aspects of their behaviour. One of the working papers associated with the NHS reforms (*Working Paper No. 6 – Medical Audit*) made self-audit by the medical profession mandatory, but did not stipulate exactly which procedures within which specialties were to be audited: that was to be a matter for local choice.

- As control of medicine by management increased rapidly following the implementation of the NHS reforms, medical audit became in some cases a focus for discussion in the contracting process between purchasers and providers (health authorities and hospitals in the main). Furthermore, medical audit (involving only doctors) became generalized in some instances into clinical audit (involving a range of professions, especially the nursing profession, and sometimes management as well). Nevertheless, in the main medical audit *per se* is a separate activity for doctors, whereas clinical audit is a broader aspect of the managerially driven 'quality assurance'.

- It can be argued that various forms of medical audit in the broadest sense have been conducted throughout the history of

the National Health Service. More recently, in the 1980s, the Confidential Enquiry into Perioperative Deaths (CEPOD) considered the results of operations in a search for avoidable deaths. Participation in enquiries such as this was itself, however, voluntary.

- There are various semi-systematic means of conducting quality assessment, based on analysing the structure of process and outcome of the health-care process. While it is difficult to measure outcome directly, process is often used as a surrogate – with varying degrees of success.

- An important aspect of audit is not simply investigation but change in both clinical and arguably managerial practice in order ensure that quality assessment becomes incorporated into a wider process of quality assurance – to investigate and maintain quality, through change of behaviour where appropriate. These 'behavioural' aspects have often proved the most difficult to tackle.

- Clinical research concerns the investigation of how different types of intervention produce different types of results. Medical audit, on the other hand, may be considered to be at the other end of the continuum: in other words, once the process has been agreed, audit investigates whether or not it is being appropriately carried out. This is, however, a simplistic distinction between research and audit – or rather, a definition of two ends of a spectrum, which contains intermediate points. One of these points may usefully be termed 'audit research' (a phrase coined here). This refers to a stage after which basic clinical research has been conducted, but when it is still uncertain as to which interventions are most effective in which circumstances, and so forth. As a result, one is not simply auditing practice but is conducting research into appropriate processes and their links with different outcomes.

- In many cases this type of audit research has less credibility simply because it deals with smaller samples and is based on small studies using local 'medical audit monies'. Generalizing such research into regional and national databases is an important challenge for the future.

- As well as audit within particular specialties (whether within the hospital or within community services), it is important to conduct audit of the whole care process – for example, involving audit at the 'interface' between primary and secondary care. The chapter discusses some of the issues involved in this process.

- If the outcome of care is being audited, audit can become linked to questions of resources and economists can seek to draw relationships between different outcomes (measured in terms of utility) and costs. However this is not a simple process. It is difficult to agree on appropriate measures of utility and value judgements are often involved in mediating between different actors' views of utility (for example doctors, managers and patients). It is not simply a question of using averages and other means of mediating between different views. Basic value judgements often 'get in the way' of simple answers and simple rankings of different procedures in terms of their relative utilities and costs – whether between specialties or even within specialties.

For example, different procedures for tackling patients with similar symptoms may differ in terms of likely risk and benefit. One procedure may produce a better average outcome (across all patients) but be riskier (for example, involving death for some). Another procedure, on the other hand, may have a poorer average outcome but be less risky. If these procedures have different costs, there may be an attempt to standardize within a hospital (or a clinical directorate), yet difficulty in securing the agreement of different clinicians to one procedure rather than the other – for perfectly good reasons, rather than the more traditional reasons, in 'audit', of lack of information or unwillingness to change conservative practice. Additionally, different groups of patients – such as the elderly, or even patients with different characteristics – may benefit from different procedures, techniques or 'clinical pathways'. This makes the QALY a suspect device: it assumes (too much) standardization, both of medicine and of social choice.

What we are in effect saying is that there is disagreement about the utility of the different procedure – and the disagreeing clinicians may be unwilling simply to have their views 'averaged out' in a kind of opinion poll – whether of doctors or of all participants in the process. Recourse to patient choice may be possible in some circumstances, but is not always possible – and in any case, cost considerations may prevent patient choice without reference to resources involved being used as the gold standard of decision-making. In these situations, it would be unfortunate if the audit process were used by management to force a contentious solution: this would be an illegitimate assault upon clinical freedom. There is no easy answer in such situations, and sensitive local management is required. In the era of the purchaser/ provider split, such negotiations will involve doctors within a clinical directorate or specialty, the trust management if necessary and purchasers.

ACKNOWLEDGEMENTS

I would like to thank Anne McBride for co-authoring this chapter, which draws on much of our effort together on this topic and on three audit projects conducted in Staffordshire under the aegis of the local Medical Audit Committee and the Medical Audit Advisory Group of the Family Health Services Authority.

APPENDIX 1: AUDIT OF DAY-CASE SURGERY

STRUCTURE, PROCESS AND OUTCOME MEASURES

Patient characteristics

- Age
- Gender
- Social circumstances
- Time taken to travel home
- Medical characteristics
- Past medical history
- Social habits
- Pill/HRT
- Family – anaesthetic
- Fixtures and fittings
- First GA
- Worries
- Living arrangements

Measures of structure

- ASA grade
- Surgeon grade
- Anaesthetist grade

Measures of process

- Duration of operation
- Duration of anaesthetic
- Administration of premedication
- Administration of anaesthetic
- Pre-op discussion with surgeon
- Pre-op discussion with anaesthetist
- Blood pressure test
- Pulse test
- Urine analysis
- Weight check
- Written information before stay
- Explanation before stay
- Explanation of treatment during hospital stay
- Warning of departure

Measures of satisfaction/perception

- Worries
- Aspects of hospital
- Person most helpful in explaining operation
- Information given about treatment
- Recommendation of day case/ inpatient

Measures of outcome

- Post-op experiences at 1–4 hours
- Need for painkillers at 1–4 hours
- Readiness to go home at 1–4 hours
- Post-op experiences at 24 hours
- Need for painkillers at 24 hours
- Post-op painkiller
- Sleep patterns
- Breakfast taken
- Post-op painkiller
- Days of post-op painkiller
- Complications
- Recovery time
- Activities
- Self-perception on speed of recovery
- Re-admittance
- Use of services
- Need for more help from services
- Need for more help from others

Additional outcome measures for adult day cases

- Time patient left hospital following operation
- Necessity for patient to have wheelchair
- Administration of drugs on discharge

APPENDIX 2: AUDIT OF POSTOPERATIVE PAIN RELIEF

STRUCTURE, PROCESS AND OUTCOME MEASURES

Patient characteristics

- Age
- Gender
- Ethnic origin

Measures of process

- General preoperative discussions
- Pain control preoperative discussions
- Premedication (drug, dosage, time given)
- Anaesthetic drugs (time of induction, drug, dosage, technique, duration)
- Postoperative painkiller (analgesia: time to first dose, drug, route, frequency; antiemetic: drug, route, frequency)
- Postoperative advice from staff
- Asking patients (post-op) if they have pain

Measures of patient satisfaction

- Helpfulness of preoperative discussion with nurse/surgeon/anaesthetist (helpfulness categorized: in general, with regard to postoperative pain, in reducing anxiety)
- Satisfaction with pain relief after operation

Measures of outcome

- Experience of pain in the recovery area: extent to which pain relieved
- Experience of pain on the ward: extent to which pain relieved
- Degree of vomiting
- Ability to pass urine
- Degree of itching
- Request for postoperative painkiller
- Administration of postoperative painkiller to patient

REFERENCES

Audit Commission (1990) *A short cut to better Services: Day Surgery in England and Wales*, HMSO, London.

Baker, R. and Presley, P. (1990) *The Practice Audit Plan*, Severn Faculty of the Royal College of General Practitioners, Bristol.

Beech, R. and Morgan, M. (1992) Constraints on innovatory practice: the case of day surgery in the NHS. *International Journal of Health Planning and Management*, 7, 133–148.

Berwick, D. M. (1989) Continuous improvement as an ideal in health care. *New England Journal of Medicine*, 320, 53–56.

Berwick, D. M., Enthoven, A. and Bunker, J. P. (1992) Quality management in the NHS: the doctor's role – I. *British Medical Journal*, 304, 235–239.

Black, N. (1990) Quality assurance of medical care. *Journal of Public Health Medicine*, 12, 97–104.

Black, N., Petticrew, M., Hunter, D., Sanderson, C. (1993) Day surgery: development of a national comparative audit service. *Quality in Health Care*, 2, 162–166.

Black, N. and Sanderson, C. (1993) Day surgery: development of a questionnaire for eliciting patients' experiences. *Quality in Health Care*, 2, 157–161.

Bowden, D. and Walshe, K. (1991) When medical audit starts to count. *British Medical Journal*, 303, 101–103.

Brice, J. (1989) On introducing medical audit. *Journal of Management in Medicine*, 4, 179–183.

British Thoracic Society (1990) Guidelines for management of severe asthma in adults: II – Acute severe asthma. *British Medical Journal*, 301, 797–800.

Brook, R. H. and Appel, F. (1973) Quality of care assessment: choosing a method for peer review. *New England Journal of Medicine*, 21 Jun, 1323–1329.

Buck, N., Devlin, H. B. and Lunn, J. N. (1987) *The Report of a Confidential Enquiry into Perioperative Death*, Nuffield Provincial Hospitals Trust, London.

Campling, E. A., Devlin, H. B., Hoile, R. W. and Lunn, J. N. (1992) *The Report of the National Confidential Enquiry into Perioperative Deaths 1990*, HMSO, London.

Cartwright, A. and Windsor, J. (1992) Outpatients and Their Doctors: A Study of Patients, General Practitioners and Hospital Doctors, HMSO, London.

Cochrane, A. L. (1972) *Effectiveness and Efficiency: Random Reflections on Health Services*, Nuffield Provincial Hospitals Trust, London.

Coulter, A. (1990) Patterns of hospital referral, in Griffin, J. (ed.), *Factors Influencing Clinical Decisions in General Practice*, Office of Health Economics, London.

Colleges of Surgeons and Anaesthetists (1990) *Pain After Surgery*, Royal College of Surgeons, London.

Deming, W. E. (1982) *Quality, Productivity, and Competitive Position*, Centre for Advanced Engineering Study, Massachusetts Institute of Technology, Cambridge, MA.

Deming, W. E. (1986) *Out of the Crisis*, Centre for Advanced Engineering Study, Massachusetts Institute of Technology, Cambridge, MA.

Department of Health (1989a) Working for patients, *Cmnd 555*, HMSO, London.

Department of Health (1989b) Medical audit, *Working Paper No. 6*, HMSO, London.

Department of Health, Welsh Office, Scottish Home and Health Department, Department of Health and Social Security, Northern Ireland (1991) *Report on Confidential Enquiries into Maternal Deaths in the United Kingdom 1985–87*, HMSO, London.

Department of Health (1994) The Patient's Charter Hospital and Ambulance Services Comparative Performance Guide 1993–1994, HMSO, London.

Donabedian, A. (1966) Evaluating the quality of medical care. *Milbank Memorial Fund Quarterly*, 44, 166–206.

Donabedian, A. (1980) *Explorations in Quality Assessment and Monitoring – vol. 1: The Definition of Quality and Approaches to its Assessment*, Health Administration Press, Ann Arbor, MI.

Eddy, D. M. (1990a) Clinical decision making: promoting the jump from theory to practice. *Journal of the American Medical Association*, 263, 279–290.

Eddy, D. M. (1990b) Clinical decision making: the challenge. *Journal of the American Medical Association*, 263, 287–290.

Eddy, D. M. (1990c) Anatomy of a decision. *Journal of the American Medical Association*, 263, 441–443.

Eddy, D. M. (1990d) Practice policies – what are they? *Journal of the American Medical Association*, 263, 877–880.

Eddy, D. M. (1990e) Practice policies –- where do they come from? *Journal of the American Medical Association*, 263, 1265–1275.

Eddy, D. M. (1990f) Practice policies – guidelines for methods. *Journal of the American Medical Association*, 263, 1839–1841.

Eddy, D. M. (1990g) Guidelines for policy statements, the explicit approach. *Journal of the American Medical Association*, 263, 2239–2243.

Eddy, D. M. (1990h) Comparing benefits and harms: the balance sheet. *Journal of the American Medical Association*, 263, 2493–2505.

Eddy, D. M. (1990i) Designing a practice policy: standards, guidelines and options. *Journal of the American Medical Association*, 263, 3077–3084.

Eddy, D. M. (1990j) Resolving conflicts in practice policies. *Journal of the American Medical Association*, 264, 389–391.

Eddy, D. M. (1990k) What do we do about costs? *Journal of the American Medical Association*, 264, 1161–1170.

Eddy, D. M. (1990l) Connecting value and costs, whom do we ask, and what do we ask them?

Journal of the American Medical Association, 264, 1737–1739.

Eisenberg, J. M. (1986) *Doctors' Decisions and the Cost of Medical Care*, Health Administration Press Perspectives, Ann Arbor, MI.

Ende, J. (1983) Feedback in clinical medical education. *Journal of the American Medical Association*, 250, 777–781.

Fowkes, F. G. R. T. (1982) Medical audit cycle. *Medical Education*, 16, 228–238.

Frankel, S. and West, R. (1993) *Rationing and Rationality in the National Health Service: The Persistence of Waiting Lists*, Macmillan, London.

Hill, R. D. (1991) Paper delivered to the Conference of the Royal College of Physicians, London, 4 July 1991.

Holland, W. W. (1983) *Evaluation of Health Care*, Oxford University Press, Oxford.

Hopkins, A. (1990) *Measuring the Quality of Medical Care*, Royal College of Physicians, London.

Irvine, D. (1990) *Managing for Quality in General Practice*, King's Fund Centre, London.

Jennett, B. (1988) Balancing benefits and burdens in surgery. *British Medical Bulletin*, 44, 499–513.

Jones, N. P., Lloyd, I.C. and Kwartz, J. (1990) General practitioner referrals to an eye hospital: a standard referral form. *Journal of the Royal Society of Medicine*, 83, 770–772.

Juran, J. M. (1964) *Managerial Breakthrough*, McGraw-Hill, New York.

Juran, J. M., Gryna, F. M. Jr and Bingham, R. S. Jr (eds) (1979) *Quality Control Handbook*, McGraw-Hill, New York.

Kentish, R., Jenkins, P. and Lask, B. (1987) Study of written communications between general practitioners and departments of child psychiatry. *Journal of the Royal College of General Practitioners*, April, 162–163.

Krasnick, A., Groenewegen, P. P., Pedersen, P. A. *et al.* (1990) Changing remuneration systems: effects on activity in general practice. *British Medical Journal*, 300, 1698–1701.

Kuhn, Cooke, Collins, *et al.* Perceptions of pain relief after surgery. *British Medical Journal*, 300, 1687–1690.

Light, D. (1990) Medical house arrest. *Health Service Journal*, Nov, 1648–1649.

Lembcke, P. A. (1967) Evolution of the medical audit. *Journal of the American Medical Assocation*, 199.

McBride, A. (1992) Medical audit: a critical review, in McVeigh and Wheeler (eds), *Law, Health and Medical Regulation*, Dartmouth Publishing, Aldershot, pp 193–213.

McBride, A., Goldie, D., Lee, K. *et al.* (1993a) *Waiting for Health Gain*, Staffordshire Medical Audit Advisory Group, Stafford.

McBride, A., Goldie, D., Lee, K. *et al.* (1993b) *Communicating for Health Gain*, Staffordshire Medical Audit Advisory Group, Stafford.

McBride, A., Goldie, D., Lee, K. *et al.* (1993c) *Purchasing for Health Gain*, Staffordshire Medical Audit Advisory Group, Stafford.

McColl, I. (1979) Medical audit in British hospital practice. *British Journal of Hospital Medicine*, 22, 485.

Marinker, M. J., Wilkin, D. and Metcalfe, D. H. (1988) Referral to hospital: can we do better? *British Medical Journal*, 297, 461–464.

Maxwell, R. J. (1984) Quality assessment in health. *British Medical Journal*, 288, 1470–1472.

Maynard, A. (1992) At our own disposal. *Health Service Journal*, 25 Jun, 21.

Mitchell, M. and Fowkes, F. G. R. (1985) Audit reviewed: does feedback of performance change clinical behaviour? *Journal of the Royal College of Physicians*, 19, 251–254.

Mooney, G. and Ryan, M. (1991) *Rethinking Medical Audit. The Goal is Efficiency*, Health Economics Resource Unit Discussion Paper 06/91, HERU, University of Aberdeen, Aberdeen.

Mugford, M., Banfield, P. and O'Hanlon, P. (1991) Effects of feedback of information on clinical practice: a review. *British Medical Journal*, 303, 398–402.

Nelson, A. R. (1989) Orphan data and the unclosed loop: a dilemma in PSRO and medical audit. *New England Journal of Medicine*, 295.

Ovretveit, J. (1992) *Health Service Quality*, Blackwell Special Projects, Oxford.

Packer, G. J., Goring, C. C., Gayner, A. D. and Craxford, A. D. (1991) Audit of ankle injuries in an accident and emergency department. *British Medical Journal*, 302, 885–887.

Pfeffer, N. and Coote. A. (1991) *Is Quality Good for You? A Critical Review of Quality Assurance in Welfare Services*, Social Policy Paper No. 5, Institute of Public Policy Research, London.

Rice, T. H. (1983) The impact of changing Medicare reimbursement rates on physician-induced demand. *Medical Care*, 21, 803–815.

Rogers, B. (1983) *Diffusion of Innovations*, 3rd edn, Free Press, New York.

Roland, M. O., Porter, R. W., Matthews, J. G. *et al.* (1991) Improving care: a study of orthopaedic outpatient referrals. *British Medical Journal*, 302, 1124–1128.

Rosenfeld, L. S. (1957) Quality of medical care in hospitals. *American Journal of Public Health*, 47.

Sanders, D., Coulter, A. and McPherson, K. (1989) *Variations in Hospital Admission Rates: A Review of the Literature, Kings Fund Project Paper No. 79*, King's Fund, London.

Schoenbaum, S. C. and Gottlieb, L. K. (1990) Algorithm based improvement of clinical quality. *British Medical Journal*, 31, 87–91.

Shaw, C. D. (1989) *Medical Audit – A Hospital Handbook*, Kings Fund Centre, London.

Standing Committee on Postgraduate Medical Education (1989) Medical Audit: The Educational Implications, Standing Committee on Postgraduate Medical Education, London.

Steffen, G. E. (1988) Quality medical care. *Journal of the American Medical Association*, 260, 56–61.

Van 't Hoff, W. (1986) Medical audit. *Midlands Medicine*, 17, 28–30.

WHO Working Group (1989) The principles of quality assurance. *Quality Assurance in Health Care*, 1, 79–95.

Williams, E. I. and Fitton, F. (1990) General practitioner response to elderly patients discharged from hospital. *British Medical Journal*, 300, 159–161.

Williamson, C. (1992) *Whose Standards? Consumer and Professional Standards in Health Care*, Open University Press, Buckingham.

FURTHER READING

Bell, D., Layton, A. J. and Gabbey, J. (1991) Use of a guideline based questionnaire to audit hospital care of acute asthma. *British Medical Journal*, 32, 1440–1443.

Bowling, A. (1991) *Measuring Health: A Review of Quality of Life Measurement Scales*, Open University Press, Buckingham.

Bradlow, J., Coulter, A. and Brooks, P. (1992) *Patterns of Referral*, Health Services Research Unit, Department of Public Health and Primary Care, University of Oxford, Oxford.

Bunker, J. P. (1990) Variations in hospital admissions and the appropriateness of care: American preoccupations? *British Medical Journal*, 310, 531–532.

Cartwright, A. and Windsor, J. (1989) *Outpatients, General Practitioners and Hospital Doctors, Report of a Feasibility Study*, Nuffield Provincial Hospitals Trust, London.

Corrigan, P. and Evans, K. (1993) *A Practical Approach to Quality Improvement: A Guide for*

Nurses and Health Professionals, Chapman & Hall, London.

Coulter, A., Noone, A. and Goldacre, M. (1989) General practitioners' referrals to specialist outpatient clinics. *British Medical Journal*, 299, 306–308.

Coulter, A., Seagroatt, V. and McPherson, K. (1990) Relationship between general practices' outpatient referral rates and rates of elective admission to hospital. *British Medical Journal*, 301, 273–276.

Crombie, D. L. and Fleming, D. M. (1988) General practitioner referrals to hospital: financial implications of variability. *Health Trends*, 20, 53–56.

Crombie, I. K., Davies, H. T. O., Abraham, S. C. S. and du Florey, C. (1993) *The Audit Handbook: Improving Health Care Through Clinical Audit*, John Wiley & Sons, Chichester.

Dingwall, R. and Fenn, P. (1992) *Quality and Regulation in Health Care – International Experiences*, Routledge, London.

Donabedian A (1981) Advantages and Limitations of Explicit Criteria for assessing the quality of health care, Milbank Memorial Fund Quarterly, 59, No. 1.

Donabedian, A. (1982) Introduction, in *Explorations in Quality Assessment and Monitoring, vol. 2: The Criteria and Standards of Quality*, Health Administration Press, Ann Arbor, MI.

Dowie, R. (1983) *General Practitioners and Consultants: A study of Outpatient Referrals*, King's Fund, London.

Emmanuel, J. and Walter, N, (1989) Referrals from general practice to hospital outpatient departments: a strategy for improvement. *British Medical Journal*, 299, 722–724.

Farrow, S. and Jewell, D. (1993) Opening the gate: referrals from primary to secondary care, in Frankel, S. and West, R. (eds) *Rationing and Rationality in the National Health Service: The Persistence of Waiting Lists*, Macmillan, London.

Fletcher, C. M. (1972) *Communication in Medicine*, Nuffield Provincial Hospital Trusts, London.

Frankel, S. and Robbins, M. (1993) Entering the lobby: access to outpatient assessment, in Frankel, S. and West, R. (eds) *Rationing and Rationality in the National Health Service: The Persistence of Waiting Lists*, Macmillan, London.

Gonella, J. S., Louis, D. Z., Zeleznik, C. and Turner, B. J. (1990) The problem of late hospitalization: a quality and cost issue. *Academic Medicine*, 65, 314–319.

Griffin J (1990) Factors influencing clinical decisions in General Practice, London, Office of Health Economics.

Griffiths R (1983), NHS Management Enquiry Report, DHSS, London.

Ham, C., Dingwall, R. *et al.* (1988) *Medical Negligence, Compensation and Accountability*, King's Fund, London.

Harvey, I. (1993) And so to bed: access to inpatient services, in Frankel, S. and West, R. (eds) *Rationing and Rationality in the National Health Service: The Persistence of Waiting Lists*, Macmillan, London.

Hopkins, A. and Costin, D. (1990) *Measuring the Outcomes of Medical Care*, Royal College of Physicians, London.

Hughes, J. and Humphrey, C. (1990) *Medical Audit in General Practice: A Practical Guide to the Literature*, King's Fund, London.

Jost, T. S. (1992) Recent developments in medical quality assurance and audit: an international comparative study, in Dingwall, R. and Fenn, P. (eds) *Quality and Regulation in Health Care – International Experiences*, Routledge, London.

Koch, H. (1992) *Implementing and Sustaining Total Quality Management in Health Care*, Longman, Harlow.

Lawrence, M. S. (ed.) (1993) *Medical Audit in Primary Health Care*, Oxford University Press, Oxford.

Light, D. (1991) Effectiveness and efficiency under competition: the Cochrane Test. *British Medical Journal*, 303, 1253–1254.

McBride, A., Goldie, D., Lee, K. *et al.* (1993) *A Primary–Secondary Care Interface Medical Audit Project – Executive Report*, Staffordshire Medical Audit Advisory Group, Stafford.

McIver, S. (1993) *Obtaining the Views of Health Service Users About Quality of Information*, Kings Fund, London.

McKee, C. M., Lauglo, M. and Lessof, L. (1989) Medical audit: a review. *Journal of the Royal Society of Medicine*, 82, 474–477.

National Health Service and Community Care Act 1990, HMSO, London.

Patrick, D. L. and Erickson, P. (1993) *Health Status and Health Policy: Quality of Life, Assessment of Health, and Allocation of Resources*, Oxford University Press, Oxford.

Royal College of General Practitioners (1992) *The European Study of Referrals from Primary to Secondary Care, Occasional Paper 56*, Royal College of General Practitioners, London.

Scottish Home and Health Department, Clinical

Research and Audit Group (1990) *Confidentiality and Medical Audit – Interim Guidelines*, HMSO, London.

Shaw, C. D. (1980) Acceptability of audit. *British Medical Journal*, 14 Jun, 1443–1446.

Stocking, B. (1992) Promoting change in clinical care. *Quality in Health Care*, 1, 56–60.

Stone, D. H. (1990) Proposed taxonomy of audit and related activities. *Journal of the Royal College of Physicians of London*, 24, 30–31.

Walshe, K. and Bennett, J. (1991) *Guidelines on Medical Audit and Confidentiality*, Brighton Health Authority, Brighton.

Weale, A. (1988) *Cost and Choice in Health Care – the Ethical Dimensions*, King Edward's Hospital Fund for London, London.

Wilkin, D. and Roland, M. (1992) *Waiting Times for First Outpatient Appointments in the NHS*, Centre for Primary Care Research, University of Manchester, Manchester.

Wilkin, D. and Smith, T. (1986) *Variation in General Practitioners' Referrals to Consultants*, Centre for Primary Care Research, University of Manchester, Manchester.

Wright, C. and Whittington, D. (1992) *Quality Assurance: An Introduction for Health Care Professionals*, Churchill Livingstone, Edinburgh.

WHAT IS THE PURPOSE OF RESOURCE ALLOCATION?

The first point to remember about resource allocation conducted on a systematic and equitable basis is that very few health-care systems in the world undertake such a challenge. Three characteristics of health-care systems are associated with such a policy.

- The system should be public, raising revenue centrally which can be allocated through a clear methodology.
- Systems involve cash limits, such that there is a need to allocate systematically rather than simply reimbursing whatever people want.
- There is a desire to meet a principle of equity in making allocations; in the UK this principle has (since 1976) involved allocating resources to promote equality of opportunity for access to care for those at equal risk or with equal need.

It could be argued that the beginnings of systematic resource allocation in the UK, with the RAWP (Resource Allocation Working Party) formula in 1976, represented the beginning of what would now be called 'purchasing' in its broadest sense. This is because the formula sought to measure needs across geographical areas – and to make a distinction between such areas' need for services and existing distributions (provision). In other words, a distinction is made between current provision and hypothesized need. Of course, before 1989/1991, planning to meet this need meant direct control of providers to seek to ensure that services were in line with the formula – not by a dogmatic or one-to-one correlation between components of the formula and service plans, but to ensure a broader compatibility of money and services in line with need. There was thus a balance between central criteria of need and local choice as to services, as inevitably there will be in any system. It is a question of the extent, and also the mechanism used to link central and local choices.

Chapter 4 discussed briefly the possibility that, on the one hand, resource allocation can be undertaken prior to planning and, on the other hand, planning can be undertaken prior to resource allocation. That is, one can have resource-led plans or plan-led allocation of resources. The 1976 RAWP methodology, translated into a specific formula as discussed below, in effect instituted a system whereby resources were allocated to regions, ensuring that regions' plans were resource-led. When it came to allocations from regions to districts, however, different approaches were taken. Some regions sought to have resource-led plans, by simply replicating the national formula (or something similar to it) in allocating money to districts. The districts were then left to plan services (other than those provided through top-sliced money by regions) – not necessarily directly in line with the assumptions of the resource allocation formula, but at least constrained by it.

Other regions, however, sought to take a more strategic approach to planning, at the regional level (also briefly discussed in Chapter 4) and thereby moved more in the direction of plan-led resource allocation. This meant that districts received funds on behalf of the services for which they were responsible, but not necessarily only for their own population. That is, they received catchment allocations rather than residential population allocations.

Chapter 7 discussed different approaches to purchasing and commissioning – and the underlying assumption in that chapter was that districts or health authorities, in whatever form, would receive funds on behalf of their residential populations. The basis for this allocation is, of course, need as measured by some broad methodology, translated into a specific formula. The pages below discuss the evolution in thinking from 1976 to the present day in how such a formula ought to be constructed. Here, more generally, it should be noted that there was actually a belief that districts (even with populations of 250 000) were often too small to allow coherent global resource allocation – and it was more sensible to plan according to need and desired patient flows across the region. It is within such a context that one can understand the extremities of difficulty in allocating directly to GP fundholders – especially when there are different types of fundholders, ranging from 'total fundholders', who hold the budget for most care, to small-scale fundholders, who hold only the budget for limited types of care. Although one can understand the importance of allocating either to health authorities on behalf of the residential populations or to fundholders on behalf of specific patient groups, in order to ensure that the money is actually spent on those identified as having the need, the paradox is that in practice this can lead to less ability to allocate on

the basis of need across all purchasers – and also to difficulties in ensuring the most appropriate distribution of services. In other words, decentralization of purchasing beyond the optimum level can lead to suboptimal services.

Recent research has suggested that allocation to fundholders on a formula basis, using a formula that is both sensible and simple, is very difficult if not impossible. Glennerster and Matsaganis (1994) have suggested that individual patient indicators may be the best means of moving towards such a formula. The huge costs of using such an approach to allocate across the National Health Service on an equitable basis would be likely to make it prohibitive, even if desirable. More to the point, a more fundamental consideration arises from the fact that finding a methodology that equitably applies formulae to both health authorities and to fundholders – on an equitable basis both within and between – is almost impossible. We have already seen the misallocations and political haggling which has followed from allocations to fundholders in different regions. Such behaviour undermines the stability and indeed tenability of global resource allocation formulae and therefore arguably the noble tradition that began with RAWP in 1976.

One could argue that, if fundholders club together into consortia and cover large areas of population – for most services, what is more – then the problem would be overcome. But this is merely a solution at the definitional level. For such fundholders would have become new health authorities in all but name – with the important proviso that only doctors would be 'members of the health authorities'! (The question then arises, why be a fundholder – the original motivation has gone.) At the time of writing the problem is that the Government is leaning both ways as far as fundholding is concerned: it wishes to encourage it but wishes also to discourage the unevenness in planning and uncertainty for providers that fundholding can create. As a result the new (post-April 1996) health authorities are to have a responsibility for fundholders. It remains to be seen which wins in aggregate when conflicts mount. At the end of the day, in 1995, it was a political question – the Conservatives wanted to see fundholding 'bedded-in' to make it awkward for Labour to oppose it at the following general election; yet they also (behind closed doors) feared the consequences of 'universal fundholding'. That is because doctors holding specific budgets and using cost per case contracts on a large scale would fully expose the relative underfunding of the National Health Service and – via the role of the media – rationing would be placed more firmly at the door of the politicians. Currently, one of the major objectives of the NHS reforms is to devolve responsibility and deflect attention away from debates about overall levels of funding.

Another fundamental question for resource allocation is, resources for what? Is it resources to combat ill health, to fund the health service or both? Obviously the ideal is to maximize health status – or to reduce inequalities; or whatever strategy is chosen to have the maximum impact on health, not just health services. One can disagree about the ethic or norm lying behind the outcome adopted. For example, utilitarianism – the greatest good for the greatest number – suggests a maximization of health status; whereas egalitarianism would suggest equality of health status as an alternative or at least additional value. Nevertheless, having agreed on values or having found a mechanism for deciding which values to adopt, resources ought to be allocated for a broad health strategy. The question is, should this broad health strategy be left to the NHS? There is a role for prevention of ill health and promotion of good health on the one hand and for curing disease and caring for those who cannot be cured on the other. The NHS undoubtedly is the agency for the latter. For the former, although the NHS will have a complemen-

tary role alongside other agencies, broad social and economic policy, and a variety of social and environmental factors generally, help to determine the health status of the nation. Using a formula to measure the need for health care may in effect be to measure the generalized causes of an absence of better health in society than would otherwise be possible. That is, such a formula may be of use in allocating across a whole range of social budgets (housing, relief of poverty, etc.) as well. At the very least there ought to be coordination between NHS formulae and other, multi-agency attacks upon ill health (Judge and Mays, 1994).

To put it another way, even the ideal formula may measure the social and economic characteristics correlated with ill health – to put it bluntly, if social inequality is linked with ill health, as we know it is, a formula may reflect social inequality. This is not to argue that the formula is inappropriate for allocation within health services. For – in the absence of wider social action – relieving ill health on such a pattern, and concentrating resources where most needed, may be even more urgent. It does, however, militate against assuming that the NHS is the agency to 'do everything'. The NHS alone cannot be responsible for both improving health generally and for curing and caring. A political trend of the 1980s and early 1990s has been to assume that the avoidance of ill health is an individual responsibility. While this is part of the story, the social and environmental causes of ill health must also be tackled if one is serious about prevention. The *Health of the Nation* targets unfortunately favour the former – and there is an assumption that, wherever people are on the social spectrum, they should be equally motivated to look after their health. This is sometimes not only patronizing but also cruel. An approach which is both egalitarian and libertarian would involve greater redistribution and more active social policy, and then a dissemination of knowledge, rather than 'nannying', in encouraging people in more relaxed social circumstances to take responsibility for their own health where appropriate.

An interesting political characteristic helping to determine reaction to formulae to distribute and redistribute resources to areas in greatest need, is that such formulae will be most embarrassing to governments that are least concerned with inequalities of income and social conditions on the one hand and inequalities of health status between classes on the other. That is, such formulae will mandate significant moving of money from Conservative seats to Labour seats! As a result, Conservative governments will be less willing to implement such formulae, and will seek – if not to reject them openly – to moderate their effects. This occurred with the RAWP Review in 1988 and in 1994/5 when the Government was considering the latest research (from York University), which sought to improve the basis upon which genuine need for services was measured (Carr-Hill *et al.*, 1994; Smith *et al.*, 1994; NHS Executive, 1994).

One question of policy concerns whether a formula measuring the need for access to the National Health Service should take into account the existing supply across the country of private sector facilities. If it does, then it could be argued that any government – Conservative or Labour – ought not to object to a redistribution to 'poor areas', as the impetus to seek private care in the better-off areas (from which resources would then be directed away) would then be enhanced. This depends on diminishing universality of the National Health Service, however, and – given its popularity – even a Conservative government is unlikely to wish to do so overtly. Although taking account of private sector facilities, furthermore, can lead to targeting on areas of direct need in the short term, such moves can also institutionalize a greater role for the private sector than advocates of an universal NHS might wish. This issue has been discussed in Chapter 2.

A more technical point concerning the existence of the private sector and its possible contribution to meeting need (especially for care of the elderly, in the south) concerns how any formula seen to measure the need for National Health Service care ought to 'control for' the existence of private supply. This relates to the more general point about how to 'control for supply' in a formula. There is a difference between supply that has been created in order to respond to identified need or legitimate demand, on the one hand, and supply that seems more arbitrary or simply variant across the country or across regions due to historical factors or less need-related factors. The new research from York University is more ambitious in making a more sophisticated control for supply, in seeking to measure usage of the National Health Service as a surrogate for need. But all in all it is a thorny area, both conceptually and technically. For example, while access to acute care – especially emergency care – can be modelled more accurately due to its greater measurability and due to the more standard uptake of such care, palliative care and, for example, care of the elderly may only be able to be modelled as to 'appropriate supply' by making heroic assumptions or value-laden assumptions – at the very least assumptions about norms. Yet the existence of such care can affect the supply of acute care. It is therefore an intricate area as to how one controls for existing supply – and indeed chooses between appropriate use of acute and non-acute facilities for certain client groups.

This reflects the more general point that, although formulae can help in allocating within categories of care (e.g. non-psychiatric acute care), it is a value-laden choice as to how much is spent generally upon different forms of care (e.g. care of the mentally ill and handicapped, care of the elderly, care in the community, and so forth). Neither the total quantum of care nor allocation across the various categories and client groups within the National Health Service is susceptible to purely 'scientific' analysis.

Overall there is a danger that, while research on resource allocation formulae becomes more sophisticated, the salience of such formulae altogether is diminished – as commitment to an equitably funded NHS, with global budgets allocated to health authorities on the basis of need, is diminished.

Another option is, of course, to leave decisions on spending to local assessment, and thereby to water down or abandon a commitment to national criteria of need and national allocation to health authorities for a different reason. The discussion sections of Chapters 1 and 13, however, point out some of the disadvantages of such an approach, in, for example, giving responsibility for health-care spending over to local government.

Another aspect of local choice, even within a centrally funded National Health Service, is that, of course, some health authorities may choose to spend less on hospital care – and therefore will have less usage and apparent need when compared with other areas. That makes it all the more important that attempts are made to gauge relativity within health authorities as well as between health authorities and feed such information into a formula capable of abstracting from such local choice in order to measure the need for the purposes of national allocation. Again, the new approach from York University is effective at doing this by comparison with previous approaches.

Finally for now, it has been argued in the past that resource allocation by need is not the same as resource allocation by need for effective services. That is, simply recognizing morbidity may allocate money to areas of clinical care where effective services are not (yet or ever) possible. Against this, however, it can be claimed that resource allocation formula do not mechanistically translate into exact service plans – the correlation between resource allocation and service planning is broader. Furthermore, identifying need in the absence of the possibility of effective clinical intervention is nevertheless important, as it identifies aspirational need and potentially allocates resources for care when cure is not possible. Recognizing only the present state of knowledge is damaging to a research-oriented NHS. Decisions as to effective care, and where money ought to be allocated, are better taken within allocated budgets rather than in providing the criteria for allocation to budgets. Thus inevitably resource allocation will involve rough justice as well as fair shares – what is important is to avoid sophisticated injustice and unfair shares, as the increasingly complex system of allocation to an increasingly complex array of fundholders and other agents is threatening.

THEORETICAL PERSPECTIVES ON RESOURCE ALLOCATION

There are many different ways of measuring 'need' for health care. Indeed, the relevance or otherwise of the concept of need, in considering appropriate provision of health care for populations and individuals, has long been debated. The creation of a National Health Service in 1948 embodied the principle that services ought to be 'free at the point of use' and at time of need. Economists, of course, distinguish between demand and need. While some would define demand as expressed need, it might be argued that not everything that is demanded is 'needed'. Equally, not everything that is 'needed' is demanded. And not everything that is demanded by the public is financed.

If not everything that is 'needed' is demanded, how do we define need? In a now standard article, Bradshaw distinguished between felt need, expressed need, comparative need and 'expert-defined' need (Bradshaw, 1972). Without debating further the validity of different approaches to the concept and indeed application of need, it is clear that – in a publicly financed National

Health Service funded centrally from the public purse – criteria for meeting 'need' will be necessary.

In 1976, the report of the Resource Allocation Working Party (RAWP), adopted the definition of 'equal opportunity of access (to health care) for those at equal risk' (Resource Allocation Working Party, 1976). This embodied a principle of equity which argues that there should be equality of opportunity for care for those with similar 'needs'. In itself, the formula does not make a distinction between the importance of cure, prevention, care or rescue. It seems to embody the principle whereby there should not be differentiation on social grounds, or grounds of ability to pay, between different members of society in terms of their access to health care. Implicitly, the implication presumably was that avoidable differences in health status in individuals, groups, classes and so forth, ought to be diminished or ideally eradicated. (Paton, 1985).

The proxy measures of need for health care adopted by the RAWP are by now familiar (if fairly contemporary) history. Broadly speaking, it was argued that the best available proxy for morbidity was derived from mortality figures. This contention was debated increasingly throughout the 1980s, and the RAWP Review reported at the beginning of August 1988 with the recommendation that a slightly different approach be taken to gauging the need of populations. (NHS Management Board, 1988).

The original RAWP report had argued that an appropriate formula for allocating resources to health authorities ought to take account of population, a weighting for morbidity (based on mortality) and a weighting to translate an 'objective' measure of need into quantified financial allocations. The last weighting was achieved by using national average specialty costs, weighted by age group within the population and applied to each region's age cohort by specialty. The 'need' measure itself, however, was unrelated

to existing supply and demand. The RAWP Review (1988) argued that an alternative way of conceptualizing the need for health care is to look at which variables best explain **usage** of health care. Naturally, to prevent this simply being an inappropriate measure which measured existing supply (in other words, provision and location of hospitals and other services) a 'control' for supply had to be built into any such model. Otherwise, it would not be need so much as the existing distribution of services which would generate demand – as health care has its own flourishing Parkinson's Law.

In current language, provision would not be the result of deliberate overt purchasing, but instead provision would **determine** consumption, and the gauging of 'need' and therefore would constrain purchasing plans.

Such an approach, of course, conflates need and expressed need, if not demand. Nevertheless, sophisticated work was done which led to the conclusion that a combination of death rates and various social measures provided the 'best' predictor of need. A basic question, however, arises: if 'usage' is to be used to allocate monies, why not just allocate in line with usage figures themselves, having adjusted for supply?

In the end, the national formula for allocating from the Department of Health to NHS regions in England was amended to diminish the import of the standardized mortality ratio (SMR) but without including social measures (such as the Jarman Score, which is a composite measure of eight or 10 'deprivation factors').

Another important issue concerned the distribution of regional monies to purchasing health authorities or other purchasers. Before the 'NHS reforms' based on the White Paper *Working for Patients* and the NHS and Community Care Act 1990, district health authorities were in effect responsible for both purchasing and provision. Regions planned ('purchased') capital projects, in coordination with districts. Districts then allocated revenue (recurrent) monies to their hospitals (and other providers) – but with an adjustment made (in theory, for districts' targets) for flows of patients, i.e. retrospective reimbursements used to determine future targets for districts. In other words, when one talked of allocating from regions to districts, one was talking of allocating to districts as catchment areas responsible for the provision of health care within their boundaries – whether or not for residents living within these boundaries. That is, the old pre-White-Paper RAWP formula sought to take account of what were then known as 'cross-boundary flows'. But this process worked slowly, as moving from current allocations to target was difficult when money was scarce. Also, targets were for the parent district, not the provider.

Attempts to improve this situation generated a number of options: (1) direct allocation to providers by regions, based on patient flows and what would now be called 'purchasing decisions'; (2) creation of catchment populations, based on inflows and outflows to districts (involving a choice of complicated methodologies and yet still the problem that one was allocating to districts on behalf of providers); and (3) the idea of the 'internal market', whereby contracts for care were made directly rather than by formulas.

Following the NHS reforms, resource allocation by regions is to district purchasers – with districts now responsible for the residents contained within their boundaries. Patients treated within one district who live in another no longer automatically adjust a resource allocation formula which takes account of such cross-boundary flows, but have to be the subject of specific contracts made between the host district within which they live and the providers from which they receive care. Additional to this system are the GP fundholding practices, who receive money from the region as a separate allocation from that which goes to the district – for certain stipulated services, now including community services. Thus, regions generally allocate to two purchasers – purchasing districts (or consortia of districts) and GP fundholders. After 1995, allocation will be directly from the Department of Health to districts and fundholders.

This follows the review of 1993 and 1994 (of manpower and functions), involving the replacement of regional health authorities by central regional offices of the NHS Executive.

A new formula was proposed, for this purpose, taking a more sensitive account of the relationship between need, supply and demand and drawing on mortality data **and** socioeconomic data (see a series of articles in the *British Medical Journal*, 22 Oct 1994, pp 1031, 1046, 1056 and 1059).

The question for regions was whether to replicate the national formula (based on death rates, to a more limited extent than before the NHS reforms) or to devise their own formula. There is the further question of what is the most appropriate means of resourcing GP fundholders, who have the added problem of dealing in much smaller populations and for only certain specific services, than districts. Currently, the Department of Health is investigating some types of capitation formula for GP fundholders.

Different regions have taken different approaches to allocating to their purchasers. Some have used full standardized mortality ratios, as was done nationally after 1976. Some have copied the (post-NHS 'reforms') national approach, diminishing death rates but not building in anything else. Yet other regions have sought to allocate on the basis of a different way of measuring 'need'. Various approaches have used socioeconomic data as an alleged predictor of demand/need, unemployment rates and various devices such as the ACORN (a classification of residential neighbourhoods), which seeks to categorize small area populations in socioeconomic terms.

More recently still, the replacement of regions by regional offices of the NHS

Executive (the renamed ME) within the Department of Health will, as stated, lead to a direct allocation from 'the centre' – not only to districts but also within them to GP fund-holding purchasers (no doubt heavily advised by regional offices in the latter case!). Districts and family health services authorities will be merged (subject to legislation as with the regional change). As a result, large purchasing 'commissions' – and GP fundholders – will purchase most care. There may well be a significant problem in allocating appropriately to myriads of different 'purchasers'.

THE SMR – HAS ITS TIME COME OR GONE?

Intermittently since the 1980s, various regions have investigated alternative methodologies and formulae to the national RAWP for allocating to districts. The broad thrust has been to suggest the replacement of the standardized mortality ratio (SMR) – death rates adjusted for the age and possibly other characteristics of populations – as the weighting for health need, with an alternative based upon a measure of need which is directly correlated with hospital workload.

Such measures of need involve statistical correlation between a variety of 'social factors' (normally known as social deprivation) and hospital admissions in a standardized form (adjusted for age and sex). Other options, rather than adding to or replacing the SMR with social measures, could have involved setting targets for health states and longevity, and allocating according to districts' distance from them, e.g. using 'years of potential life lost' (YPLL) or by 'adding in' assumptions about improvement in quality of life that were attainable as opposed to merely desirable.

In summer 1988, the RAWP Review recommended that, at the national level, the formula for allocation to regions ought to reflect – as the main measures of need – an SMR diminished in salience and 'a social deprivation weighting' based on the Jarman score. In the end, following the White Paper *Working for Patients*, which also discussed the updating of the RAWP formula, the new weighting for need became the square root of the SMR and there was no separate calculation for social deprivation (justified on various grounds).

In allocating to districts (and now GP fundholders as well), the NHS Management Executive allowed flexibility in the methodology used. Criteria that must, however, be obeyed are 'simplicity, stability, sound empiricism and consultation with the DHAs'.

Traditionally, there has been a 'divide' in approaches to measuring need by formula for resource allocation purposes within the NHS. Advocates of the SMR have argued that it is simple and robust, and that it is indeed correlated with more general morbidity. As a result, the argument that many of the health service's 'priorities' are in areas where death rates are not significant or irrelevant is not necessarily a valid one. That is, the relationship between the SMR and either directly measured morbidity or 'social factors' is a statistical one. It does not matter if 'counterintuitive' examples exist (e.g. the argument that a system relying on death rates rewards services leading to a high level of mortality or removes funds from areas which have been successful in reducing their death rate).

At the time of the creation of the RAWP formula, although there was an attempt to correlate SMRs to morbidity to other measures of need, there was no attempt to do sophisticated regression analysis relating SMR and usage of hospital or other services.

This was not an omission so much as a recognition of the theoretical point that seeking to measure existing usage is not necessarily the best means of measuring need – if indeed it is a means of measuring need in a pure sense at all. It may be a means of measuring demand. It may further be a means of measuring supply, especially if there is no attempt to control for location of services. We all know that an increase in the quantum or proximity of health services leads to an increase in usage of them (Parkinson's Law applied to the health service).

The SMR was therefore an allegedly independent measure of need. It of course had the problem that it did not **quantify** the need for health services, especially service by service. As a result, the original RAWP formula weighted crude populations by SMR, but also by the age (and originally, sex) structure multiplied by the national average costs of providing services by age group. This allowed a quantification in practical terms of need.

The alternative approach is to argue that, in order to gauge need in any practical sense, it is important to test any measure of need against usage of health services. Hence there has been an proliferation of research, leading up to the RAWP Review in 1988 and in the 5 years since, relating various social factors to usage of health services. If there is an attempt to 'control for' supply (i.e. eradicate or diminish the bias produced in any such research by the fact that the existing configuration of health-care facilities will determine usage patterns to some extent), then it can be argued the most significant factors affecting expressed need can be determined.

It can, of course, be argued that there is more to need than expressed need. For a start, there is unexpressed need, which may or may not be 'expert'-defined need. There are various normative and comparative criteria for determining need – based on judgement or both national and international comparison.

Furthermore, if the attempt is to find the best possible explanation of hospital and general health service activity, it might be asked, somewhat sceptically, whether or not a measure of relative activity itself should not simply be used. In other words – subject to cash limits – 'demand' should be met – or at least the basis of the formula!

Such a reflection illustrates the fact that paradoxical situations can be detected amid the rationale for virtually any methodology or formula. Certainly one can point out that death rates perhaps illustrate areas where health services are relatively impotent, as well as areas of need. Additionally, death rates may reflect iatrogenic causes.

Mortality data can, of course, also be used as part of an audit of performance as well as for other 'provider-based' purposes – as recently allocated (but not implemented) when 'league tables' for hospitals were created (see Chapter 11). These are, however, fraught with theoretical and practical difficulties, and also create unfortunate incentives for providers. They can be used more profitably, in a more aggregate sense, as a correlate of need for different reasons and in different ways. Likewise, one can be sceptical about usage data as reflecting something other than need. In other words, such 'debating points' do not answer the question, what is the best approach?

Arguing that one approach or another can reward one type of service or another (i.e. services involving high mortality, whether in hospital or not, are best rewarded by an SMR approach) may also be based on a misunderstanding. The function of a resource allocation formula is to provide an aggregate allocation to a purchaser. This allocation should recognize aggregate need in as appropriate a manner as possible, always recognizing that such a manner will be imperfect. What one is in effect doing is identifying a rough and ready measure of relative aggregate need, district to district; region to region; or whatever. It is then up to the purchaser in the post-reform NHS) (or indeed the health authority in the pre-reform NHS) as to what purchasing and planning priorities are made through a more disaggregated needs assessment process, in line with GP referrals and complementary (or alternative!) criteria for using resources.

While it is naturally appropriate that the overall formula indirectly leads to a rewards of services which are 'needed', a confusing of the macro- and micro-levels is always possible. If one is seeking a global measure of need for a population, it is inevitably going to be the case that – service by service – the correlation of the need measure in the formula and (either) usage of hospitals or other measures of practical need may vary. Indeed one can see this in the case of the many formulae: different approaches (such as the Townsend correlation of social factors with a number of health factors including SMR, and others) (Townsend, Phillimore and Beattie, 1988) explain usage differentially for different groups of the population and – towards the end of the paper – for different specific disease groups.

Having said all this, it is nevertheless the case that the Townsend approach (Townsend, Phillimore and Beattie, 1988) is one example of a robust, and well argued methodology, which incidentally incorporates the SMR in a coherent manner. If it is possible to have an approach which gets the 'best of both worlds' (in the sense of fulfilling intrinsic criteria of need and also relating such criteria to usage of services), then the Townsend approach is probably as good as any. Previous regional attempts to replace the SMR as a result of regression analysis linking social factors and usage have been less valid, in the present author's view, than this approach. That is not least because they have often used tools derived for other purposes, such as ACORN – originally a marketing tool – and 'Jarman scores', derived from a desire to measure causes of GP workload, especially in inner cities.

An important issue is whether it is hospital services or the whole gamut of services that can be incorporated into an allocation procedure using such a methodology. In the spirit of finding allocation procedures which seek greater simplicity than previously, it is appropriate that a global measure is found. It is likely that the Townsend score can predict need more generally than for hospital services.

An important task is indeed to extend the analysis beyond the hospital. That is, the difficulty in both designing research and finding accurate disaggregated data to allow analysis of community service use (and so forth) to be correlated with social factors is a moot point. Work has, however, been done in a number of regions to inform their allocation procedures. The Mersey Region, for example, was for some years increasing the sophistication of its disaggregated studies relating social factors to 'need' for a whole range of health services. Here, of course, a problem exists, in that, if an increasingly 'rationed' NHS is to exclude certain types of service, then a global formula which seeks to 'predict' all need will be less useful – or rather will be politically inconvenient!

In other words, what business in the NHS in? Is identifying need in the broadest sense identifying the challenge for the whole range of social policy and not just for the health service? This point itself can be argued two ways (as can most theoretical issues).

On the one hand, some may argue that social need as accurately measured by regression analysis and so forth is in fact a measure of something beyond the scope of the NHS. On the other hand, it can be argued that, if such need exists, it will inevitably be the job of the NHS to 'pick up the pieces' created by either social structure or (the lack of) other social policy. It may be that bad housing produces ill health – but the ill health still exists. It may be that unemployment creates psychological problems – but they will still be registered. And so forth.

This is analogous to the debate about whether general 'health gain' is the NHS's responsibility, or whether other social policy should seek this while leaving the NHS as a robust health service for curative and caring services as well as appropriate prevention. The danger of using the NHS for general health gain is that overall social spending is reduced, the NHS is left to 'do everything'. Instead, a multidepartment strategy, including Environment, Social Security and others as well as Health, should allocate particular responsibilities to particular departments – which would ensure that the NHS kept its core responsibilities for cure and care. Currently, care – in particular, long-term care – is often being ignored, under the pseudo-progressive rubric of 'more attention to prevention'. It would be better if the Government tackled the causes of poverty and ill health, including pollution and bad housing, rather than relying on a nannying approach to individual health. The truth is, individuals pay more attention to their health when they are secure.

It can also be pointed out that the exact nature of the formula is less important than the rigour and indeed speed with which targets created by the formula are met. In other words, one can play around with as much mathematics as one likes. If, however, the politics of resource allocation (at both national and regional levels) mean that targets remain indistinct or are interfered with for political reasons, then one may legitimately ask the question, to what end hyper-sophistication?

THE NHS REFORMS

Three main changes to resource allocation procedures heralded by the NHS reforms were:

- firstly, a new formula;
- secondly, an allegedly faster route to achievement of targets (since modified);
- thirdly, an end to provider allocations (as with the old RAWP) and a move to purchaser/residential allocations.

The last phenomenon – and the means of managing this transition by region, as it has transpired – is arguably much more salient than the nature of formulae. (Indeed the similarities as well as differences between certain different 'formula' approaches ought to be emphasized. Professors Peter Townsend and Brian Jarman co-signed a letter in the *British*

Medical Journal a couple of years ago which argued that the challenge was not to 'nit-pick' over minute differences but to agree an approach and get on with it.)

Turning to a sensitive issue, some regional attempts to replace a reliance on SMRs would have disadvantaged their peripheral, non-urban districts. It is not, of course, the case that any approach seeking to incorporate analysis of social factors will have this effect. In the absence of details as to the effects on purchasing districts, it is likely that the application of a 'Townsend' approach (whether to hospital data or across the board) would have a less disadvantageous effect upon the 'deserving, non-urban' than previous attempts by various regions to diminish or change the role of the SMR. It is, however, difficult to predict such effects – especially in the absence of knowledge as to how much of the global allocation would be determined by such a procedure (whether hospital services or wider). In the spirit of the post-RAWP resource allocation methodology throughout the NHS, it would be very strange if a disaggregated approach to allocations were selected. The national formula, for example, after 1988 no longer differentiated between a number of categories of Health Service expenditure (six – or seven including maternity – in the old RAWP system, embracing non-psychiatric inpatients, psychiatric inpatients, community, and so forth). Instead, crude population was weighted by the square root of aggregate SMRs (for the under-75s) and by a weighted average cost for age cohorts.

GP FUNDHOLDING

Firstly, if one wishes to move away from 'funding the current costs' of GP fundholders, plus or minus increments here or there, it is important to have an approach by which the initial budget available for GP fundholders (as opposed to district purchasers) is determined. In other words, fundholders should really be treated as mini districts and allocated accordingly on this principle. The problem, of course, is that the small numbers involved (except in exceptional cases of very large consortia), and the partial nature of GP fundholding, make this an exercise that is neither methodologically nor statistically sound.

Secondly, given the (likely) political unacceptability in any case of such an approach, once the pot of money available to GP fundholders (in the aggregate) in the region has been determined, it is still the case that most GP fundholders purchase only certain (limited) services on behalf of their patients. Moving to a formula approach is devilishly difficult in this circumstance. Again, if the initial allocation to fundholders is determined, one can use deprivation weightings to allocate amongst the fundholders – for whatever purpose.

But the exercise is less valid if the specific service mix the GP fundholders are purchasing directly is less correlated to the general deprivation weighting. A different weighting might be necessary or desirable (unless fundholders purchase all care, as in some pilot projects, e.g. in Bromsgrove). But this is not the answer – it further diminishes coordinated planning for populations' needs.

Further complication arises now that three separate types of fundholder have been created, after October 1994: 'total fundholders', standard fundholders and limited fundholding for small practices.

Current research is suggesting that a more sensitive approach is provided by a methodology based on **individual patient indicators**, which can be applied statistically to calculating GP fundholders' budgets. This research is primarily motivated by an attempt to avoid what is known as 'cream-skimming' (either indirect or implicit 'patient-dumping') by GP fundholders.

OVERALL

The best approach is likely to be one that incorporates the SMR into a more sophisticated measure which is correlated with usage of service, rather than rejecting it. Arguably, using a broad brush approach, need and demand are therefore combined – and existing supply can be reasonably effectively 'controlled for' by aggregating small geographical areas such as electoral wards with (say) similar Townsend scores (similar levels of deprivation) in order to make the statistical correlation with hospital activity. This diminishes the likelihood that supply factors are predominating. To put it another way, different wards with similar scores are being grouped. These wards will vary in terms of the proximity to hospital and health services, in terms of the referral habits of GPs dealing with the ward's patients, and so forth. In consequence, such an approach is a pragmatic and quite useful means of diminishing the 'supply bias' and also the 'referral bias' whereby differential use of health services simply reflects different behaviour patterns (by autonomous GPs in the pre-reform NHS and by a combination of GP decision-making and purchasers contracting in the post-reform NHS). Once correlations are established, allocations can be made to overall districts rather than electoral wards themselves, which are far too small for such purposes.

SENSITIVE PURCHASING

Following the White Paper *Working for Patients* and the 'purchaser/provider split' inherent in the NHS reforms, much attention has been given to the need to develop an effective purchasing function in health care. The institutionalizing of a purchaser/provider split can in certain circumstances give more rather than less power to the provider, *vis-à-vis* the purchaser or allocator of funds, and it is therefore all the more important to ensure that contracts for health care, in line with purchasing priorities, reflect the needs of communities.

As purchasers and providers seek to gain power *vis-à-vis* each other, moreover, there may well be a trend to larger providers, merging in search of a 'monopoly', and larger purchasers, coming together to act as a counterweight to provider power. The blunt reality is that, given increasing financial constraints under Conservative governments, contracts have to be made to realize economies of scale. 'Local purchasing' is just a myth, in such circumstances (Chapter 11).

In such a scenario, purchasing sensitively for the needs of local communities may become more difficult – for the reason that contracts are made on behalf of large populations with reference to basically economic criteria. Where finance dictates a different solution to 'local voices', finance will tend to win. Furthermore, 'local voices' may not be internally consistent; nor consistent with experts' views of need.

Leaving aside for the moment the question of the GP fundholder, the district purchaser will typically have different types of population within its boundaries for which needs have to be accurately assessed. Existing services may not be the best means of meeting such needs, nor may the location of services be most appropriate for encouraging equity in access and other desirable objectives.

It is important, despite current frustrations, to look to the future and consider how effective large-scale purchasing can be combined with small-scale locality inputs.

In consequence, it is important to compare how small populations within district boundaries are currently 'provided for' – that is, the current expenditure on such small populations, and the services provided within such expenditure – with alternative means of assessing the needs of these small populations.

As a result, finding a criterion for assessing the need of small populations – independent of current expenditure or service mix provided for these populations – becomes an important task, as it has always been recognized to be at 'higher levels' within the National Health Service (at national level, in allocating to regions; and at regional level, in allocating to purchasers). There are, of course, significant problems in using 'top-down' resource allocation formulae for allocating to small populations. Some of these problems are concerned with appropriate measurement of need, others with the 'statistical problems' of dealing with small populations.

It can be argued that – once a district or other purchaser has received its allocation – the translation of purchasing priorities into contracts ought to reflect a number of criteria. The formula used to produce the purchaser's allocation may, for example, be based on death rates or a composite of death rates and other measures. This does not mean that the district's purchasing priorities ought to reflect only the criteria used in assembling the formula. For example, if there is a lot of 'death from cancer' registering significant weight in the formula, which therefore affects the size of that district's allocation *vis-à-vis* others, it may nevertheless be the case that that purchasing district wishes to use its funds primarily for other purposes.

This opens up difficult questions. Can a national service allow local priorities if these challenge the national criteria for allocating money? Up to a point, yes, but beyond that money, local revenue may be required. And how will the centre adjust that revenue, to ensure equity between rich and poor areas if there is no one criterion for spending money?

In other words, central criteria for resource allocation – valid and worthwhile as they may well be – may be an incomplete or only partial determinant of local purchasing priorities. The ideal picture of purchasing would suggest a judicious mix of criteria – effectiveness, equity and so forth – being used to make priorities in health care. Such criteria would reflect national, regional and local priorities in all likelihood. What in the pre-reform NHS would have been known as 'plans' can then be sorted out with providers. This glosses over the above problem but such a pragmatic compromise in the NHS will always be likely.

Otherwise, local choices will themselves degenerate to individual choices. For example, should limited money be spent on 'curing' a compulsive smoker? Why not give vouchers to individuals to spend as they like? But then all the efficiency and equity problems of quasi-privatization arrive (third-party reimbursements of private provision, as vouchers are used to buy insurance; 'top up' with private money; and so on. It is better to use the public purse for all reasonable health needs.

An important challenge is to ensure that those small populations for whom services are intended are those who actually receive the services. In other words, it is of limited use to place contracts as a result of purchasing priorities – and even to gear up providers to fulfilling these contracts effectively – if the patients do not 'turn up at the door' who are assessed as having the need! To that end, monitoring the take-up of services by intended small populations is important. The smaller one's geographical area of focus, the more homogeneous small populations become. The electoral ward, for example, will have greater homogeneity than the district – although even within an electoral ward there may be variation in socioeconomic and other categories.

In consequence, looking at how the populations of different electoral wards 'benefit from' current arrangements – and comparing that with what a different way of allocating resources on their behalf would achieve – is important. It should be stressed that such an exercise is not intended to imply that purchasing ought to be made directly by 'small-population health authorities' or indeed that purchasing ought to be rigidly defined in terms of, for example, the use of services by inhabitants of electoral wards. It is merely a case of comparing 'current spend'

with what different means of assessing relative need would imply the spend ought to be.

It is a fact of life in the evolving National Health Service that the health authority and other purchasers will be purchasing on behalf of populations of 250 000 and above, in the main. In consequence, purchasing on behalf of small areas or localities will mean sensitivity to local needs when placing contracts. The paradox is that, in order to purchase effectively on behalf of large enough populations, the particular needs of small populations may be ignored.

To counteract this possibility, contracts made by health authorities ought to reflect input from localities and also from general practitioners operating within localities, whether fundholding or not. (Fundholding GPs ought – by this perspective – to be 'integrated' into overall health authority purchasing to ensure that their priorities do not undermine global purchasing priorities, and render it impossible for providers to indulge in long-term planning to ensure that purchasers' priorities are met.)

In consequence, the particular needs of small area populations (such as those within electoral wards, or aggregations of electoral wards) should be assessed in making contracts and, once such contracts have been placed, individual providers in small areas (general practitioners, district nurses, health visitors and others) ought to indulge in 'social marketing' to ensure that the people on behalf of whom contracts are made actually are the ones who take up the services. Otherwise contracting – just like planning in the pre-reform NHS – will fall into disrepute as a means of meeting needs on an equitable basis.

The challenge exists to reconcile the aggregate needs of health authorities' populations with the particular needs of subdivisions of these populations – in electoral wards and aggregations of electoral wards. In this context, one can compare current expenditure upon 'small area' populations with the expenditure implied by certain criteria for measuring the needs of small populations.

There are two – arguably, diametrically opposed – methods of assessing the needs of such populations. One is the 'top-down' method, which seeks to apply formulae that measure need by population statistics, to small area populations. The other approach, the 'bottom-up' approach, conducts direct surveys of need among local populations. The problem in reconciling these two approaches is naturally to reconcile a requirement for a common measure of need that allows comparison of populations, whether small or large, with direct 'needs assessment'.

'Needs assessment', generally conducted by survey techniques, may produce a lot of valuable health and social data concerning local populations. What it does not do is translate such data into an agenda for the provision of health services to meet such need effectively. Subjective – or direct – needs assessment may therefore be an input into the process of assessing need for health services rather than the linchpin of such assessment.

The countervailing problem of 'top-down' approaches – building formulae to assess need across populations with different characteristics – is that the particular needs of particular populations may be ignored, inadequately gauged or inaccurately gauged by measures that are best applied to larger populations as an aggregate measure of need for broad resource allocation purposes. In other words, applying formulae that are suitable at national – or even regional – level may be less appropriate when considering allocations made by districts on behalf of local populations.

The challenge therefore is to consider how 'current demand' (as measured by current expenditure on local populations) compares with the amount which such populations should be allocated on the basis of 'need' implied by a formula, and in turn how these compare with the relative quantum of need implied by more direct means of needs assessment for both health and social care.

It is important to be modest about the purposes of such comparisons. It is not suggested that contracts are placed specifically on behalf of local populations within health districts. In particular, it is inevitable that the contracts placed by districts (or GP fundholders) will set the overall quantum of need against which providers have to offer generally available services. On the other hand, if there is any purpose at all to assessing need, it is in order to meet the needs of both particular local populations and indeed particular individuals. The alleged advantage of meeting such needs through a public health-care system is to combine equity with efficiency. In consequence, it is the task of responsive public authorities to make decisions on behalf of individuals which the latter would make themselves if they combined adequate knowledge of their needs with adequate finance to meet these needs.

It is up to purchasing health authorities to ensure that local populations benefit from services according to their need. Local health providers (GPs, nurses and others) ought therefore to 'market' available services to local populations to ensure that those whom 'the planners' desire to take up services do in fact take them up. In other words, large-scale contracting ought to be rendered compatible with locality purchasing.

If there is a philosophical basis to reconciling resource allocation and local need, that is surely it.

Appendix 1 outlines an actual project which compared current expenditure with what a formula approach would have mandated, for a health district's electoral wards.

FROM RESOURCE ALLOCATION TO RESOURCE MANAGEMENT

Hitherto, we have talked of allocating the money. But what about more direct service planning and management, which relates resources to programmes and services? In the UK, this area has – since 1986 – been known as resource management.

A HISTORICAL NOTE

Resource management has existed as a formal initiative in the National Health Service since 1986, when the so-called resource management initiative (RMI) was instigated. Its stated aims were 'to build on the involvement of doctors, nurses and management; to bring together clinical and financial information about treatment activity; and to put clinicians and managers in a position to monitor outcomes of health care'. The resource management initiative itself had 'taken over' from an earlier exercise known as clinical budgeting. This, however, had allegedly fallen into some disrepair on account of a supposed stress upon 'data and systems' rather than the broader behavioural changes necessary to achieve effective management of resources. The National Health Service has, of course, been seeking to manage resources since 1948, albeit in different ways. Early experiments in what latterly became known as 'specialty costing' began as early as the 1950s. Different regions, and different areas of the country, have over the years seen different experiments in costing and budgeting. These have ranged from broad programme costing, through specialty costing, through disease costing, to individual patient costing.

The Griffiths Management Enquiry, which reported in October 1983, naturally provided a major boost to 'resource management'. The institution of general management itself was at least in part geared to creating a mechanism and cadre of general management responsible for financial control while pursuing clearly identified objectives.

The 'NHS reforms' have subsequently taken the service in a number of different directions. The formal institution of a purchaser/provider split has created a situation in which provider units, whether self-governing trusts or not, are responsible for the management of their own resources. In such an environment, whether or not it is fairly described as a market, resource management can in fact mean the inevitable responsibility for managing resources which financial survival necessitates. That is, rather than simply being a 'top-down' requirement within a public bureaucracy, resource management may be a component of the inevitable business planning and financial control which any enterprise operating at the 'sharp end' must adopt.

In this connection, clinical directorates are a mechanism by which individual specialties and departments can be responsible for managing their own resources, again employed in pursuit of specific objectives. These objectives may be 'bureaucratically' ascribed by the provider unit, or the clinical directorate – more radically – may in effect be a firm within a firm, responsible for defining and acquiring its own business at least to a significant extent. Whatever point on the continuum occurs, resource management is naturally a *sine qua non*.

A BASIC DEFINITION

Resource management may be defined as programme budgeting in a health-care context. Of course the concept of resource management has been applied widely throughout the public sector, borrowing from private sector ideas in many cases, and is not uniquely a health service activity. However, for present purposes, resource management can be considered to be a procedure which addresses 'two sides of the equation': desired outcomes and the management of available resources to achieve these outcomes.

Programme budgeting is, analytically understood, an alternative to the earlier functional budgeting – whereby budgets were provided for inputs such as materials and labour. Programme budgeting ascribes total budgets for the achievement of objectives, and assumes that inputs will be planned, or 'bought in', within these total budgets. (A political aspiration here is often to cut labour costs, whereas ascribed functional budgeting often guaranteed labour remuneration and conditions.)

A distinctive feature of resource management in community services, or for specified client groups, is that it is conducted within a complex environment of 'chronic and continuing care' (perhaps within a client group for which acute care is only one small component). That is, resource management in a context of community-based health care for – say – elderly people may pose different, or at least more complex versions of, problems than acute-based resource management. The methodology outlined below will be accompanied by discussion that seeks to identify the particular features of resource management in this environment.

'Community resource management' is, of course, an activity which developed throughout the National Health Service from the late 1980s onwards. Particular issues involved in defining desired outcomes and mobilizing resources – often from different agencies with different budgets – in order to achieve outcomes will be alluded to below where necessary.

Overall then resource management is a behavioural activity as well as a technical or 'data-oriented' activity. It involves creating structures and devising mechanisms whereby different professionals can work together to achieve jointly agreed objectives. It would, however, be naive to assume that it is all about behaviour and nothing to do with money! Naturally the resource management initiative is part of the administration's attempt to ensure that existing budgets are, at the very least, used to the full before requests for more money are made. To that end, it is also a task of resource management to identify the necessary trade-offs between quantity and quality of service, if indeed trade-offs exist. There may be examples of cost improve-

ments which are also quality improvements. It would, however, be naive to assume that such are other than discrete examples. In consequence, agreeing acceptable levels of quality within available resources may be an important challenge within a resource management framework.

Already, this discussion reveals that resource management may be a procedure 'carrying a lot of baggage'. In New Zealand, the British approach to resource management was renamed 'service management' to take account of objections that the procedure is now broadened beyond the technical exercise which the earlier policy of resource management was, at least in part, geared to addressing. The name itself is not, however, of such great consequence, except possibly for political reasons. What in essence 'resource management' concerns is the mobilization of resources, from whatever source, to achieve agreed objectives in an agreed manner. Discussion of the roles of different agencies, different personnel and different structures are therefore introduced with this understanding.

RELATING NEEDS TO RESOURCES

A key hypothesis underlying the operation of this methodology is that the basis for resource management is provided by the needs assessment process. In other words, one is asking the question: for what end is one mobilizing, let along managing, resources? In the language of the purchaser/provider split, the purchasing strategy, based on the choice of priorities and the purchaser's service plan which results, must be assembled from an agreed consensus between subjective needs assessment, professional assessment and their translation into an affordable strategy.

Priorities refer not only to priorities within a particular client group's needs but across the needs of all those clients or potential clients for whom the purchaser (or joint purchasers), are responsible. Do clients perceive their needs as being met; and, if not, can resources can be further mobilized? To put it bluntly, are there unmet needs? And if so, can available resources cope? And if so, how? In practical language, resource management asks these questions and seeks to provide answers.

THE BASIC METHODOLOGY

Resource management can concern:

- how to meet currently met needs differently (more economically, more efficiently, or whatever);
- how to meet different needs from the same pool of resources;
- how to meet additional needs from the same pool of resources;
- how to meet current plus additional needs by pooling resources in a new way or by mobilizing new resources;
- how to make 'hard choices' about which services will have to 'go by the board' in order to meet needs which are considered to be more important, whether by the criterion of the epidemiologist, sociologist, economist or philosopher.

RESOURCE MANAGEMENT FOR COMMUNITY CARE

Much has been written on resource management, for the acute services in particular (Perrin, 1994). Less has been written on resource management for community services, and even less on multi-agency collaborative resource management for community care for the so-called 'priority groups', e.g. the elderly, mentally ill, handicapped and physically disadvantaged. I therefore focus on this group.

In the context of needs assessment and 'resource management' for care in the community, community services and/or client groups requiring a mix of services including community care, a major challenge for resource management is likely to be consider-

ation of a hierarchy of needs alongside the **total** available resource, involving a need to consider the total quantum of resources, across the following agencies:

- general-practice-based services, including:
  - GPs;
  - District Nurses;
  - Health Visitors;
  - and others, such as auxiliaries;
- community health services other than those attached to the general practice;
- local authority social services;
- voluntary services;
- private and personal services;
- hospital services;
- long-stay nursing or residential services.

Looking at how resources are currently used is in effect to look at the current supply or availability for supply of services. This supply is likely to condition demand. In looking at the current configuration of resources we are likely to be looking at how available resources currently translate into available services, and how these services are taken up.

Appendix 2 provides a practical example. Meanwhile, the implications for policy and management of effective linking of resources to needs for a particular client group are set out.

NEEDS AND RESOURCES: A POLICY FOR THE FUTURE

In judging whether total resources are adequate or not, it is necessary to:

- enumerate all resources across all relevant agencies;
- decide whether it is possible to expand the total resource for a particular client group within the total agency budgets, or within one or more particular agency budgets in line with appropriate care protocols;
- decide, in the absence of such being possible, whether it is possible to change priorities within the current budget for the particular client group, without deleteri-

ous effect upon statutory responsibilities, the health status of needy groups, or the legitimate conditions of staff.

For example, one of the three practices surveyed in the project detailed in Appendix 2 was revealed to have significantly greater needs, by our criteria, than the other two. A naive assumption could be that too much time is being spent on the care of other client groups within the total workload of the professionals attached to that practice or within the area generally. Before one can even begin to substantiate such a hypothesis, however, it will be necessary to demonstrate, that, as far as other client groups were concerned, the picture was in fact 'better' than in the other two practices. Even then, this might represent a deliberate local choice. There are therefore no easy answers. Instead, the challenge is to develop a consensus as far as possible amongst the different professional groups, and it is then less likely that rash decisions will be justified in the name of priorities or efficiency.

In the acute sector, the clinical directorate has increasingly been seen as the orthodox location for resource management, in that each clinical director is responsible for a programme (or series of programmes) which is clearly identifiable, and is therefore the best locus for budget holding. The analogy in areas such as the one tackled by this project to a clinical directorate is the 'care team'. Whether or not this means that there ought to be one identified person (the 'clinical director') who leads the team is a point worthy of discussion. In this case, the 'clinical team' presumably comprises the GP, district nurse, health visitor, physiotherapist, occupational therapist, social worker, voluntary worker and so on. The methodology underpinning resource management would encourage the definition of objectives to which all the team must subscribe. In a pure sense, there ought to be one budget held by such a team, which itself ought to be operating within one

agency. That is naturally not the case currently as regards either community care generally or care of a group such as the over-75s substantially in the community. Instead, the challenge might be to improve joint planning without formal reorganization or formal merging of budgets.

The historical problem naturally concerns the existence of different budgets, operated by different agencies, for sometimes different but sometimes overlapping and indeed sometimes similar purposes. The problem for the client has often been that the care received has depended upon 'whom in the system one has first bumped into' rather than upon any rational basis. This is the policy environment into which the Audit Commission's report *Making a Reality of Community Care* (December 1996) and subsequently, of course, the Griffiths Report *Community Care: Agenda for Action*, published in 1988, made their entry.

What is now known as 'community care', which was implemented formally in April 1993, in essence concerns a merging of local authority and social service budgets and what were formally Department of Social Security 'welfare' budgets, in order to allow monies to be merged and decisions to be taken rationally as to care in the community within such as budget.

What is known as 'Griffiths 2' – after Sir Roy Griffiths' report on community care, following his earlier report on general management *per se* – is, of course, only a framework for care which is unequivocally to be paid for from that newly merged budget. The project reported in Appendix 2 concerns the need to consider general-practice-based budgets and also National Health Service community health service budgets – arguably, these are much more significant in the realm of 'community services' of the sort identified in this project. GP budgets may be held directly by the practices, in the case of fundholding practices, for certain categories of care beyond those traditionally managed by family health services authorities and their predecessors family practitioner committees. Where GPs are not fundholding, health authorities naturally hold budgets. Both fundholding and non-fundholding practices naturally have responsibilities for **non-**'hospital and community health service' budgets to the FHSA.

Ideally therefore, a budgetary unification bringing together all the budgets relevant to this project would unify GP budgets generally, community health service budgets generally, local authority social service budgets and social security money – as well as informal and voluntary resources, and of course hospital and other long-stay resources.

We are, of course, experiencing considerable change in structure and therefore financial incentives at the present time. As well as the Griffiths 2 partial unification of budgets, we have a trend to encourage GP fundholders to hold budgets for certain community services. In the context of the purchaser/provider split, we may therefore be moving to two significant purchasers: on the one hand the GP fundholder and on the other hand the local authority Social Services Department.

In the context of these two purchasers with relevance for community care for groups such as the over-75s, it is necessary to identify the relevant providers. In such an environment, community health services – whether or not organized as trusts or whether 'employed' by GPs – are likely to grow in importance and the decisions that joint acute/community trusts were generally not welcome encouraged free-standing, albeit larger or merged, community trusts.

The argument is that, standing alone, these are less likely to be 'swallowed up' by acute sector priorities. On the other hand, it is less easy, in the sense of formal planning, to arrange for the 'seamless' care of individuals whose problems require a continuum from acute to community service care. Additionally, separate trusts have a tendency to 'shift costs and responsibility' to each other

for financial reasons. This is the antithesis of 'seamless' care, and a better idea would have been separate management structures for hospital and community units without making them 'financial' trusts.

As it is, the purchaser must ensure that incentives offered to providers are compatible with appropriate continuums of care for both individuals and populations.

This will often be a very difficult task in the context of autonomous acute and community trusts facing different financial incentive. Lessons from abroad, as well as theoretical reflection, suggest that the greatest danger consists in 'cost-shifting' from one providing institution to another. In consequence, it is important for purchasers to work closely in the realm of community services with their providers, to ensure that the advantages of local or 'autonomous' management by separate acute and community institutions are not offset by financial or other behavioural obstacles to cooperation.

The creation of discrete purchasing budgets for community care, as well as community services, opens the door to formal rationing of such services, as has been experienced with the social fund in the realm of social security. As yet, given the preoccupation with the fall-out from the NHS reforms generally, strict guidelines as to priorities have not yet been devised in the community care field for local purchasers. A major opportunity therefore exists for local purchasers to set out examples of good practice in order to inform the national debate. In particular, it is important that the new policy agenda is not simply seen as one of rationing (or denial of care) as opposed to needs-based planning. Unfortunately, this has been part of the 'welfare agenda' of the Conservative government, which has thereby – and ironically – discredited some good non-partisan ideas.

NHS hospital provision is of course free to the patient. This has ironically produced a source of fragmentation in planning the care of 'priority groups', such as the elderly. For traditionally, a rational decision as to the best location of care – in hospital, or out of it (as the fundamental decision) – is more difficult if one type of care is free and the other is means-tested, as with certain local authority types of provision, benefits which allow the purchase of supportive care and so forth. Interestingly, given the purchaser/provider split, it is possible to conceptualize a 'level playing field' for providers of relevant care for groups such as the elderly, given that they are charging a public purchaser and not the individual patient.

The stumbling block is that there is **not** a unified purchaser covering all conceivable forms of care for (for example) the over-75 client who requires assessment to determine the best form of care. The Griffiths 2 purchasing budget is a partial one; any (even extended) GP fundholding purchasing budget is also a partial one. The ultimate conceptual challenge is to devise a unified programme budget, within which all available care is to be purchased. This, however, runs into the problem of the policy inheritance, which is that some forms of care for some people are free and others are not. Making all such care the responsibility of the public purchaser would therefore be financially untenable, to the present Government at least. Such a global purchasing budget would require to be augmented through individual/private contributions, arranged through means testing.

An important challenge is to think in terms of types of care rather than in terms of the agency which historically provided care (or indeed, in the language of the purchaser/provider split, the agencies which are either responsible for providing care or for purchasing it). Thinking instead in the generic terms of primary secondary and tertiary care, the following framework emerges.

- Primary care is defined as holistic, first contact care.
- Secondary care is defined as specific, second contact care.

- Tertiary care is defined as specialized referral from secondary care.

In this context, one can conceptualize the following:

- primary, community care (involving GPs, community services, community care of various sorts);
- secondary community care (involving various types of home care, ambulatory care and so forth);
- primary hospital care (comprising prevention and promotion programmes, for example, based in and around the hospital);

and – more conventionally –

- secondary hospital care.

In terms of coordinating care for priority groups such as the one identified in address of this project, one may conceptualize a 'primary care authority'. This would hold the budget for all the above, while being directly responsible also for the provision of primary community care and secondary community care. From its total budget, it would be responsible for purchasing both primary and secondary hospital care. Such an authority would therefore supersede DHAs, the FHSA, GP fundholders and separately organized community services. The purchaser/provider split would only be maintained for hospital care. Concerning community-based (i.e. non-hospital) care, purchasers would employ providers and the **functional or conceptual** purchaser/provider split would remain, in that providers would be allowed to manage themselves with as much autonomy as was reasonable, but the **practical** purchaser/provider split would not remain.

In particular, one must consider:

- if and how a 'directorate' or 'committee' can manage the total budget, derived from different agencies for care of particular client groups;
- how the most appropriate care for particular clients within such a total budget can

be decided and, therefore, if and how particular budgets should be managed, i.e. by the traditional budget holders or by joint decision-making.

In particular, it might make sense to consider 'locality management teams' based on GP practice catchment areas with as much virement between separate budgets as possible. That is, instead of spending 'functionally' within the different agency's budgets, it might make sense to allocate all relevant monies to particular geographical areas in the light of agreed needs. In the context of the purchaser/provider split, this would mean all relevant purchasers agreeing on the location and degree of spending for particular client groups and then engaging providers – such as community service trusts – to 'do the necessary'. Such 'rational planning' is, however, full of potential difficulty in an era of compartmentalized budgets and 'enthusiastic local decision-making' (as with GP fundholders).

DISCUSSION

- Different methodologies for allocating resources to health authorities (and now GP fundholders as well) have been debated up to and since 1976, when the Resource Allocation Working Party (RAWP) set out a blueprint for allocating resources to (in those days) regions, and indirectly to districts.
- The basis for a resource allocation formula is the relative needs of populations within the country. We have a **national** National Health Service, funded centrally, and this is the best means of ensuring allocation of funds in respect of relative need (however contentious the measurement of that relative need may be). The alternative, of having at least partly self-funding local government units allocating resources, could lead to different services being made available in different localities – which might be an element of 'local choice' but it would end the national

nature of the National Health Service. Furthermore allocation from the centre to 'top up' the needier local authorities could be based on political wrangles as much as need; and additionally a 'revenue equalization' formula that sought to allocate from the centre to different local authorities on the basis of partial relative need would be difficult to arrive at. This is because it would not only be a question of measuring the relative poverty of different local authorities (based on firstly their local tax base and secondly their relative need) but because different local definitions of relative need would make such a formula potentially open-ended; and it would be to arbitrary central choice as to what to subsidize and what not to subsidize.

- Measuring the need of populations is of course a question of measuring the relative morbidity of different populations. It is the difficulty of measuring morbidity directly across all services (although it is possible for some, for example through cancer registration) which leads to the need to find a surrogate measure of morbidity. This has traditionally been mortality – and now there are moves to supplement mortality with various gauges of social deprivation and other factors which condition the 'need' for health services, or at least the legitimate demand for these services.
- There is a problem here both in methodology and measurement: how does one find the factors responsible for affecting need? Is need to be defined in terms of existing demand? Are differences in supply of services (based on historical patterns as well as upon need) to be taken into account? Refining methodologies which seek to correlate influences upon ill health with use of services is an important task, but is fraught with methodological difficulties. Nevertheless, consensus is beginning to emerge about a number of means of so doing, briefly referred to in the chapter.

• Having defined population need, it is of course important to translate the resources therefore supplied to health authorities into actual services provided by hospitals, community services, and indeed GP practices under the new unified system of health authorities incorporating the former family health services authorities. In other words, one is moving from relative population need to the specific needs of specific client groups and population groups within the health authority's boundaries. Making these planning decisions in the light of available resources is perhaps the broadest definition of resource management – relating desired services to resources and making the appropriate choices where necessary.

ACKNOWLEDGEMENTS

I would like to thank Stockport Health Authority and the Steering Group of 'Project Orange' for sections of this chapter respectively – Appendices 1 and 2 – on 'small area' resource allocation in Stockport and resource management for care of the elderly in Cheshire. (Both these projects were funded by what was then the Department of Health Management Executive.)

APPENDIX 1: A METHODOLOGY FOR COMPARING ACTUAL EXPENDITURE WITH A FORMULA BASED ON ALLEGED NEED – THE STOCKPORT PROJECT

CURRENT EXPENDITURE

The first task is to calculate the actual expenditure on health services in each of the 21 electoral wards. The approach taken was as follows:

Hospital expenditure

Stockport residents (total population to be split into 21 wards) may be treated either in Stockport hospitals or in hospitals outside Stockport.

The calculation of expenditure on Stockport residents using beds in Stockport hospitals was based upon patient data stored on a DHA database. This data consisted of details of all patient episodes in all Stockport hospitals for the period from 1 April 1991 to 31 March 1992. The next section provides the detail on how, and what, data was acquired; and what was done with it.

Naturally, information on the postal ward of patient was necessary in order to 'map back' to electoral ward of origin, in which the patient was resident. Information also had to be sought on length of stay, specialty of admission and diagnostic code within specialty.

Using statistical software, the independent data were broken down into number of patient days per postal ward. This calculation for each of the 21 Stockport wards was then expressed as a percentage of the total number of patient days. Furthermore, the percentages of patient day totals allotted to postal wards (percentages of total Stockport patient days) were then transformed into 'spend upon each ward' by calculating the effect of the individual specialty costs accounted for within each ward percentage.

While carrying out this analysis, it was of course important to exclude residents from outside Stockport being treated in Stockport hospitals.

The next stage was to estimate the number of patient days spent by Stockport residents in hospitals which were not within the Stockport district. Again, the next section explains how this was done.

The information on Stockport residents treated in hospitals outside the district was provided for all specialties.

Hospital outpatients in Stockport

The data to provide the required information in this category is much less developed than for inpatient analyses. In particular, a sample for a 6-month period was the approach taken. In consequence, the expenditure upon each ward had to be calculated by applying specialty costs to each ward's percentage of activity derived (as an estimate) from this information.

Family Health Services Authority (FHSA) expenditure

The patient lists of all GP practices in Stockport were broken down by number of patients in each of the 21 postal wards. As a result, figures were derived to produce the salience of each ward in individual GP patient lists, and therefore the contribution of each practice list to the total number of GP patients in Stockport. Naturally, non-Stockport-residents registered with a Stockport GP were excluded. Separate breakdowns of fundholder practice lists were made. In consequence, three categories for 'primary care' were derived:

(a)   drug costs and general medical services payments in FHSA administered practices;
(b)   non-cash-limited expenditures (plus administration costs);
(c)   data deriving from GP fundholders.

In the case of GP fundholders, the 'fund' includes traditional FHSA costs as well as the budget for limited categories of hospital care (and now community services). The expenditure involved in the cases of the two GP fundholders was naturally relatively small.

Community services

Ideally, an information system would have been available to allow workload by ward by various categories of community service to be derived or fairly accurately estimated. In other words, different budget-holders (real or nominal) and professionals involved in community services (such as district nurses, health visitors and others) would have had their workload broken down ward by ward.

In practice, such information was not available. Another option would have been to undertake a survey of the key professions to see what the relative workload in different wards was. This, however, was not at all feasible within the confines of the current project.

There was therefore no alternative, for present purposes, to simply averaging community service expenditure over wards by population. (Arguably, given the lack of significant variation between wards in terms of population, simply attributing one-21st of the community service budget to each ward would have been a 'rough and ready' way to proceed.)

Such a simple procedure – inevitable in the circumstances – at least allows the total budget (for hospital and community health services, and also FHSA expenditure) to be attributed to the 21 wards – with varying degrees of sophistication depending on which category of patient and data one is dealing with. As a result, a total figure is available that can be compared with the 'target' figure suggested by the application of a resource allocation formula, to be discussed just below.

Another approach would be to exclude community services data – which is, of course, significantly smaller in salience than hospital data as a total. If this is done, it is necessary to derive each ward's current expenditure as a percentage of the total district expenditure (across all patient categories for which information is available). Then this percentage can be compared with the percentage of the available finance to which each ward would be entitled as its 'target' as produced by the resource allocation formula.

In other words, one is assuming 'flat rate' apportionment of community services, in the absence of better information. Community services expenditure would therefore not alter the percentages, and therefore the comparison. Refining this part of the analysis is important, if difficult for now, and would go hand-in-glove with an attempt to relate community workload (*via* a COMWAY system, for example) to 'needs assessment'-type estimation of community need across the district.

APPLYING A RESOURCE ALLOCATION
FORMULA

The North-Western Region applied a simple 'mortality-based' formula, in allocating to its districts. The challenge here was to derive data on population (broken down into the usual age cohorts) for each ward, aggregate SMRs for each ward (which had to be compiled from condition-specific SMRs, available from OPCS data) and age weightings in order to quantify in terms of expenditure per head per age group, so that the objective measure of need (the SMR) could be augmented by a practical estimate of likely call on health services resources per age group. This is, of course, what national and regional formulae do, in order to quantify simple and 'independent' measures of need such as the SMR.

To sum up, it was necessary to acquire the population for each ward, an age-cohort breakdown for each ward, a (Department of Health-derived) expenditure per head per age-group estimate and an SMR for each ward.

This data was provided by the North-Western Regional Health Authority Finance Department, which undertook the progressive, step-by-step weighting of population to produce weighted population targets for each ward. The same methodology was used as when the region produced district targets. This weighted population can then be translated into financial targets by taking each ward's weighted population as a proportion

of the new artefactual total population, and applying for each ward that percentage to the available total budget (total revenue budget).

When one allocates from the centre to regions, one takes national averages around which regional figures vary, in order to calculate SMRs. Similarly, in allocating from regions to districts, one takes regional averages around which district SMRs vary. The same procedure was applied in calculating ward targets: ward SMR rates were based on the district as baseline comparison. (In other words, ward SMRs varied around a district average.)

An 'under-65' SMR was chosen reflecting increasing consensus that, if the SMR is to be an effective measure of 'need', data should not be biased by deaths among the elderly. In this way, the SMR is closer to alternative measures of need such as Years of Potential Life Lost.

While this varies slightly from national practice, the data was most easily available in this form in any case. Furthermore, the aim of this project is not to compare a **current** national formula (likely to change in any case before very long), and what it implies for ward expenditure, with actual ward expenditure, so much as to compare an **appropriate** formula with current ward expenditure, in order to 'throw up' useful indicators to be interpreted cautiously (see conclusion).

A significant caveat has to be entered, as briefly discussed in the opening theoretical section. One cannot simply use 'death rates', standardized or not, to suggest that the need for services for each ward is accurately gauged by such a procedure. Arguably, it is inappropriate to do this in allocating from region to district, in that the smaller the population one is dealing with the less (and less stably) simple mortality measures are correlated to need for health services. Indeed, at the national level, it is argued by some that the SMR is no longer as appropriate as it once was, originating as a one-to-one measure of need in the days when other sources of data were less available and when other theoretical approaches to gauging need were less well developed.

In consequence, aggregating electoral wards into groups – such that the Stockport residential district was, for example, divided into four or five (rather than 21) 'small areas' – would provide more reasonable populations to which death rates could be applied. However, in the context of this project it is not necessary to do this – as naturally the aim of such information is not to allocate to 'ward purchasers' nor to suggest that the expenditure generated by such a formula is the expenditure which should occur on behalf of ward populations in some precise manner. It is merely an indicative guide to whether current expenditure is 'on the right track'. Other criteria for deriving need for such small areas are necessary. In this context, a needs assessment exercise being undertaken in parallel with this research project is expected to produce useful data which in the long term might be able to be incorporated into a sensitive needs-weighting for community services (not hospital services), which the district might wish to use for planning, prioritizing, purchasing and contracting purposes.

The aim of supplementary indicators of need is not to build a mechanistic formula so much as to provide sensitive information for purchasing for the needs of localities. And, as pointed out in the theoretical section above, if such an approach is to produce fruit, it is necessary that the needs identified are met – in other words that the clients who produce the statistics on need are the ones who benefit. There is therefore much behavioural work in the 'social marketing' of health services to be done to achieve such ends. Naturally such work is well outside the remit of this project.

The information provided here allows one to compare current expenditure with what a formula approach (with all its inadequacies at small area level) might imply. The research

agenda stemming from this information is to explore differences and to look for more sensitive measures of need which might validate one approach or the other – current expenditure or targets derived from the formula – or indeed neither. In other words, the information generated by this project should be considered as part of an ongoing attempt to derive more sensitive measures of need for small areas in the context of purchasing strategies. This task is all the more important when larger purchasers (such as consortia) have somehow to be 'kept in touch' with specific locality needs.

INTERPRETING ACTUAL EXPENDITURE AND FORMULA RESULTS, AND FURTHER WORK

An important caveat should be remembered: the formula weights populations by mortality rates – which may well not reflect local need, in any direct or clear relationship between such rates and implied need for (all) services. Furthermore, very small populations will have widely varying death rates. The ones provided, for one year, may not be typical.

Nevertheless, comparison is illustrative: wide discrepancies may suggest that current expenditure is leading to unmet need in certain wards (those with significantly lower actual expenditure than that provided by the formula as a target). This is a complex matter. Which is more important: 'expert-defined need' or 'actual demand'?

Furthermore, actual demand may be conditioned by supply: some ward populations may have better access than others.

At least death rates are not 'contaminated' by existing supply of services, as are some criteria of 'need' for allocating resources, which use actual admission rates as part of the analysis (for example, Jarman scores are used in 'RAWP-like' formulae according to their ability to predict admissions).

Further work should therefore target the following.

- Allocations suggested by formulae other than those using (only) mortality rates – the NW region formula is only one approach. Formulae-using 5- or 10-year averages of mortality and other data can also improve reliability of data.
- Direct 'needs assessment' and wider interview-based and questionnaire-based surveying of populations to see if (for example) discrepancies reflect real problems or if (for example) a 'needs assessment' exercise can provide data by which community services expenditure can be better targeted. The ongoing 'needs assessment' work in Stockport should be investigated as to its potential for incorporation into a formula. This is a delicate matter, however, as such 'bottom up' survey data may be difficult to use for 'top down' allocation purposes. Little has been done in this realm. An exercise such as the latter would not, however, 'answer the question' as to whether the current acute/community proportions overall are appropriate: such a judgement depends on a number of factors, for instance:
  - whether 'health gain' from either or both is measurable;
  - whether 'health gain' should override local (or indeed district, regional or national) wishes and subjective priorities;
  - whether 'prevention and promotion' in the community can be set – in outcome and cost terms – directly against 'acute expenditure saved' (if any); again, the importance of this topic is in inverse proportion to the quantification achieved in this realm.
- Conceptual elucidation of:
  - how to compare different approaches;
  - how to use monies locally to meet needs identified through locality-sensitive purchasing;
  - how to balance different considerations both in compiling the most satisfactory approach and moving to targets;
  - how to balance the need to 'target' on the basis of data with the need not to have rigid 'purchaser targets' for small areas in a service (the NHS) which should 'meet need at the time of asking' (for which, read demand!).

Overall, this research is an input to what ought to be a growing debate.

APPENDIX 2: A SPECIFIC EXAMPLE OF RESOURCE MANAGEMENT IN COMMUNITY CARE – CHESHIRE'S ELDERLY CARE AND 'RESOURCE MANAGEMENT'

METHODOLOGY

It was decided to undertake a survey of workload across the relevant community services. Ideally, all services catering in any way for the over-75s would be surveyed. The focus of this project was, however, upon community services, and the needs assessment concerns the elderly living in the community. To that end, those in long-stay institutions (hospital or otherwise) were discounted. A challenge for the future would be to enumerate and consider this population also, and the additional services it receives. It should also be emphasized that the methodology is geared to enumerating the salience of care for the over-75s by the relevant agencies, and in particular the professionals working within those agencies. It is not an exhaustive survey or prolonged piece of research which seeks to enumerate everything that is done, nor is it a full cost analysis – let alone a cost-effectiveness analysis – concerning care of the over-75s. To that end the data is purely illustrative, and it would be wholly illegitimate to use it in an attempt to pass judgement upon the contribution of the personnel being surveyed. It is capable, however, of providing data of the 'snapshot' variety in order to illustrate how different professionals are currently involved in care of the elderly over-75s and the extent to which such care is salient in their overall workload.

The basic premise is that human resources are the most significant cost component involved in care. To that extent, the basic premise of the survey is that it is important to acquire an impression of how different professionals working in different agencies currently are involved in care of the elderly.

A picture of one month's activity in care of the over-75s was sought as follows. Forms were provided to the participating personnel intended to enumerate, for each participant in each category of staff: the number of contacts; the date of contact; the purpose of contact; the diagnosis and related information (if relevant for the personnel – for example the general practitioner); and the duration of the contact.

The aim was to enumerate direct patient care time allocated by the various staff to the over-75s, as a proportion of their total direct patient care time. Furthermore, for each participating member of staff in each category, an estimate of hours worked in an average week was made, as was an estimate of the percentage of the working week spent on direct contact with clients and patients.

The following categories of staff at the following agencies were surveyed:

- general practices:
  - GPs;
  - district nurses;
  - health visitors;
  - other attached practice staff, such as auxiliaries;
- NHS community services;
  - community psychiatric nurses;
  - diabetic nurses;
  - chiropodists;
  - health promotion officers for the elderly;
  - others as applicable, such as stoma care nurses;
- local authority social services;

- social work teams;
- community occupational therapists;
- home care organizers and carers;
- voluntary organizations.

Anonymity of staff being surveyed was possible in that, for each practice or agency, the total staff time for a particular professional group (such as district nurses attached to the general practice) was used as the denominator, with the numerator being the sum of staff time spent on the over-75s, derivable from the survey. It was assumed that non-patient-care time (such as administration, travel and so forth) could be apportioned proportionately. In other words the fraction derived from our numerator divided by our denominator was unchanged, in that if one quarter of the working week (for example) was spent on the over-75s, it was assumed that non-patient-care time could be similarly apportioned.

To do a full cost analysis, one would survey or estimate all the time of all the carers spent on the relevant population, i.e. the over-75s in the three general practice catchment areas in this case. Human resource costs would then be estimated. An important task for the future would be to survey, estimate or calculate: the total budgets for relevant agencies in caring for the client group; the percentage of that budget which can be attributed or apportioned to care of the particular client group; and therefore the total derivable as an estimate of the total money involved in care of the relevant client group.

In our case, we were not seeking at this stage 'a figure with a pound sign in front of it'. The aim was to look at the salience of care of the over-75s in a number of agencies, over a range of professional providers.

The results obtained are summarized in Tables 10.1–10.4.

Table 10.1 Proportion of total community service provision to over-75s by individual service (based upon 6-month period) (illustrating for each practice the proportion of time spend by each of the listed professions in face-to-face contact with the over-75s – i.e. the denominator is the time spent in total by all community services on the over-75s; the numerator is the time spent by each profession as a proportion of that denominator)

Practice 1	%	Practice 2	%	Practice 3	%
District nurses	71.1	District nurses;	70.2	District nurses	71.2
Chiropodists	20.4	Chiropodists	13.7	Chiropodists	19.9
Physiotherapists	5.5	Physiotherapists	9.3	Physiotherapists	5.4
McMillan nurses	1.7	Mental handicap nurses	2.6	Continence nurses	1.2
Health visitors	0.6	Speech therapists	1.1	Speech therapists	0.9
Speech therapists	0.3	McMillan nurses	1.1	Health visitors	0.5
Continence nurses	0.2	Stoma nurses	0.9	Dental nurses	0.4
Dental nurses	0.1	Continence nurses	0.5	McMillan nurses	0.4
Diabetes nurses	0.1	Health visitors	0.4	Stoma nurses	0.1
		Diabetics nurses	0.1		
		Dental nurses	0.1		

Table 10.2 Average time in minutes allocated to each over-75 person on the practice register by community services (based upon 6-month period) (the numerator is the total time spent by each community service on over-75s in that 6-month period, the denominator the number of over-75s on each practice list, thus providing a measure of salience of care of the over-75s)

	Practice 1 (n = 690)	Practice 2 (n = 780)	Practice 3 (n = 1010)
District nursing	45.9	58.1	46.3
Chiropody	13.1	11.4	12.9
Physiotherapy	3.5	7.7	3.5
Continence nursing	0.2	0.4	0.8
Speech therapy	0.2	0.9	0.6
Health visiting	0.4	0.3	0.3
Dental nursing	0.05	0.04	0.2
McMillan nursing	0.07	0.09	–
Mental health nursing	–	2.2	–

Table 10.3   Percentage of time spent by selected professionals based at GP practices on care of over-75s (face-to-face contact with over-75s/face-to-face contact with all patients, based upon a 1-month period of staff activity)

	% of total working time spent on home visits	% of this time spent with over-75s
Practice 1		
District nursing team	50.7	60.6
Health visitors	10.1	5.9
Practice 2		
District nursing team	57.2	75.7
Health visitors	33.9	4.6
Practice 3		
District nursing team	35.8	68.9
Health visitors	23.1	4.7
	% of total working time spent on patient contact	% of this time spent with over-75s
GPs	70	15.0
(Contact with over-75s at home = 69.0; contact with over-75s in surgery = 31.0)		
Practice nurses	80.0	8.8

Notes: (1) Data on GPs and practice nurses available for Practice 3
(2) We are taking as our denominator actual client contact time. Our assumption is that time not spent with clients (e.g. administrative or travel time) can be apportioned to client time in a straightforward manner.

Table 10.4   Proportion of Social Services staff time spent on the over-75s (face-to-face or telephone contact with over-75 clients/face-to-face or telephone contact with all clients) (based upon 1 month staff activity for two Social Services 'patches' – these are not coterminous with GP practice catchment areas: the two patches sampled are areas with a close overlap to two of our three practice areas)

	% of time spent on the over-75s	No. of staff
Patch 1		
Social work team	26.7	3
Community occupation therapy	16.3	1
Home care team	–	–
Patch 2		
Social work team	37.9	2
Community occupational therapy	–	–
Home care team	69.0	7

The ultimate aim of a resource survey would be to provide an estimate, or actual calculation, of the total budget available for care of a particular client group – what might therefore be termed a **programme budget**. This programme budget could be broken down into a variety of subheadings, and for present purposes we chose three areas identified from the needs assessment phase of the project – the **physical**, **emotional/psychological** and **social isolation** categories.

However the data on activity is classed almost wholly as services provided to address physical needs. It may be that a wider social purpose is served by some of these visits. The data does not allow this to be quantified. Our conclusion, with this caveat, is nevertheless that social isolation represents a potential unmet need.

Alternative methodologies exist for enumerating resources. As in this project, the percentage of the time of particular professionals geared to the relevant 'programme' can be estimated. In consequence, given knowledge of salaries plus on costs for these professionals, a money equivalent can be derived if necessary. (It was not considered relevant to do so within this phase of the project, and might legitimately be perceived as threatening in the absence of further explanation or cogent demonstration of reasonable use of such information.) Other costs from each of the agencies concerned with care can be estimated or discovered.

These costs can be broken down into fixed versus variable and/or direct versus indirect. For example, direct costs of care might be the transport and utility costs directly related to care of the elderly over-75s. Indirect costs might be administrative costs of agencies overall which had to be apportioned, in proportion to the salience of over-75 care within that agency.

Fixed costs concern, for example, salary costs of all agency personnel either directly or indirectly involved in care of the over-75s. Variable costs might include consumables such as drugs prescribed to the over-75s, which again would have to be distinguished from general prescription costs within the practice.

For the meantime, the aim was to provide a picture of the salience of effort from each professional group in caring for the over-75s. Limiting the survey of resources to the human resource dimension is justified by the overall salience of the human resource dimension, but also by the fact that the major management challenge following from the survey derives from a joint consideration by the different professions of appropriate ways of meeting identified needs not currently met or adequately met. The first step in meeting needs, of course, is to agree them. There is, however, no point in agreeing abstract 'care protocols' for caring for clients' particular needs unless a picture of the current activities of each professional group and the salience of care of the relevant client group within that workload is provided. In other words, setting out ideal care packages for individual clients to meet needs identified in projects such as this one may be an impractical and therefore frustrating exercise if it does not take account of 'the art of the possible'. To that end, intra- and interprofessional dialogue has to take account of possible changes of priorities within the relevant client group, as well as between different client groups.

A workshop was held, for all participating professionals as well as the project team. Whereas an earlier workshop had been concerned with discussing the implications of a needs assessment exercise which had been conducted for the population of the elderly, to set against this 'resource management' exercise, and introducing the second phase of the project concerned with resource management, this second workshop was concerned with presenting the overall methodology that the project had used and with developing the implications for individual general practices – as well as for more general management and policy concerns. Important issues were identified, as follows.

- It was important to consider the degree of match or mismatch between needs identified in the needs assessment phase of the project and needs by implication being tackled as a result of the activity revealed in the workload survey in the 'resources' phase of the project. It should be pointed out that an apparent 'mismatch' might mean that resources were currently being directed to other important activities, which therefore did not show up as 'unmet' needs in the needs assessment phase. Were resources to be diverted to meeting these identified needs, it might be that currently met needs would no longer be met and that therefore other needs would show up at a future needs assessment phase! In other words, one can consider the need for an 'audit cycle' of activities as follows: needs assessment, resource survey and then needs re-assessment – say 2 years later, surveying a similar population or the same population. with allowance made for the fact that it was older. In other words, one takes the needs assessment as a starting point, agrees priorities and 'care packages' to meet these priorities, interprofessionally, as the next stage (taking into account available resources) and then 're-audits' needs in the hope that a later phase of needs assessment reveals that there are fewer outstanding needs. In other words, one is tackling outcomes through resource management.
- The main substantive need identified was the need to 'care for' the consequences of social isolation or to 'prevent' social isolation as far as possible. The most appropriate ways of caring for such a need were discussed at the workshop.
- How can people suffering from social isolation be helped through more visits; who ought to make these visits; how often; and at what cost to current programmes?
- One should consider specific care packages to address specific needs. It is always

a question of striking a balance between arbitrariness and unacceptable variation, in caring for people with similar needs in different locations on the one hand and over bureaucratic 'care protocols' on the other hand which remove legitimate professional autonomy. In between these two undesirable extremes lies consensus between different professionals – allied to a sense of what is practically possible in terms of resources and time – as to acceptable care packages for individuals with particular needs. For example, one can consider the following: how can more effective continual relief of chronic physical pain be provided, and what is the different role over what periods of time and at what particular times, of different professionals?

- How should programmes be assessed as to outcome? In other words, the need is to **plan**, **programme**, **implement** and **evaluate**. And finally, what are the best forms of management, organizational collaboration or even change in structure and policy to achieve agreed objectives?

It can be seen that this list varies from the specific to the general. For example, practices can be responsible for auditing and re-auditing the achievement of outcomes for particular audit groups, using needs assessment and resource evaluation methodologies as above. On the other hand, the policy environment is at the end of the day the responsibility of the Government, especially in a centralized state such as the UK. In consequence, working within current structures may not mean working within best available structures. The challenge therefore is to mobilize resources informally as well as through formal collaboration or merged agencies.

REFERENCES

Audit Commission (1986) *Making a Reality of Community Care*, HMSO, London.
Bradshaw, J. (1972) in McLachlan, G. (ed.) *Problems*

and Progress in Medical Care 2, Nuffield Provincial Hospitals Trust, London.

Carr-Hill, R. *et al.* (1994) Allocating resources to health authorities. *British Medical Journal*, 309, 1046–1049.

Griffiths, R. (1988) *Community Care: Agenda for Action (Griffiths 2)*, HMSO, London.

Glennerster, H. and Matsaganis, M. (1994) *Implementing GP Fund-Holding: Wild Card or Winning Hand?*, Open University Press, Buckingham.

Judge, K. and Mays, N. (1994) A new approach to weighted capitation. *British Medical Journal*, 309, 1031–1032.

NHS Executive (1994) *Review of Weighted Capitation – New Formula*, Resource Allocation and Funding Team, Finance and Corporate Information Directorate, Leeds.

NHS Management Board (1988) *The RAWP Review*, Department of Health, London

Packwood, T. *et al.* (1991) *Hospitals in Transition: The Resource Management Experiment*, Open University Press, Buckingham.

Paton, C. R. (1985) *The Policy of Resource Allocation and its Ramifications*, Nuffield Provincial Hospitals Trust, London.

Perrin, J. (1994) *Resource Management in the NHS*, 2nd edn, Chapman & Hall, London.

Resource Allocation Working Party (1976) *Sharing Resources for Health (The RAWP Report)*, HMSO, London.

Smith, P. *et al.* (1994) Allocating resources to health authorities. *British Medical Journal*, 309, 1050–1053.

Townsend, P., Phillimore, P. and Beattie, A. (1988) *Health and Deprivation*, Croom Helm, London.

FURTHER READING

Mays, N. and Bevan, G. (1987) *Resource Allocation in the NHS*, Bedford Square, London.

Sheldon, T. *et al.* (1994) Attempt at deriving a formula for setting general practitioner fund-holding budgets. *British Medical Journal*, 309, 1059–1064.

PART THREE

UNDERSTANDING AND LEARNING

THE GOALS OF HEALTH POLICY

The purpose of this chapter is to consider the most important challenges in devising an improved national health policy for the future. It focuses on the **structure** of health policy, the institutions and changed framework required to improve purchasing and planning, and strategies for coordinating purchasing and provision to meet agreed needs. The chapter is about more than 'structural fixes' or organizational issues, although these form part of the focus. In essence, it is about how to improve upon current policy at the national level, and therefore upon strategic management of and within the National Health Service, in order to provide a better framework within which to pursue health objectives.

Policy can refer either to the process by which laws and regulations concerning health care (and its provision) emerge or the effect of such 'outputs' upon society – in terms of health status and wellbeing. This book has assumed the relevance of both, in that auditing or monitoring the latter is very likely to involve a critique of the former. Policy analysis, in turn, in its broadest sense, consists in understanding the policy process and then seeking to influence it to achieve desired goals.

Policy analysis, in other words, is concerned with both process and outcome, in investigating how to achieve desired goals.

The primary goals of British health policy are, or ought to be:

- to ensure effective health-care provision for the whole nation, in pursuit of health for all;
- to ensure that equity in access to care is pursued in conjunction with an aspiration of equity of outcome in health status, across classes, regions and groups (the idealistic nature of the outcome not undermining the endeavour);
- to institute the most appropriate structures and incentives to achieve these objectives.

The premise from which the chapter begins is that 'the NHS reforms' currently embrace contradictory agendas as well as many inappropriate policies (Paton, 1992). It is also clear that, if and when a Labour government (whether a majority government or not) can be elected, it will be inappropriate simply to 'abolish' the NHS reforms *in toto* or to work against the grain of **all** – increasingly established – management structures and practices. That does not mean that significant new policies ought not to be adopted or that significant planks of the current agenda ought not to be repealed. In short, a radical and yet also pragmatic approach is required, by which it is meant that advocacy of significant change to current policy should be combined with workable proposals.

The challenge for any future Government, say a Labour government, whether or not supported by Liberal Democrats, is threefold: (1) to remove damaging aspects of the 'reforms'; (2) to improve on the best elements of the pre-reform NHS; and (3) to do so with the minimum of yet further 'reorganization', given the Conservatives' rather clever forcing of so much 'reform' that the NHS staff and public are too exhausted to change even the bad!

All in all, this tripartite challenge means improving incentives, without the retrograde move to a market and even (quasi-)privatization (Chapter 13).

THE POLICY ENVIRONMENT

INTRODUCTION

This first part of the chapter considers the policy environment within which the 'NHS reforms' are being implemented. The changing nature of the NHS is part of an environment that is hostile to public health services, coordinated to achieve public goals. Finance is, of course, at the heart of the Government's approach to the public sector. Hard choices in financing the NHS – and targeting its programmes – are outlined at the general level. It is argued that the form of centralism in NHS policy and management pursued by this Government (against the prevailing rhetoric) is a consequence of political didacticism and economic constraint.

THE NHS REFORMS

The chapter examines certain key aspects of the NHS reforms and asks how they might be changed, superseded or repealed in order to produce a better coordinated health policy. To summarize, key elements of the reforms, at the general level, are considered to be:

- the institution of a contracting process through a purchaser/provider split;
- creation of self-governing trusts ('opted out' providers);

- the creation of a fragmented and unclear purchasing structure, including both a haphazardly demarcated GP fundholding and a failure to determine priorities – or clear criteria for priorities – in purchasing. The failure to determine the relative priority (or salience) to be given to district health authority purchasing on the one hand and GP fundholder purchasing on the other hand is but one example in the last category.

It is now over 6 years since the Prime Minister's Review of the National Health Service reported, in the form of the White Paper *Working for Patients*. Within that time the NHS and Community Care Act was passed in 1990, and various stages of the NHS reforms have been implemented since April 1991. In fact the 'managerial' side of the reforms – including the creation of the NHS (Management) Executive to replace the NHS Management Board, for example – predated legislative change. The key components of the NHS reforms are now well known – on paper.

In practice, the agenda was so broad and so hurriedly concocted that many of the current problems emanate from a failure to think through the consequences of particular policy initiatives and a failure to ensure the compatibility of different strands of the NHS reforms. Implementation has thus involved policy-making – not *ipso facto* a bad thing, but dangerous if policy is made 'on the hoof'.

Furthermore, the later emergence of the White Paper *The Health of the Nation*, and the Patient's Charter as part of the Citizen's Charter for public services, has meant that later policy also has been cobbled on to an already complicated agenda with – again – a failure to think through ultimate objectives or the compatibility of different initiatives.

The purpose of this chapter is not solely to present a critical review of these episodes, from the viewpoint of contemporary history. Instead, while drawing attention to the consequences of emerging policy, it seeks to suggest alternative routes, where these are considered to be necessary. Some lessons from abroad are also considered pertinent. Comparative insights are especially important when the 'export' of the NHS reforms is seen as something of a growth industry.

PRIORITIES

At the level of national policy, the following ought to be priorities:

* the coordination of 'purchasing' into coherent service planning;
* an end to fragmentation and 'perverse incentives' in provision;
* clearer delineation of national, regional and local responsibilities for planning and provision;
* a translation of the 'rationing' debate into an equitable strategy for provision of health care, with both national and local contributions;
* the rendering compatible of greater democracy in health policy-making with effective management.

There are many important challenges beyond those; likewise, there are significant overlaps in the areas listed. Overall, the aim is to suggest the rationale for a more effective structure within which priorities, purchasing and provision can be tackled. Currently, policy-making and implementation of policy by management occurs 'on the hoof' – which produces some interesting local innovations but a worrying lack of coherence in health policy.

Ultimately, the political context of health policy-making must not be ignored. What John Kenneth Galbraith has called the politics of the 'contented majority' (Galbraith, 1992) may be considered to have a long-term effect upon the evolution of British health policy, priorities developed therein and the means by which conflicts are settled, under Conservative governments. The UK's failure

to spend on health care commensurate with our European neighbours – both in terms of total expenditure and in public health-care spending – coupled with the economic crisis confronting the UK, means that expensive care for the less economically productive may be a longer-term casualty of the overall economic and political environment. Some specific consequences of 'the NHS reforms' which may hasten this trend are outlined, and – by way of a number of caveats – the need for an alternative approach is identified.

THE CHANGING NATURE OF THE NHS

Recent changes increase pressure to ensure that the NHS workforce – especially at the poor end of the spectrum – is paid as little as possible for as much effort as possible: for two reasons. Firstly NHS providers are now behaving commercially, and therefore seeking to maximize the productivity of the workforce at minimum cost. Secondly, NHS providers are funded (mostly) from state sources (channelled through health service 'purchasers') and the increasingly tight budgets available from the state to purchasers mean that a squeeze is put on providers and their workers. A centralist agenda thus lies behind the eulogy of 'local bargaining'.

In essence, the NHS is arguably becoming a support service for the economy as a whole. Making health priorities according to individual and social definitions of 'health gain' is bound to be influenced by economic criteria such as productivity restored to workers, using the human capital approach. This means that companies, tax payers generally and the state are pooling resources in as efficient a manner as possible in order to finance health care as a 'support service' to the economy. The status of community care *inter alia*, within such a scenario, would of course be a cause for concern.

This is a two-edged sword. On one interpretation, this is a source of economy and efficiency being compatible with (some) equity. On the other hand, it allows (mis)use of the NHS by right-wing governments, exploiting cheap labour under the guise of 'decentralized, individual bargaining'.

Certainly key workers in short supply are able to be paid more, as local bargaining (whether collective or individual) is sought by self-governing trusts. The other side of the coin is, however, less frequently advertised in official circles.

FINANCING

Recent evidence has shown that spending on the National Health Service has fallen even further behind health service spending by other 'Western democracies'. The percentage of gross domestic product spent on health care (public and private) in the UK is lower than nearly everywhere else in Europe; the percentage spent on **public** health care is also lower than in most countries in 'western' Europe, despite the fact that the lion's share of the UK's expenditure is on public health services and that therefore one would expect to compare the UK's total with other countries' totals (see Table 2.1). Other countries have their private spending built into the system (as with most European countries) and therefore the first set of figures is the most useful. For example, in the Netherlands, much 'private' spending is integrated into the national system. In the UK, any greatly increased private spending would make it more difficult for the better-off to redistribute to the poorer, who are dependent on the NHS. This is because private care is more expensive, in aggregate (when not subsidized from the public purse, as with the provision of medical staff at marginal cost!). As a result, boosting private finance in the UK would not boost the total spending significantly, if at all.

The primary reason for the figures given in Table 2.1 is that, as health expenditure has grown to cope with changing and increasing needs for health care throughout the 1980s and early 1990s in Europe, Conservative governments in the UK have strictly limited increases in expenditure on the NHS to the minimum required to allow the political claim that 'real' growth has occurred. Commentators who point out that there has been 'real' growth during this period miss the point that the increase in the UK has been significantly less than in most comparable European countries.

Major trends in NHS policy during this period have included:

* a diminution in commitment to 'priority' care (i.e. 'chronic' and social care) on the NHS, accompanied ironically by an increase in the volume of rhetoric hailing this as a priority; for example, only 10% of 'chronic' beds are now in the NHS, as opposed to 30% in 1979. Despite evidence that public (NHS) nursing homes are a cost-effective answer to the need for an 'intermediary' tier between the expensive hospital and home, the Conservative government has not been interested. Despite lessons also on 'hospital hotels' for aftercare being more efficient than either bed-blocking or inappropriate discharge, there has been little progress here either (in the UK);
* significant increases in total waiting lists despite targeting of certain, less urgent waiting times;
* an increasing exploration of devices such as the 'quality adjusted life year' (QALY) and its methodological soulmates in an attempt to 'ration' (or deny) care.

These trends make it easier to depict the NHS, as a result, as a very tightly funded service geared increasingly (on the basis of various rationing devices devised by economists) to meeting the needs of the more productive people within the British economy. In effect, the state may be beginning to justify its role in health care as taking limited tax money on behalf of industry and the economy as a whole and using it, in as parsimonious a manner as possible, to meet needs defined with negligible reference to equity, let alone equality. Equity, one hears it stage-whispered in the Department of Health, is a very '70s' concept!

In the 1970s, certain (so-called) Marxist commentators such as Vicente Navarro seemed to imply that public health services in capitalist societies exhibited the feature of extracting surplus value from public sector workers on behalf of the economy as a whole. This was often too simplistic an argument in that value for money was not distinguished from exploitation. The NHS as a 'noble and cost-effective socialist island' was also a plausible portrait. Today, however, it seems intermittently as if the Conservative government is determined to bear out a Marxist partial truth.

Devices such as the QALY can easily degenerate into excuses for de-emphasizing priority, care or protection for the less productive, the older and socially less valued.

A CHANGING SOURCE OF FINANCE

Another major trend throughout the 1980s has been the rendering less progressive of the taxation system. Direct (income) taxation has been significantly reduced for the better-off, with the abolition of higher rates of tax; indirect taxation (principally VAT) has been significantly increased (from 8–17.5%) under the Conservative government, which places a greater burden on those who consume a greater proportion of their income – the poor. As a consequence, funding the NHS from general taxation means making the responsibility for paying for the NHS a greater relative burden upon the poor.

As a result, it might ironically be more equitable to consider moving to a 'national health insurance'/'public health tax' system whereby particular contributions were paid by the individual, the employer and the state. This might, if designed in a particular manner, ensure that the richer in fact paid more by way of their contribution – whether

we are talking of employers or richer individuals. It might also mobilize more resources for the health-care system. Since an earmarked tax (call it public insurance, if you like) would be guaranteed to be spent on health care, it might be more possible thereby to generate extra revenue. But a caveat should be entered: at time of recession or economic downturn, any source of finance is diminished. Earmarking a tax does not guarantee the maintenance of revenue.

A CHANGING ROLE FOR THE NHS? – UNIVERSALISM VERSUS TARGETING

In early 1995, both major political parties are rethinking the role of the welfare state. The Conservative government has found itself with a rapidly increasing public sector deficit, owing principally to a combination of cuts in direct taxation throughout the 1980s and the continuing recession. As in the United States (although with a less severe deficit than there), the dictates of fiscal policy are forcing a rethink about both the extent and structure of welfare. The Labour Party set up a Commission for Social Justice to consider priorities in welfare policy, among other things, which reported in October 1994. The fundamental nature of the NHS has been its universalism – the service is available, broadly free at the point of use, to all citizens. Any radical or iconoclastic thinking, under the rubric of the debate about universalism versus targeting of welfare programmes, is even more controversial and – to many – unwelcome when applied to the NHS, which is an institution whose core values are subscribed to by the vast majority of the population.

Nevertheless a basic question exists, at least at the level of theory: can the more disadvantaged in society best be helped through a public health-care system that focuses on their needs or one that is universal? If there is an increasing need to ration health care, the argument might go, it would make more sense to give the poor all they need and others only some of what they need from the public purse. Otherwise, rationing by service rather than by population group (or social class) would allow the better-off to purchase, or insure themselves for, excluded services, whereas the poor would be less able to do so without financial hardship. In other words, such rationing is denial of care to the poor but not to the better-off. It is therefore a progressive argument for targeting – if demand and need outstrip supply or finance to create supply – geared to favouring the poor, whether or not on a sliding scale.

There are, however, severe difficulties with such an approach. Programmes which are 'for the poor' may be poor programmes: they are likely to fall victim to spending cuts, especially by right-of-centre governments representing 'the contented majority'. Such programmes become 'welfare wedges' like Medicaid in the United States unless strong political correctives are available to prevent this. Furthermore, there may well be a poverty or unemployment trap created, whereby one loses benefits (such as health care) as one raises one's income.

Nevertheless, if the 'politics of the contented majority' are rampant, even a universally provided service, available to all irrespective of means, is also subject to cheese-paring or diminution. In other words, the NHS as currently available may be able to meet (relatively) less of society's expectations. In such a context, the worse off may be those least able to benefit from such a service, or to have their needs met fully from such a service, again in the absence of strong political correctives.

Specific aspects of the 'NHS reforms' may exacerbate such a trend. GP fundholders may have an incentive to 'cream-skim' (exclude the most expensive patients), if formulae reimbursing them are not meticulously devised. Both district purchasers and trusts may seek to exclude the 'awkward' patients – respectively through contracts and admissions policy.

It is an empirical question – whatever one's ideology or policy preference, in the first place – as to whether targeting or universalism will in practice help the poor (however their needs are defined), whether in health or in welfare policy generally. What can be asserted is that targeted programmes will be more effective if they are allied to an established set of substantive 'health rights', whether constitutionally protected or not, to prevent such programmes being susceptible to gradual erosion or Government cuts at times of financial difficulty.

Likewise, in the context of a universal National Health Service, overt rights – to update the 1977 Health Services Act, which is vague on the matter – might usefully be tailored to protecting the interests of the most needy in terms of those currently with the worst health outcomes, well known to be strongly correlated with lower socioeconomic groupings. Unfortunately, the present government is only interested in relatively superficial 'process' rights of a minimal sort, as in the 'Patient's Charter'.

Maintaining the universal nature of the NHS – if not, naturally, of all welfare programmes – is judged by the present author to be the best means of ensuring that the NHS is protected both politically and economically. This does not, however, prevent priorities being established within the financing and provision of such a service which favour those least able to exit to the private sector when their needs or demands are not available (or available in a timely manner) through public health services. That is, national, regional and district purchasing priorities can reflect a 'bias to the poor' that walks a tightrope between favouring the poor on the one hand and maintaining middle-class allegiance to the NHS as a service capable of meeting most of its needs on the other hand. To say this is easier than to achieve it. In practice, it may be argued that the NHS is trying to achieve such a balance at the moment. The rest of this chapter, however, points to some trends developing from the 'NHS reforms' which may threaten the service's ability to favour the worse off in society. A major challenge for a future left-of-centre government is to establish a coherent set of priorities, justified by social and epidemiological data capable of being audited as time goes on, which seeks the equalization of health status across the nation to a much greater extent than is occurring at present – or would be capable of occurring as a result of bland initiatives such as *The Health of the Nation*.

Since public finance and public provision are both – in British and international evidence – more cost-effective than private, a mildly progressive tax system can encourage all citizens to get benefit from the NHS (rather than opting out), as well as redistributing 'a bit' in the name of equity. As a result, greater NHS spending should be politically possible.

A problem with encouraging – overtly or indirectly – middle-class 'exit' from public health services is, of course, the fact that their need to insure themselves to have their care provided in a more expensive private sector will create pressures for tax relief and tax reductions, which in turn might threaten the remaining public health services targeted allegedly more effectively at the poor. In consequence, maintaining universalism in a National Health Service whose international and national characteristic is efficiency as well as effectiveness is likely to be the most sensible policy.

Seeing privatization, or private finance, as 'inevitable' is simply to reflect the reality that after-tax income is now more unequally spread. As a result, more can be spent on private care.

In order to demonstrate value for money for all social groupings and classes from publicly financed and publicly provided health service, a hypothecated health tax may be an appropriate means of relating costs to benefits in health care. This could comprise contributions raised in a tripartite manner from the individual, employer and the state; from existing taxation sources; or even from a single tax earmarked for the health-care system. The danger of such an approach is that, like all direct and indirect taxes, allying the prospects for generous health-care provision to revenue available from a particular tax may make fluctuations in health service spending greater than at present. In other words, during the downswing of the economic cycle, there is less money available – as fewer people are employed if direct taxation is used, or as less revenue is garnered from indirect taxation. If the NHS is financed from general revenues, it can perhaps be more easily protected, if it is seen as a priority, at the expense of other social programmes. Whether this is considered a good thing or not is a different question, but for defenders of the National Health Service it is likely to be. That is, the smoke-filled room of the cabinet's Star Chamber or of the Public Expenditure Review may have its advantages, despite the often arbitrary nature of such centralized decision-making.

A hypothecated tax, however, as an additional source of revenue rather than a total source might be promising – additionally as it would not have the disadvantage of encouraging the public to resist unpopular taxes (in areas other than health) even when necessary.

PRIVATE FINANCE

Another significant trend is the growth in private care, or rather – to diagnose the trend at its source – the growth in private financing. As society becomes more unequal, then even if the proportion of GDP going to public expenditure or the proportion within that going to health care does not diminish, what is 'left over' in private hands is to a greater extent in the hands of the better-off. In consequence, the growth in private care ought not to be a surprise. There is therefore nothing 'inevitable' about this phenomenon (as again some commentators have blandly assumed): it is in fact the (not always visible) result of a general redistribution of wealth. The consequence of such a trend for the public/private mix in health is not necessarily planned to evolve in this manner by conspiracy – but when it does so evolve, it becomes seemingly acceptable as a 'fact of life'. It is in fact a Tory fact of life.

In this context, it is somewhat ironical that so-called 'radical' ideas such as those pursued by David Willetts to encourage private capital, private finance, private provision and private management are fundamentally motivated by the incapacity or unwillingness of the Treasury to allow adequate public sector investment in the future of the health service – whether on a commercial basis or not. How can one expect radical and effective policies from a Government which is too weak to challenge more than incrementally the policy of its own Treasury?

There is still a significant 'bias against the public sector' in allowing it to compete on an even playing field with private investment. The essence of schemes such as the much-touted one which would allow Marks & Spencer and Tesco to build and equip hospitals in return for the proceeds from selling land and sites from closed hospitals, is that the public sector does not have access to bridging loans. They can only close a hospital once the new one is opened; but they can only afford to open a new hospital once the proceeds from the closure and sale of land and property of the old one have been obtained! David Willetts specifically acknowledges that the motivation of his various schemes is disillusionment with Treasury rigidity, based to some extent on his own experience as a junior Treasury official in the early 1980s (Willetts, 1993).

In 1994, the 'private finance initiative' was rigorously promoted within the NHS; but many managers found it a bureaucratic obligation (to search formally for private finance)

rather than an aid. Private need for profit often leads to limited interest in the NHS. More worryingly, it *distorts* the NHS. Hospitals have to seek income to 'pay off' their private 'partners'. The purchaser/ provider split, and internal trading, allows hospitals to seek masters other than public need. Even 'public borrowing' from private markets would be better than the crazy PFI. It *is* privatization – as assets are owned by private partners.

STRUCTURE: CENTRALISM?

It is in the above overall context that a changing structure for the NHS ought to be perceived. It is hardly surprising that, given a strategy of employing meagre resources to achieve what ought to be complex social ends, centralization should be increasing within the National Health Service. Nor is it surprising that such centralization should be accompanied by rhetoric pointing the other way, to 'decentralization' and 'devolution'. Control of resources and regulation of rationing approaches in particular (or rather, procedures for denial of certain types of care) have to be a responsibility of 'the centre' if the centre's objectives are to be met and political accountability for the NHS is to remain. Increased operational devolution is therefore accompanied by increased strategic centralism.

This may not be a bad thing, of course. Operational devolution may increase efficiency, while strategic centralism may ensure that national priorities are met, or at least sought – and indeed in the most cost-effective way (for example, as regional offices ensure that 'rival' or neighbouring purchasers do not cancel out each other's intentions) – for example, as regards concentrating services in the name of either economy or clinical quality. As with all questions about centralism, and whether it is a virtue or a vice, perhaps the most honest question asks, whose centralism? The left is less likely to complain about 'centralism' during the ascendancy of Labour governments; but right-wing centralism, as characterized many aspects of Thatcherism in the 1980s, naturally creates a desire for a new politics of decentralization on the left. It would certainly be a challenge for future Labour governments to ensure that central priorities are reconciled with scope for additional local priorities, in making purchasing and planning decisions for health care. A fair degree of cynicism is justified concerning the Conservative government's centralist approaches, purely because they are often justified as being the opposite – but perhaps also because such centralism reflects a desire to make national priorities that do not reflect the social mission of the NHS as understood traditionally by the left. In other words, current central priorities are not redistributionist or egalitarian.

It is interesting to note that, if the state is to represent the whole community more effectively in health care, it has to be the 'democratic' representative of the whole community rather than the agent of a particular economic interest or political function. We are currently witnessing the promulgation of 'democratic' local initiatives (for example, in making purchasing more democratic) encouraged from the centre (as in the NHSME's document *Local Voices*) in the context of increasingly 'undemocratic' national priorities.

The Patient's Charter reflects nationally – and arbitrarily – determined priorities on what might be termed the window-dressing side of the support services for health care. That is not to decry the need to reduce outpatient waiting times or the need to provide useful information to patients/consumers. If there is to be devolution of decision-making as to certain priorities to purchasers, however, why not let them decide what the most important issues are locally, in these, if not in more important, areas?

The Health of the Nation, equally, is a document which is uncontroversial in some respects but limited. In other words, many priorities which might have been established simply are absent, especially adequate targets for socioeconomic equalization. Green and White Papers so far have not faded the relevance of the Black Report (1980), nor the 'blacker' report (*The Growing Health Divide* – Whitehead, 1987). What is more, rhetoric favouring 'primary care' ignores the adverse effect of social policy in the 1980s upon health status, especially of the poor. A stress on 'prevention and promotion' which is geared to individual action (even in conditions of adversity) and not enough to social and environmental causes of ill health (let alone genetic causes) is a con. In any case, even **successful** primary care calls for more secondary care, as people live longer and fall ill in more complex ways! There is a suspicion that 'primary care' rhetoric is often just to soften up the public for bed closures.

Such a national picture does not, of course, invalidate local initiatives, such as innovative purchasing strategies by districts on the one hand or innovative means of cooperating between different purchasers (districts, GP fundholders, local authorities and others) on the other hand. But it does severely hamstring them.

THE CONSEQUENCES OF THE NHS REFORMS

ASSESSING THE REFORMS

A major problem in assessing the NHS reforms is that they have become 'all things to all men'. To the Government, everything good that has happened is because of the reforms; everything bad is somehow nothing to do with the reforms. As a result of this, it is probably impossible – given also the constantly changing and evolving plethora of initiatives subsumed under the continuing reforms – to attribute cause and effect in an empirical and scientific manner, in order to say 'the reforms have worked' or 'the reforms have not worked'.

That said, one can point to some trends that are associated with the changed NHS. If the linchpin of the reforms is a market-oriented purchaser/provider split, then one can look at the consequences of operating a market; the consequences of the purchaser/provider split as implemented from 1991 to 1995; and factors such as changing power relationships and growth of bureaucracy within the National Health Service.

One can outline a set of *desiderata* for the NHS, based on concepts such as equity, efficiency and effectiveness in the sense of appropriate services provided with adequate quality in appropriate locations. One can then ask, what is the best means of meeting these objectives – by market means or by alternative means? Simply outlining the necessary conditions for a market to work (and the regulation which may be needed to try to get the market to work, where the market breaks down and creates monopoly – i.e. creating the quasi-market) and seeking to fulfil these conditions in practice does not mean the market was the best route in the first place! It may be more expensive, bureaucratic and disruptive of other objectives, even it does, on its own terms, 'work'.

Another important component of the NHS reforms is to decentralize operational decision-making while centralizing political control of the National Health Service. This political control is often justified as effective management from the centre, but in fact the setting of political objectives for the National Health Service has increased with the reforms, as the management side of the NHS reforms has been characterized by a tightening of accountability to the centre. This is of course paradoxical, given the rhetoric of decentralization and the market (not the same thing): nevertheless what is on paper greater autonomy for self-governing trusts is often countermanded by greater stipulation of their activity through the purchasing function, itself accountable to central government.

In any case, if the 'problem' with the pre-reform NHS was too much autonomy within providers (for example allegedly on the part of doctors), why create a formally greater autonomy for providers unless there is an ideological belief that the market is the means to bring professions to heel?

Unintended consequences of decentralizing purchasing in an operational sense have, however, accompanied the more politically motivated agenda behind the NHS reforms. For example, in planning services providers, and often individual doctors, often have to deal with a plethora of purchasers – from a range of districts to a stack of GP fundholders – in order to mobilize the money for either a new service, or even a new drug. *The Independent on Sunday* (29 Jan 1995) quoted a paediatrician suffering from work-related stress, whose observation was that

> The NHS 'reforms' have created a bureaucratic bog, which you have to wade through to get anything done. For example, we are using a new drug for some patients which is very expensive. I put in a report to the regional health authority requesting payment for it. They said I had to put it to the fourteen district purchasers in the region separately.

> The purchasers are so inept and ignorant that you have to write a simplistic report for them, as if you were writing for *Tomorrow's World*. At 7 pm and after a long day and often having been up much of the night, I do not want to start doing that.

While proper evaluation of new drugs and technologies is to be encouraged, it is nevertheless the case that the **means** of mobilizing resources may be more bureaucratic and cumbersome as a result of the NHS reforms.

An alleged advantage of the market is that it allows innovation by providers and a 'marketing process' whereby purchasers can then adjudicate amongst rival tenders – not only for the efficient running of agreed services but for proposals as to new or alternative services.

This can occur in terms of competition between hospitals, or between hospitals and community units concerning different modes of delivering care. One problem, however, is that there are significant costs attached to investment not only to provide a new service but even to tender for a new service on a tenable basis, by demonstrating its benefits. Such a process would require the prospect of long-term contracts, financial advantage to the bidder and enough money to run a system whereby there are winners and losers both in bidding and in running services. The high start-up costs and characteristics of the health-care market (not conducive to competition in the medium and long term) make this a dubious means of using scarce public money.

The lesson from other privatizations in the British economy is that tenders will require an adequate mix of profit and security. This may be neither ethically nor economically tenable for the National Health Service, if indeed for other sectors. Such a process also requires free access to capital, as in a properly functioning market. Yet despite the language of capital charging and the market, capital investment is still heavily centrally controlled in the NHS – as indeed it probably needs to be. In practice, 'the market' is simply a language whereby bids are made by providers to purchasers for capital – and you do not normally go to your buyer for capital investment in a market! Ideas to make the region or even the centre 'the banker' are a means of solving this dilemma on paper, but in practice this simply means that 'the Ministry' decides who gets the investment and who doesn't. Doing this in a roundabout means is neither transparent nor, probably, efficient.

Arguments in favour of the purchaser/provider split are quite familiar by now and boil down to three major ones.

- Needs can be assessed separately from provider interests.
- Decisions can be taken in a global manner alongside consideration of resources, rather than simply through what has been called 'planning by decibels'.
- GPs and patients can gain power which has been redistributed away from the alleged 'hospital barons'.

However assessing needs does not require a market, as pointed out in previous chapters; nor does incorporating cost-effectiveness into choices as to type and location of services to be provided within available budgets. While illegitimate power by hospital consultants may, of course, be an occasional problem, a 'doctor-bashing' agenda, bolstered by a deliberate policy of divide and rule (between, for example, fundholding general practitioners and hospital consultants) is a less productive means of proceeding than managing hospital performance in a stable and planned manner.

The existence of even formally self-governing trusts indeed makes closures and reorientation of services a more difficult process. Separate boards for every trust mean a process of politics lying behind even rational decisions to close and merge hospitals and either transfer services to other locations or choose different services as a new and greater priority. Additionally, regulating a competitive market into existence, where it is both difficult to do so and indeed counter-productive *vis-à-vis* other policy objectives (as discussed at the end of Chapter 4), is an expensive means of proceeding.

The disadvantages of the purchaser/provider split, understood as an institutional split to run a market as opposed to merely a functional distinction between needs assessment and the management of services, are also significant. Later sections of this chapter discuss these. Admittedly a purchaser/provider split without a market is not necessarily subject to the same degree of inter-provider gaming, nor the same extent of provider marketing to distort purchaser objectives. Nevertheless an institutional purchaser/provider split *per se* may often have all the other disadvantages listed below under Damaging aspects of the NHS reforms, even although a market in any meaningful sense is not involved.

All systems have their disadvantages. For example, more liberal systems, which simply reimburse care chosen by patients or general practitioner, have the disadvantages of what economists call 'moral hazard' ('overconsumption' due to care being free at the point of use, such that individuals consider only the benefits and not the cost, and do not trade off cost and benefits); and of 'the problem of the third-party payer' whereby the reimbursing agency does not have an integral part in shaping the services.

However in public as opposed to private reimbursement systems, these disadvantages can be avoided – through (respectively) cash limiting and incorporation of patients' and doctors' perspectives into planning. A public planning process, linking capital planning with funding of services, can diminish the disadvantages of private reimbursement systems, which often amount to a failure to make priorities due to the absence of a public planning function.

That is, a system which combines liberal reimbursement (in the sense of funding services which people want to use) with public planning can achieve much. It is also important to note that another problem with private insurance – adverse selection, whereby, in the absence of expensive regulation, both providers and insurers have an incentive to screen out expensive cases – may actually have been exacerbated by the NHS reforms. This is because both purchasers and providers have a clearer financial nexus, and therefore a clearer incentive to avoid expensive cases which make it difficult for them to meet their financial targets.

The short-termism of financial targets (for example annual 'break evens' for trusts, on an individual basis, rather than longer-term financial stability of the whole district's service mix) will also exacerbate such factors.

Annual financial targets for purchasers also militate against sensible planning, as – for example – purchasers fail to invest in services with a long-term benefit yet invest in short-term high cost (for example, specialist services in mental health).

Finally in this section, in comparing alternative systems and indeed alternative ideas for reform of health-care systems, it is important to remember that lessons from abroad should be taken account of where possible. Comparing different health-care systems is fraught with difficulty and is a complex task (the full complexities of which cannot be discussed here). Nevertheless, an important lesson from the United States, from the 1960s to the present day, is that assumptions that competition will cut costs – in the absence of top-down Government pressure to do so – are dubiously founded. For example, in the United States, it was alleged that the planning legislation of the 1970s, which sought in a very tentative way to control both quantum and price of service provision, was unnecessary, in that the market could do a better job. The reality was, however, very different: the surplus of providers necessary to run a market may mean both greater cost and a subversion of what in the UK would be known as purchasing priorities.

DIFFERENT MODELS OF PROVISION

One can distinguish between various possibilities for providing health care as follows:

- **free market**, by which is meant a private market of providers without significant regulation;
- **competitive market**, by which is meant attempts to use regulatory powers to ensure that markets become and/or remain competitive (not the same thing as free markets, which have a tendency towards monopoly or oligopoly, especially in health services);
- **managed markets**, whereby markets are managed not – or not only – to create

more competition but to ensure the achievement of public or managerial objectives which neither free nor competitive markets may achieve;

- **planning models**, which may use costing and other managerial mechanisms but which do not use market mechanisms.

Alongside this typology of theoretical possibilities for providing health care, one may consider the following policy options, which are being used in the public sector and former public sector more generally in the British economy:

- replacement of public service with national private monopoly or near-monopoly (as with British Gas or British Telecom);
- replacement of public service with either local 'public' monopoly or near-monopoly or local 'public' competition (as with NHS hospitals – examples in both categories);
- replacement of public service with a hybrid model of private monopoly and private competition (as originally attempted in theory with British Rail, before political compromise);
- maintenance of public service but with improved incentives to providers (signally unattempted in recent British experience!)

The most significant distinction is between public service on the one hand and use of the market mechanism – whether or not competitive markets and whether or not public or private. Failure to make appropriate distinctions between different policy options has led to a lot of confusion both in commentary on recent public sector reform in the UK, including health-service reform.

One should distinguish between industries or sectors of the economy in which something resembling adequate (if not perfect) competition can occur – such as the retail trade in food, cars and the like – and sectors of the economy where adequately competitive markets either do not occur naturally (as with public utilities

such as gas, telephone and so forth) or where competitive markets soon yield up their opposite. This occurs where winners in the marketplace establish themselves as local monopolies or oligopolies and more generally where the conditions for perfect competition do not apply to ensure the maintenance of competitive markets. In the latter category come hospitals – as once one hospital has 'beaten the competition', it is difficult for entry to the market by new competitors (except in atypical circumstances) to provide a natural competitive force in the long term.

The main reason for advocating competitive markets in hospital and general health-care provision has been the statement, whether true or false, that such markets aid **technical efficiency** – that is, greater productivity for given amounts of money; 'more bang for the buck'. However, for services which are either natural monopolies (meaning that competition is difficult to establish and even more difficult to maintain for economic rather than political reasons) and/or where allowing competition is wasteful of public money (as with the hospital sector in many instances), a policy problem soon arises. This can be described as follows.

On the one hand, it is desired to have competitive markets (whether public or private) for reasons of technical efficiency. Yet what economists would call **allocative efficiency** is not necessarily aided by the existence of competitive markets. For example, in the hospital sector, it may make sense for particular hospitals to provide local or even regional services. In other words, 'competition for its own sake' is not sensible: it may make sense to identify 'preferred providers' geographically and functionally (for example by hospital specialty). That is, the alleged advantages of technical efficiency may come into conflict with the demands of allocative efficiency. In a public sector where funds are tight, such as the National Health Service, it may make even more sense to ensure that finance is used in specific hospitals and other service providers for specific services and to ensure that money is not wasted keeping open surplus beds as possibly fictitious sources of competition purely to satisfy a text-book view of the market.

If public planning for a public service is not an option under consideration, then the policy has to fall back on the choice between a competitive market and a free market which may produce monopoly – freedom to win in the marketplace, producing monopoly. It is where competitive markets and free markets are not synonymous that the power of the state through regulation is required to maintain competitive markets.

But this may contradict other policy objectives – such as the use of scarce public money to rationalize services and only use competition as a 'last resort' to ensure that technical inefficiency does not arise over time to an unacceptable extent. The 1994 document from the National Health Service Executive entitled *Local Freedoms, National Responsibilities*, exhibits this tension, as discussed in Chapter 4. On the one hand it is concerned to ensure that competition is preserved and not merely a transitory device while winners and losers emerge. Yet the regulation required for this pro-competitive policy may be substantial – and what is known as the quasi-market (rather than the free market) consists in stimulating competition where it does not naturally occur. Another aspect of the quasi-market, however (a confusing and catch-all term unfortunately) is the limitation or regulation of competition where it works 'too well' or too quickly, e.g. puts hospitals out of business or redistributes resources between hospitals too abruptly to be acceptable in a public service, which is politically-directed and which guarantees (at least to some extent) the local availability of services. Thus the document *Local Freedoms, National Responsibilities* uses a two-edged sword in its policy prescription: stimulation of the market for some reasons and in some circumstances and restrictions on the market in other circumstances. The problem is

that, taken as a whole, it creates confusion both for policy-makers and for health managers and hospital chief executives who do not know if they are expected to win in the marketplace or only win to a limited extent compatible with longer-term pro-competitive prescriptions!

Thus the document, as well as seeking to vet contracts to ensure that competitive situations are maintained when providers make contracts with purchasers, also seeks in effect to regulate prices where competition is simply not possible or is simply not clear enough to guarantee technical efficiency through price competition on the basis of open, 'posted' prices (as opposed to vaguer relational contracts between purchasers and providers).

But the question arises, why not simply identify appropriate types and locations of services and then use public finance to fund these? The public-service model would require an end to the market in the sense of providers marketing themselves through price and other mechanisms – and would use instead performance management of quantity, cost (not the same as price) and (hopefully) quality.

Another example of the different procedures followed by the market model as opposed to the public-service model concerns the planning of services themselves – the creation or maintenance of services through capital policy. A public-service model decides upon the appropriate location of services (hopefully democratically – for example in the health service with health authorities consulting the public and general practitioners) and then the allocation of capital to create or maintain such services. The reimbursement of the necessary running costs (revenue monies) for such services then follows, and capital and revenue policy are integrated.

The market means (whether public or private) of handling this process is, however, to allow providers to have access to banks (whether private or public, such as the NHS region) in line with their ability to attract funds from purchasers. There are thus different and complex (although overlapping) business planning processes for purchasers and providers respectively – with region as both banker and arbiter of the process. This is a very cumbersome means of obeying the textbook market in the public sector and political interference with such a process, on top of all the necessary 'economic' interference, means that the costs of such an ideologically pure system are likely to be high indeed.

One can also turn to what the market would call the factors of production and their cost. In a public service, labour costs are likely to be significantly the highest element of such 'production costs'. A 'textbook' competitive market – with assumptions at the level of the macro-economy of full employment! – would ensure that labour (whether the doctor or the cleaner) was paid its marginal product. In other words there would be zero profit and zero exploitation. But we do not need to be Karl Marx to make a trenchant critique of this unrealistic model! In practice, there will be significant unemployment in the macro-economy and competitive providers (such as hospitals) will be able to bid down the cost of all but the scarcest labour. In the NHS market, examples of labour having their costs (salaries) bid up stem from the short-term and transitional situations in which one hospital trust seeks to undermine its rivals, for example, by poaching its doctors; creating a local monopoly; and then in the longer term seeking to strike a harder bargain with its prized factors of production.

Paradoxically a monopoly provider in a market (whether public or private) is able, if it wishes, to reward labour better as a result of its ability to generate 'abnormal profit' (or surplus if we are talking about the public sector). But the phrase 'if it wishes' is paramount. The recent example of British Gas, a privatized utility operating in near-monopoly conditions, is instructive. It is able to do virtually as it wishes with dividends to shareholders and massive remuneration to its senior

management, yet jack up prices to the consumer (only subject to weak regulation and weak market competition from other utilities such as electricity, at the margins) and also to force down the wages of its less fortunate employees. This is often dressed up as the operation of the market, but it is simply monopoly power: wages can be forced down through direct fiat: and chief executives can be given massive salaries out of proportion to their need for job satisfaction (or perhaps ironically as a compensation for diminished job satisfaction in the new environment). It is argued that recruitment necessitates such salaries, but it is more likely that such salaries are a means of 'vanity signalling': 'We are the sort of company that pays our top managers huge amounts'.

The question arises for health services, do we really want to be making the choice between the devil and the deep blue sea; between competitive markets (expensive to create and maintain) or weakly regulated monopolies? It would be more sensible to allocate capital and revenue funds to providers in line with desired public objectives and to manage performance through the sophisticated information systems now available which are not intrinsically to do with a market but are a lot to do with effective public management.

REGULATING THE MARKET

It is important to distinguish between regulating the structure of the free but uncompetitive market to make it more competitive; regulating prices in either the free or competitive market or both (and especially the monopolistic market) to prevent excessive 'profit' or to achieve other public objectives, as central regulation about pricing in the NHS seeks to do; and 'managing the market' in effect to diminish it and ensure – by the back door – the maintenance of public planning in a political culture where the language of the market has become *de rigeur*.

The National Health Service 'market' has elements of all these three – and all three are confusingly named the 'quasi-market'.

In this sense, the purchaser/provider split – widely believed to be the best aspect of the British reforms – is actually problematic in itself. If the point of creating a purchaser/provider split is to allow providers to market themselves using price mechanisms, in most cases in a public service, the perverse incentives outweigh the advantages. It is more sensible to allow providers to be self-managing yet to allocate resources for quantified purposes, costed appropriately, directly from the parent health authority.

If, for example, one considers a region of the country – a large city such as Birmingham or an area such as the Black Country – the different health authority purchasers will require to coordinate their purchasing (what in the old days would have been called service planning) to ensure that achieving the desired services in an efficient manner does not lead them into a beggar-my-neighbour policy or zero-sum game *vis-à-vis* each other. If one health authority decides to concentrate its services in a number of hospitals (for reasons of both appropriateness of service and efficiency), this decision may depend on other health authorities making compatible decisions. There is a need therefore for the region to 'manage the market' – although the transactions costs of 'knocking purchasers' and providers' heads together' are likely to be great, by comparison with more straightforward planning. If pro-competitive regulation is, however, used in practice, this may undermine such sensible planning, as hospitals not favoured by the plan are stimulated to compete with the sensibly favoured hospitals. There will thus be conflict between different policy objectives – and it would be naive to assume that senior management or central government will resolve these in a rational manner as opposed to the short-term politically expedient manner!

In practice, the likely outcome would be that the favoured services would win but a lot of time and expense would be wasted in regulating their prices through a system of semi-fictitious market testing and repeated re-tendering against semi-fictitious opposition! This occurs both when hospitals compete with hospitals and when hospitals compete with community services to prove similar services to the purchaser.

DAMAGING ASPECTS OF THE NHS REFORMS

INTRODUCTION

This part analyses central elements of the NHS reforms in terms of their damaging, and potentially damaging, aspects. This is not to deny that there have been improvements consequent upon other aspects of the reforms. Firstly, however, such improvements often stem from a generalized 'Hawthorne effect' – whereby a culture of change stimulates innovation and achievement – or even a 'Dunkirk spirit' – whereby immense pressure creates resilience and survival through improvisation. Secondly, some of the technical or managerial changes loosely associated with the reforms (what might be termed the less political part) are promoting service improvements (such as better information systems for audit and resource management).

One legitimate question asks, why did some of the better innovations not occur before? The answer, in the present author's view, lies in the inadequate implementation of good ideas in planning and management, not the absence of markets. (Indeed, the mismanagement of markets is a much bigger problem than any previous mismanagement of planning.) There were of course some awkward incentives in the NHS before the reforms. One of the tasks of this chapter is to ensure that this section considers the problems of the reforms against such a perspective, and that the last section addresses them in its recommendations.

The following are selective but important examples of adverse consequences of the NHS reforms.

THE PURCHASER/PROVIDER SPLIT

On some occasions, in practice, the 'purchaser/provider split' has produced different results from those intended. For example, institutionalizing a split in a particular manner can give more power to the provider, rather than to the purchaser as intended. Local monopolies in provision may be created, with more autonomous power to the provider as a result of the purchaser/provider split. Purchasing strategies can easily go wrong in the uncertain configurations of an NHS quasi-marketplace. Furthermore, the phenomenon of marketing by providers in line with their preferred 'business plans' may lead to the manipulation of both public and purchaser tastes, as in any marketplace. Thus a strategy to ensure that needs are systematically defined and translated into contracts with providers may instead be thwarted.

TRUSTS

The creation of self-governing trusts in their current form has led to a dilemma. As with any income-maximizing agency (whether profit-making or not), the incentive of SGTs is to maximize income and minimize workload. This is not to cast aspersions on the motives of the individuals working for trusts – simply to point out that financial survival and financial prospering involves ensuring that income more than covers workload and therefore that the financial effects of the latter are minimized or at least strictly controlled.

Self-governing trusts refer to both hospitals and community (and other 'priority') units. Unified trusts, for example, covering the whole range of provision in a former district, have recently been discouraged, although one or two were allowed up to 1992 (for example in Macclesfield). Such arrangements tended to reflect deals with local politicians.

The creation of separate hospital trusts and community trusts may mean that cooperation between the two – in the interest of holistic patient care – is diminished. Hospital trusts and community trusts have their separate financial and other incentives.

In consequence, both hospital trusts and community trusts have an incentive to 'cost-shift' – which might mean 'patient-shift'. That is, it is in the interests of hospital trusts to minimize patient stays and move patients into the community, compatible with contracts (assuming indeed that these are capable of being policed effectively). Community trusts may have an incentive to 'cost-shift' to other units' budgets.

On the other hand, creating larger unified trusts may mean that the community is 'swallowed up' as acute financial overspends encroach on the community budget. That is, the budget for community services is not ring-fenced or specifically earmarked in a separate provider unit and as a result pressure on the hospital budget leads to pressure on the community service budget. Such pressure from the acute sector is likely to be increased as block contracts (which mandate the provision of a service, with possibly open-ended demand) and cost per volume contracts (which quantify the number of people to be treated) increase pressure on provider units in the context of limited purchasing budgets yet centrally mandated attempts to squeeze the maximum out of the system.

CONTRACTING AND INCENTIVES

As always, regulation can avoid such cost shifting or budget encroachment in theory. Nevertheless such regulation runs the risk of being either too general or too specific. General regulation may not be able to thwart the perverse incentive of cost-shifting (patient-shifting). Specific regulation may mean that the business of the provider (trust or otherwise) is so tightly demarcated that the flexibility of the 'old-style' NHS is lost. That is, the ability to make flexible decisions within an overall budget may be hampered by a tightly regulated system of detailed contracts, which spells out a 'care plan' for each particular type of patient (in order to try to prevent financially led decisions from subverting patient care).

Contracting, as it has emerged following the NHS reforms, has inflexibilities that are accentuated by the economic incentives created by aspects of the reforms. The NHS market, involving a purchaser/provider split, encourages providers to do as much as they can as quickly as they can. The original rationale for such a market was that providers had an incentive to maximize business from purchasers and then seek more if possible from other purchasers.

For the Secretary of State, therefore – in response to crises concerning 'dying patients' who could not get care – to tell hospitals to 'pace their work to ensure an even pattern through the financial year' shows a refreshing scepticism towards markets and arguably a naivete about clinical practice.

Doctors will treat deserving cases – whether urgent, semi-urgent or not – as long as money is still available, as they should. Hospital managers will seek to ensure that cases treated do not cost more than the purchaser is paying through contracts, and they will now seek to do the contracted business quickly and efficiently – because the Government tells them to! There is, in a 'block contracting' situation, an incentive to avoid expensive cases, especially late in the financial year.

But this is now a matter for the purchaser to regulate, after the NHS reforms. Waiting lists and patients turned away are the purchaser's responsibility even if the provider has the unpleasant task of saying no in practice. Ironically, what Mrs Bottomley had been requesting was that providers behave as they did in the pre-reform NHS, ignoring the

incentives her predecessor Secretaries of State were so proud of creating. This dilemma goes to the heart of the confusion in current health policy. Does the Government know whether it wants a market or not? And can contracting 'sharpen up' what is required of providers without taking away the flexibility that doctors – and providers as a whole – need in order to make sensible priorities in reaction to events?

'Semi-urgent' cases, as well as more routine cases, may be squeezed out at the end of the financial year if both underfunding and rigid contracting lead to the situation described above.

The challenge is to seek a system that encourages providers to meet priorities yet avoids overspecific incentives with (possibly) perverse effects.

Care plans for patients, of course, have their distinct advantages. But is detailed regulation to prevent patient care suffering from provider fragmentation preferable to flexibility in the light of (for example) unforeseen demand in other areas? The latter may be judged to be more important, yet may be prevented from being addressed by the need to take care of bureaucratically ordered patient-based contracts within existing resources. The comparative advantage of the NHS's planning capacity had always been its flexibility, free from finance-driven contracts.

What kind of system can prevent the creation of a direct incentive for cost-shifting, yet also prevent too loose and lax a system of planning, where the hospital and community are not adequately differentiated (as in the 'old system', when it was not working so well)? Ironically the answer is, through direct responsibility of providers to the health authority – or at least a very close relationship of accountability – such that adverse financial incentives are less, yet with adequate differentiation in mission and strategy for hospital and community units.

Devolved management to provider units – for operational efficiency – is important. Yet responsibility to the health authority may be the best means of overcoming the disadvantage of separate hospital and community and trusts (cost-shifting) on the one hand and unified trusts (conceivably 'swallowing up' the non-acute sector) on the other hand – without recourse to the hyper-regulation necessary when providers are autonomous.

Furthermore, it can reasonably be pointed out that the 'attack on the hospital' – and the uncosted advocacy of 'primary care' even when it means acute care in community settings – has gone far enough. The earlier concern to protect community budgets is now adequately dealt with.

The trouble with the NHS reforms as regards these matters is that they tended to throw out the baby of clear accountability with the rather murky bath-water, in this case, of unimaginative top-down management. No one is arguing for the recreation of that. It is, however, possible to have devolved management without self-governing trusts.

CONTROL OF TRUSTS

There has been a battle for control of trusts – between trust boards on the one hand and originally the executive arms (so-called zonal outposts) of the Management Executive (now merged with the 'purchasing arm' of the regional health authority in non-accountable regional offices). In other words, will trusts really be independent or will they be subject to central control? This rather sterile conflict is an ironical and bureaucratic outcome of an ill-thought-out policy. It would have been much better to guarantee operational devolution to the management of provider units yet to demarcate their responsibility to Health Authorities – without the hastily recognized need for excessive bureaucratic regulation to tone down the awkward incentives carelessly created by the idea of self-governing trusts in their current form.

Furthermore, the control of capital allocations by regional offices undermines the essence of the 'purchaser/provider split' at regional level. Policy is currently growing in confusion monthly: the rhetoric stresses devolution; the reality is a stage-managed market (rather than a managed market, which is an oxymoron) geared to pulling puppet-strings.

The so-called Manpower and Functions Review of 1993, and the 'follow-up' reviews of 1994 of NHS executive and regional responsibilities (as well as of the Department of Health – the 'Banks Review'), have done little of substance to clarify the situation in public, although the private agenda may well have been to 'steer' purchasing decisions and rationalize provision.

REFERRALS

The NHS reforms give an incentive to purchasers to place contracts compatible with financial limits. In consequence, referrals which were 'free' in the old system, but expensive, are unwelcome (financially at least) to purchasers in anything resembling financial difficulty. In the old system, the safety valve of unrestricted GP referral or the availability of care which was not subject to a specific contract agreed by a purchaser had significant advantages. Even if 'the money did not always follow the patient'as a result of there not being enough money in the system to pay for all need, the safety valve of free referral was institutionalized and had to be argued **against**. Now it has to be argued **for**. Indeed, now the patient follows the (increasingly centralized) contracting process, as regions control the future shape of the hospital service (i.e. cut it!) through capital policy and 'special initiatives' to cut waiting times (to 'soften up' the public for further hospital closures).

GP FUNDHOLDING: ITS PLACE IN THE SYSTEM

GP fundholders can in theory refer patients as they wish – subject to the constraints of their overall resources and limitations on services for which they hold budgets. The problem of inequity between GP fundholding practices and non-fundholding practices has grown recently, from the time when it was first noticed and discussed around Spring 1991. Non-fundholding GPs are not always allowed to refer, now, unless such referral is compatible with contracts placed by a purchasing district. Even if the old system was also underfunded, free GP referral allowed at least the initial demonstration of demand or need. Limiting waiting lists by limiting possibly legitimate demand is hardly success of the sort being claimed by the present government.

GP fundholders are in some cases purchasing private care, normally using NHS consultants (who have 'maximum part-time' contracts). Thus, as well as a 'two-tier' service, with patients' access dependent on their purchaser, we may have privatization of provision encouraged by fundholding. Only if consultants do more privately, without their NHS workload (or quality) suffering, can such arrangements increase productivity. Even then, the question may be asked: why cannot the public service respond to incentives to supply this 'extra' care? The answer must lie either in the necessity of the profit motive (a dubious assumption when applied to the majority of well meaning doctors) or the failure to allow the commensurate investment in publicly provided care.

In practice, what results is an inefficient public subsidy of the private purse – to both the private hospital and the semi-private doctor (which the hospital gets at marginal, not full, cost).

This policy fragments public services. Firstly, there is a 'domino' effect of decline in NHS hospitals, as some specialties (e.g. accident and emergency) depend on others (e.g. orthopaedics), which may disappear. Secondly, hospital/community integration – and inpatient/outpatient integration – is adversely affected. Thirdly, in the long run,

private care can jack up its prices later when the NHS facilities have been lost forever. There is a 'coal mines and railways effect' at work here.

It may well be that GP fundholding has – at best – acted as a catalyst for more appropriate behaviour on the part of hospital consultants. For example, outpatient clinics may reflect patient need more – at least as defined by GPs – than the tendency of consultants (and perhaps their junior staff, in particular) to arrange 'repeat visits' rather than leave space for 'new attenders'.

Similarly, fundholders may force 'simple but worthwhile' cold surgery to the top of the agenda. Thus overall they may provoke better prioritization within waiting lists. Advocates of fundholding generally are hostile to the 'barons' of the hospital.

Such an outcome is not, however, intrinsically due to fundholding, but to a catalyst for better management, and in particular 'management audit' for waiting lists. It is now time to generalize such benefits by subsuming fundholding within an overall health authority capable of prioritizing primary care – and GPs wishes – without the negative effects of fundholding. 'Ethical' fundholders may – in a minority of cases – organize collectively in limited geographical areas to seek to coordinate purchasing. But this is only a 'halfway house' to coordinated purchasing, unless fundholding becomes responsible for all district-based purchasing. And if it does, we have simply allowed a new form of health authority, with only GPs on it!

The initially very generous funding of GP fundholding practices will of course diminish as fundholding becomes more widespread. In consequence, tough decisions by GP fundholding purchasers will – if these purchasers become the norm within the system – raise spectres of hard choices similar to those raised currently at the level of district (or 'district consortia') purchasing.

Prior to the 1992 General Election, ministers naturally denied that the NHS reforms were about such decisions. But ironically this was the basic rationale for the NHS reforms – that decisions be taken as to priorities and contracts made (and denied) accordingly. In consequence, there have been clashes between non-fundholding GPs, whose desires for referral varied from those of purchasers making the contracts, and these purchasers.

In other words, in the new system, the patient has to follow the contract; the patient has to follow the money.

GP fundholding was a partial way out of this dilemma, which is partly why it has grown beyond the predictions of both proponents and opponents of the NHS reforms. Slipped in originally against the advice of many on the Prime Minister's Review Committee and retained in the final draft of the White Paper at the Prime Minister's personal insistence, GP fundholding allows – for those categories of care covered by fundholding, increasingly to be extended – the clinical decision and the financial decision to be taken at the same time by the same agent – that is, the fundholding practice. However, the financial nexus introduced may have adverse effects. Expensive care that is not reimbursed through a capitation formula which adequately rewards GP fundholders with (for example) socially deprived populations or populations with a preponderance of chronic need, will be unwelcome, to say the least. The short-term picture is different. GP fundholders are generously rewarded, to 'get them on board'; longer-term, the picture may be very different.

A PERVERSE INCENTIVE FOR PROVIDERS AND PURCHASERS

The incentive for providers, as argued above, is to ensure that the cost of activity does not exceed the financial reward through the contract, whether this is block, volume or cost-per-case. Expensive and complicated cases are furthermore less welcome than routine ones, in block contracts.

Extra contractual referrals are unwelcome, as the provider may have to absorb the cost of these just as some US hospitals have to absorb the cost of uncompensated care. In practice a conflict between purchasers and providers over extracontractual referrals is replicating in the UK the conflict between financiers and providers in the United States for uncompensated care. If, in the UK, episodes of care that are not 'contracted for' are characterized disproportionately by complicated or chronic care for the more socially disadvantaged, we will be replicating the US's inequity. That is, it may be that both provider power and purchaser choice, even if reflecting consumer choice, underplay the social needs of the 'discontented minority' as opposed to the contented majority. If this is so, then such needs – if translated into demands – will tend to be sought without contracts, or adequate contracts, having been placed for such care. This is of course the phenomenon of the 'NHS for the middle classes', and harps back to debates about the relative benefits of universal programmes on the one hand and targeted programmes on the other in addressing the needs of the disadvantaged.

Purchasers can of course decide for what sort of people they want to make what sort of contracts: strong, socially conscious purchasers can avoid many problems. There is always going to be an incentive, however, to contract for easily measurable episodes of care, which are not likely to have unforeseen financial consequences. It does not take too much imagination to suggest that the 'contented majority' would be better looked after in such a system.

Central *Diktat* by the Government may remove such worrying incentives from local jurisdiction. The question then arises, what has happened to a system which was allegedly founded upon decentralized decision-making in the context of an institutionalized purchaser/provider split (with the complication of GP fundholding on the purchasing side and autonomous trusts on the provider side)?

It may further be argued that the absence of democracy in local health authorities prevents a legitimate local role in making strategic purchasing decisions, and in fact deciding priorities without too much reference to central rules. The more health authorities are simply the appointed bodies of central government, the more decentralized decision-making in purchasing is likely to be an aspiration rather than a reality.

RATIONING?

One may characterize the above dilemmas as part of the question, 'who does the rationing?' In practice, it is likely to be a messy mixture of purchasers and providers. On one scenario, the UK will even replicate the 'problem of the private third-party payer'. Providers will market themselves to (especially affluent) individuals, GP fundholders and non-fundholding GPs. Under political pressures (local as well as national) purchasers will make contracts to account for these preferences. The provider and consumer will therefore collude at the expense of the 'third-party' payer. In a system such as the NHS, with such limited finance, the 'third-party payer problem' would mean that provider marketing rather than social need might swallow up significant parts of purchasing budgets. Again, this is not inevitable. It is something which extremely strong purchasing can do something about. On the other hand, the mechanics of the system – and indeed the encouragement by Government to providers to make business plans based on marketing – encourages such a process.

What strong purchasing means in practice is of course a major question both for district purchasers themselves and for the NHS Management Executive, which – alarmed about the weakness of purchasing *vis-à-vis* provision in Autumn 1992 – provided significant amounts of money to promote consul-

tancy in the realm of 'strengthening purchasing'. At one level, it may be a matter of personality and competence. Many of the so-called 'best managers' chose to be providers rather than purchasers. The strengthening of the function of public health is still an aspiration rather than a reality in many parts of the country. Again, in the absence of local purchasing strength, national rules may be the only way to ensure that both purchasing priorities and provider location and behaviour are rendered compatible.

It is indeed an irony that the problem of the third-party payer – supposedly the antithesis of what the NHS reforms are all about – may emerge. Again, in order to 'make rationing rational' it may be necessary to move to a fairly centralist system. An alternative is that local purchasers make their own decisions coherently and strongly. An alternative problem then arises. Is it acceptable in the context of a 'National' Health Service for different localities to finance different priorities on a significant scale?

OUTCOME: UNKNOWN OR UNCHOSEN?

Current problems with the purchaser/provider split include different expectations – it is 'all things to all men'. Some proponents argue that it represents an eventual chance to move away from 'provider capture' and also a bias to acute care. Others argue that is it concentrating the mind wonderfully to ensure that the NHS concentrates on its 'core business', i.e. acute/clinical rather than social care. Both predictions cannot be true!

The 'waiting-list problem' identified before the general election has often been attributed to the fact that hospital budgets grew less than family practitioner service budgets in the 1980s. This in itself does not suggest that there has been a major problem of acute care swallowing up primary care (although hospitals may have frequently swallowed up community budgets, in that the two were not specifically separated in the past).

THEOLOGY AND REALITY

The 'old system' in the UK in effect contained a purchaser/provider distinction – it is just that it was in effect regions that were doing the 'purchasing' – especially with capital monies – and districts that were the managers of providers, responsible for catchment areas rather than the residential populations strictly within the geographical boundaries of the post-reform district. Districts allocated funds to hospitals and other providers, and at best attempted to reward local workload. It was simply that 'cross-boundary flows' (some of which would now be 'extracontractual referrals') were funded differently.

That is, there was regional 'purchasing'; integrated district purchasing and provision; and 'third-party reimbursement' (in theory, to create RAWP targets) of 'cross-boundary flows' from one district to another.

In other words, the 'purchaser/provider split' is at one level a truism; an inevitability. There is finance for health care and there are services provided with that finance. That is the 'purchaser/provider split' in the way that the text book cannot deny it. It is just that in the UK the managerial responsibility for the two was not previously differentiated in any clear manner at district level. Public finance sat with public provision in a unified system.

PLANNING PATIENT FLOWS?

Patients treated outside the boundaries of their host health authority (as determined by a new, more democratic health authority in determining its priorities) can of course be catered for through contracts or plans. Regulating the basis of this and reimbursing such care provides an important challenge for a health-care system in which the disadvantages of the market are removed. For, if contracts are to be made with providers, defenders of the market argue, they must be free to compete to achieve these contracts. The degree of competition *vis-à-vis* the degree of regulation is an important issue. Stable

purchaser/provider relationships may call for stable long-term contracts/plans. Whether market discipline or performance management is used to tackle questions of cost and efficiency in placing contracts with providers is an important issue. In making both their priorities and their decisions about the placing of contracts or making of plans, purchasers will be taking hold of criteria such as effectiveness, efficiency, equity and both GPs' and patients' wishes. 'Planning and managing' raises important questions, such as criteria for reimbursement of providers and the nature of the 'performance management' of providers by purchasers. How close ought providers and purchasers to be? To ask these questions and acknowledge that there are a lot of complex issues to be sorted out is considerably more sensible than simply pretending that 'market discipline' will sort things out. This is especially so when political constraints have prevented the present government from allowing 'market discipline' to operate.

Overall, 'the market' was an ideological solution to a technical problem!

It can be argued that, if a market is to function appropriately, the consumer must have the right of 'exit', in this case to join another, more amenable, purchaser; the right of voice (to ensure that democracy in purchasing is not just a glib aspiration); or protection by a system of regulation so that the consumer/patient's rights are respected. A 'rights' approach to health care can of course exist independently of the market mechanism in health care.

It can be observed that, currently, exit, voice and rights are conspicuous by their absence. Purchasing decisions are by and large made by managers (with the exception of GP fundholders). Users of the service are by and large bound by the purchasing decisions made within the geographical area in which they live. And as far as 'rights' are concerned, constraints on available finance have been generally promoted by the

Government and (mostly) accepted by the courts as a reason for both denial of services and denial of timeliness in providing services. Even if fundholders take over most purchasing, they will become the 'managerial rationers'.

HOW MAD (IN THE US SENSE) ARE MANAGERS?

It is of course the case that many (by no means all) senior health managers identify with the present reforms. They have after all invested many sleepless nights in trying to make them work! It is important to ensure that any new policies are fully explained and justified, and furthermore involve as little restructuring or tinkering or 're-disorganization' as possible. As always, a degree of pragmatism is necessary. The increased politicization of health authorities, arguably of trust boards, and of the management process generally has, however, created a climate quite recently in which rhetoric about 'letting managers manage' and 'devolution and decentralization' is being shown to be rather hollow. In such an environment, constructive amendments and alternatives to current policy and management practices are likely to receive a more sympathetic audience. Furthermore, the need for constructive dialogue with senior management to improve rather than replace significant operational policy initiatives such as medical audit, quality management and what used to be known as 'resource management' can provide a practical means for demonstrating that 'abolition for abolition's sake' is not the objective of a non-Conservative government.

CULTURE CHANGE?

It is therefore the particular challenge for an alternative to the NHS reforms to ensure that adequate and pragmatic motivation for employees (for example by ensuring as much devolution in decision-making as possible) is encouraged in a context of 'allegiance to the whole'. Market incentives should not be set in place which have results either opposite to those intended or damaging in terms of the more intangible sources of motivation which are nevertheless crucially important in the long term. If caring, public sector workers are 'just like any other', something important will have been lost. Or, if loyalty to the firm (for which read provider unit or trust) replaces loyalty to the wider NHS (rather than being combined with it), then only if the market works as its more rigorous proponents argue it should, will the public interest be safeguarded.

Recent Conservative governments have sought to use the NHS reforms as a source of radical 'culture change' in British health services. By creating a universe of competing (economic) interests which spawns a universe of rival (political) pressure groups (such as the trust Federation and the Association of GP Fundholders), increasingly radical changes in the direction of privatization (or quasi-privatization, both in provision and financing) can be achieved through offering incentives to particular interests to accommodate them within the structure of the proposed changes.

For example, if trusts become increasingly commercial, if private provision increases in salience within the NHS, if (alongside this) social equity in purchasing is diminished in salience, 'the NHS as we knew it' may be lost. In this sense, privatization is a fair description of a commercialized NHS alongside Conservative public spending reviews and rationing according to Conservative principles and priorities.

An NHS of disparate commercial interest groups is not an NHS that can defend itself politically, and in such a situation the whole is less than the sum of the parts. More far-sighted right-wingers who saw the NHS reforms as a halfway house to something more radical always understood this. Creating loyalty to the firm rather than to the profession or to the trade union, for example, was always bound to weaken sources of opposition to either commercialization or privatization. The worker in a trust faced with worsened conditions can easily be told that market logic prevents better conditions – with some truth, at any given point in time. The other side of the coin – whereby competitive trusts rely on their workers to cooperate in order to maintain and fulfil contracts – is a more temporary one. A short-term contract can ensure that 'the troublesome' are replaced whenever possible. 'The troublesome' may mean either the shop steward or the general manager!

Such developments tend to be justified in terms of weakening 'sectional' professional interests. Professional interests may certainly be sectional and selfish from time to time. On the other hand they may also be a bulwark against the creation of an even more sectional culture. Even the Institute of Health Services Management (IHSM) fails to stand up in public for a public NHS, reflecting the Janus-face of an organization which is in part representing managers but in part reflecting the reality that NHS managers are the creatures of the Government.

REWARDING WORKLOAD AND PRODUCTIVITY

Before the NHS reforms, an alleged problem with funding of providers (through health authorities) was that they simply got an annual allocation and then had to make do with all the demand for services made by patients and doctors, within that allocation. If hospitals ran out of money before the end of the financial year, they might be bailed out by extra money or by money diverted from other purposes such as community services – if they were lucky.

A major problem with the NHS reforms, however, is that this problem is often replicated. Especially with block contracts, which fund departments and services in an open-ended manner, hospitals may well run out of money before the end of the financial year.

Indeed if they become more productive, in the specific sense of staff using the equipment and facilities more intensively and quickly, they are more likely to run out of money well before the end of the financial year. In a market which allows services to be provided and buyers for these services (purchasers) sought, an incentive to be more productive exists – in the hope that more purchasing money can be found to pay for the increased use of services allowed by greater productivity.

If this money is not found, however, the political embarrassment of hospitals running out of money well before the end of the financial year will lead to reactions such as the Secretary of State for Health's reaction early in 1993 that hospitals ought to 'pace themselves' so that the new contractual system would seemingly allow activity to continue throughout the financial year. Non-local patient care was funded differently in the 'old system' – in the sense that RAWP-based targets for (provider) districts were adjusted at full cost of the 'travelling' patients, unlike local care. But the post-'reform' NHS creates worse anomalies, as ECRs and haggles over payment affect patient care. The costs of 'marketing and contracting' – and settling purchaser/provider disputes over payments and their levels, let alone agreeing referrals bureaucratically with GPs – are very high.

The ultimate paradox is that, unlike in a normal market where providers seek to market their services in order to increase overall demand and the overall finance available (even if by redistribution from other sectors of the economy), in the Health Service, the 'quasi-market' in effect calls for more to be done within overall fixed budgets. Providers get contracts if they can do more for a fixed cost. This is not a typical market incentive: providers in this type of system are in effect getting contracts by getting more aggravation without more money! It is of course possible – given the residue of altruistic motivation in the NHS, that providers will operate on this basis. To call it a market is, however, misleading. The Government is seeking to 'do more with less' in this manner; seeking to 'strengthen purchasers' to squeeze providers.

Additionally, if providers do have some leeway to 'market' themselves to purchasers operating with fixed budgets (as argued above, in response to the wishes of the more articulate patients, consumers and citizens) then purchasing priorities may be distorted. At the very least, a quantity/quality trade-off is rendered unavoidable – as providers' preferred services may take precedence over the need for higher 'cheap and cheerful' quantity which benefits a greater number of people.

SPECIALIZED SERVICES

An important area where the purchaser/ provider split may be particularly harmful is the effect of the internal market upon specialized services. This may seem a technical area but is in fact crucial to the survival of the NHS as a comprehensive service including specialized medicine and 'centres of excellence'.

Prior to the NHS reforms, regional monies were used to protect specialized services, including tertiary services, on the basis of predicted usage and need for such services in the region. Following the internal market, such monies have been generally devolved to districts and it is difficult for such districts – even when they wish to preserve a specialized function jointly – to coordinate action to achieve this. One district quite reasonably will be unwilling to put up the money if complementary money to ensure the effective functioning of the service in a specialized location is not necessarily forthcoming from other districts. Furthermore, if districts do get together to ensure the continuation of such a specialized service, access of patients to that service will be rigidly demarcated according to which district they come from – rather

than on the basis of clinical need. The 1993 Clinical Standards Advisory Group Report highlighted this particular danger in the internal market, with particular reference to heart transplants.

What is more, inappropriate competition between specialized centres, ordinary general hospitals and other providers generally may mean that 'local' hospitals invest inappropriately in specialized services in order to try to secure a market niche for the future. (Examples exist in mental health as well as in the traditional 'high-tech' sector.) Not everyone can 'win' in such a situation – and eventually a pattern of services will emerge with winners and losers, and 'monopolies and oligopolies' arising from the ashes of competition. Meanwhile, however, the process is very damaging both to specialized services and to the priorities to other hospitals – and indeed very damaging to the public purse, as wasteful competition occurs.

Thus, services which are often inappropriately provided locally, such as specialized services, will often be provided locally in the future; whereas services which ought to be provided more locally (such as accident and emergency, maternity services) will be provided less locally. That is there will be both a levelling down and a levelling up – all in the pursuit of cost control.

Regarding hospital rationalization, there is an analogy with the 're-profiling' of the workforce, whereby more 'standard' carers replace specialized (and expensive) professionals on the one hand; and increasingly are encouraged to do more of the 'ancillary' work also, to reduce wage bills overall, on the other hand. That is, there is a 're-profiling up' and a 're-profiling down'. Changes in skill-mix driven wholly by the need for economy are dangerous both for specialized services and for hospitals generally.

If controlling and reducing cost is the main aim of the new 'contracting' system, then 'costly' patients will suffer (i.e. specialized services will suffer). Block contracts make such patients unattractive to providers, which incur large costs without extra income. Purchasing, under such a system, will seek to 'pass the buck' to providers (for expensive treatments, long-term treatments and rare illnesses). And, if 'cost per case' contracts allow such services, using individual districts to plan for what should be supra-district services leads to great practical difficulties.

Putting hospitals and units in competition with each other, and adding 'local purchasing' to that brew, leads to the decline of centres of excellence – it started in London and is spreading to cities across the country.

The Government has sought to depict rational opposition to such trends as 'vested interests' (with even the Royal Colleges often depicted as quasi-'trade unions' – the ultimate insult, it seems, to the Conservative government!). But often the Colleges are simply seeking to maintain standards at time of severe pressures to cut costs.

THE INSTABILITY OF THE 'MANAGED MARKET'

As soon as Government and the management executives of the NHS seek to manage the market (sensibly, given that *laissez faire* is much worse), there are cries of 'betrayal' from those health service actors identified with the Thatcherite revolution: those who believe the aphorism, 'private good, public bad'; disillusioned trust chairmen such as conservative right-winger Roy Lilley; former NHS personnel director Eric Caines; and even members of the Government itself. Such people depict the reforms as having reached an impasse, stymied by compromise.

As a result of all this politicization the energies of NHS leaders are often taken up defending policy against the political right instead of addressing the most important and indeed opposite challenge to that of 'extending the market' – that of reforming the reforms and re-coordinating the NHS; disposing of the perverse incentives which the

reforms have in many cases created – admittedly alongside 'a general Hawthorne effect' of improved performance management.

By seeking to manage the market rather than plan and manage the service, there is a danger of treating symptoms rather than causes; and of susceptibility to the argument that, when it comes to the managed market, it is the management part and not the market part that is causing problems.

But pushing further towards commercialization and privatization ironically decreases the scope for cost control, equity and the effective commissioning of specialized services. International, and indeed recent British, experience, on a smaller scale, teaches us this. The long-term evidence suggests that public finance and public provision are both more efficient and more equitable; and that what benefits the private sector offers stem from its marginality to the system.

A market, to be efficient, requires many things. To list only a few: plentiful and indeed surplus providers in free competition; quick and easy entrance and exit by providers, which is likely to mean low fixed costs; complete dedication to the profit motive, to derive the public good from private vice; perfect information; and transactions costs that are under control. These are the costs of negotiating, contracting and monitoring; of re-negotiating, re-contracting and marketing to GPs and others – rather than planning in an ordered hierarchy. It is these costs, incidentally, that are out of control.

The truth is that such prerequisites for a successful market are not satisfied nationally in health care. But the paradox is that trying to regulate them into existence means that you break some of the conditions in order to satisfy others. For example, you incur extra costs trying to preserve spare capacity while closing surplus capacity – 40% of our hospital beds, according to one confidential report – despite the mounting pressure on hospitals and frequent cancellations of non-urgent admissions due to no beds being available.

A major question for the future is whether in the end the costs of the quasi-market were justified by commensurate benefits, or whether an alternative means of allocating resources and planning services is better.

Political awareness of the cost of the market is demonstrated in central directives to establish league tables of trusts' management costs.

As of 1995, the NHS was facing a tough choice – the unfairness and inefficiency of a real market or the bureaucracy of what is called a regulated market but is actually a haphazardly managed system using a partial market as a politically controlled competitive tender to survive, by providers.

The essence of the market system for staff is that they have to produce more, even to earn the same in real terms; one can only get a rise at the expense of someone else's terms and conditions, or even job. At best, this is an NHS example of the 2:3:2 rule: half the people work three times as hard for twice as much.

A reasonable hypothesis is that the costs of the market – in the absence of clear allocative (service) benefits to offset them – can (only) be outweighed by a centrally steered search for 'technical efficiency', as economists call it. Are we doing more things of the measurable sort for the money? Is any increase in output due to real efficiency, or simply to economy or even exploitation?

Any further advocacy of an 'NHS market' should take account of the following dangers.

- **The purchaser/provider split can be a source of perverse incentives**. With a block contract, the purchaser often puts unreasonable pressure on the provider, faced with unpredictable workload and the knowledge that the public complains to the hospital and not to the (generally unknown) purchaser or commissioner. On the other hand, more specific contracts can encourage gaming by the provider – for example, the cost per case contract can

replicate the incentives of fee for service reimbursement. In a tightly funded NHS, this is highly problematic.

Since providers have service knowledge but purchasers have the money and depend on providers (or alternatively national clinical information) to make their purchasing plans and contract specifications, a formal split may institutionalize such gaming rather than cooperation.

- **Inequity is encouraged** as both purchasers and providers respectively have a sharper incentive to avoid expensive care in either contracting or providing. The chronically sick and those in need of what is now being called social care as opposed to health care are but the most extreme example. Providers face a direct incentive to deny admissions under district contracts yet seek business from GP fundholders, in many circumstances. This is actually destructive of good relations between clinicians and general managers.

As far as purchasers are concerned, cost-shifting from one budget to another is a threat. Fundholders may pass on awkward cases as emergencies, to get the health authority to pay. The elderly may be classified as emergencies to ensure they get a bed and do not simply get rationed out due to inadequate community care budgets.

- There is now an official extension of the GP fundholding policy, but **objectives have not been clarified**. On the one hand there is a need to coordinate purchasing such that long-term business planning by providers is possible; such that the priorities of both localities and the geographical areas covered by commissioning authorities are addressed; and such that value for money is achieved by appropriate concentration on appropriate providers. If fundholding operates in the manner it is 'sold' to GPs, it will threaten all this. So there is a need to change what fundholding means.

- **There is actually no point in purchasing at all** if it is simply a bureaucratic reproduction of referrals and services which would have been chosen anyway. Purchasing at its most creative probably occurs in developing new services for non-acute care, i.e. for those in the community. In this arena purchasing has less to do with markets than with sensitive planning.

  Purchasing overall is, however, a means of seeking cost control and, of course, the rationing which dare not speak its name. It is little to do with significant local choice and a lot to do with reconciling within the budget the acute demand that presents at the hospital door, on the one hand, and national priorities, on the other hand. To understand purchasing at all, consider the contrast with the pre-reform NHS, when there was no overt purchasing – but instead a mix of regional planning of services (via capital), district planning and also provision, and reimbursement of referrals outside the district via a formula.

  Then, at its worst, the system simply meant referral to the services which existed by GPs, without much power to change service mix or quality. In other words, in today's language, there was a mix of regional and district purchasing without much involvement of others.

  At its best, however, the old system had the potential for flexible planning in one clear sense: GPs, communities and others could feed into the planning process; and then GPs could refer to the services which resulted, duly funded in line with workload, i.e. there was a creative interplay between what would now be called purchasing and reimbursement.

  The difference between the two is clear: you purchase with money; but you refer freely, and hope it will be reimbursed or because it will be reimbursed.

  Purchasing – by managers or GP fund-

holders – means referral and use of services must follow the money. Reimbursement means the money follows the patient. But, as we now realize, in our new system of tight purchasing, the patient follows the money. Only at the margins is patient choice affordable in the new NHS.

  Local voices should actually be renamed local listening, for communication with the public is actually about selling the inevitable.

- **Screening programmes that are hospital-based – i.e. PHC in hospitals – may be discontinued** if the contracting system does not reward them overtly. This may occur if the longer-term benefits do not accrue to the hospital but to the community, in reduced morbidity.

- **There is a lack of overall accountability.** In England, for example, regional health authorities are abolished and the only legally constituted authorities – districts or commissions, including the FHSA – are losing out to fundholders. This, paradoxically, produces greater centralization of authority and power, in that there is no authority with teeth other than the Government and its regional offices. The democratic deficit which results is serious. As a result, it is proposed by some to transfer health purchasing to local government – which, in practice, would be disruptive and would bring its own disadvantages. In other words, the capacity for further destabilization is enhanced.

- Just as medical and clinical audit are being extended to link secondary and primary care (i.e. audit 'at the interface'), **relations between these two actors are being rendered competitive rather than collaborative.**

- **Marketing by trusts directly to GPs** (in the hope, even for non-fundholders, of influencing health authority contracts) and separate business plans for purchasers and providers, **may retard**

rational allocation of funds and increase transactions costs.

- **The 'rush' to advocate use of the private sector is dangerous**. Sensible 'private sector deals' depend on the private sector's marginality. The private sector rarely trains its own medical and professional staff, and its costs would rise if it did. Furthermore, it is actually the recession of the early 1990s that temporarily allowed cut-price deals with private hospitals with spare capacity. That is why on one occasion patients were sent to a formally bankrupt private hospital in Glasgow (from Birmingham hospitals built with public money).

A FRAMEWORK FOR A NEW HEALTH-CARE SETTLEMENT

If it is genuinely desired to reap some of the advantages of the better health maintenance organizations, a new type of health-care authority can do so. It would be responsible for directly providing the primary and community services required by its population. Regarding secondary care, it would enter into long-term service agreements with the main providers within its boundaries, and indeed outside where such contracts were appropriate. Such secondary providers (hospitals in the main) would be responsible for their own management – in other words, they would be managed separately from the health authority. Whether or not they are called 'self-governing' would be a matter of theology, at one level. But the main aim would be to ensure that they were responsible for meeting the needs of the health authorities with which they had long-term and stable contracts. By 1996 or 1997, it is not so much a case of 'abolishing trusts' as of making secondary providers strategically accountable to the health authorities with whom most of their business is transacted. They would be self-managing, but responsible to the new health authorities for meeting objectives set by the latter.

A KEY INCENTIVE

It would be in the interests of such a health-care authority to 'do as much as it could itself'. That is, where it was more effective, efficient and economical to provide services at the primary and community level, the authority would do so and therefore would not have to pay secondary providers through service agreements or contracts. A major advantage of the GP fundholding system in theory would therefore be retained: primary care actors would 'do what they could themselves'. It would make sense for such authorities to comprise a majority of personnel from primary health care, community health and public health – both on the authority and on any management board responsible to that authority.

I propose that such an authority should have 15 members, of whom at least six should come from primary and community/public health. The others would comprise citizens, consumers, secondary care representatives and (possibly) executive officers.

Whether or not there is an authority separate from the 'Management Executive' (of executive officers as opposed to non-executive officers) is a moot point. Currently, the policy has been to merge executive and non-executive members on to a unified authority. Management teams comprising executive officers still remain, however; and there has been recent disquiet at the ineffectiveness or role confusion of non-executive members.

HEALING THE SPLIT WHEN IT RIPS THE SEAM

The purchaser/provider split would therefore be ended. For primary and community health care there would not even be a managerial distinction. In practice, GP fundholding as it is extended under the current system is in fact re-closing the purchaser/provider gap. GP fundholders will increasingly be directly employing health visitors, district nurses and other community personnel. This may have (again) some 'micro-'advantages, but is likely to diminish the provision of such community services on the basis of geographical equity. GPs are not likely to forgo such staff because they are based in affluent catchment areas.

A purchaser/provider distinction but not split between the health authority and secondary providers may be retained at the level of managerial structure, but with the harmful effects of 'gaming' between purchasers and providers significantly diminished by the creation of long-term stable service agreements between purchasers and providers. In other words, the rationale for any purchaser/provider distinction is to ensure operational self-management by providers rather than autonomy which may lead to the subversion of health priorities. Competition is not an objective *per se*, but will occur at the margin, not as the basic dynamic of the system. Otherwise, providers will 'game' to deceive purchasers; and purchasers will seek to 'cream-skim'.

Provider autonomy in management, however, is useful – not least to ensure that regional planning of capital and finance generally rewards providers in proportion to workload, without 'fudging' by a parent health authority. Accountability **to** such an authority is not the same as financial management **by** such an authority.

TERTIARY CARE

Regarding tertiary care, much damage is currently being done by subjecting tertiary services to the vagaries of decentralized purchasing. In most cases – and this is not a rigid rule – tertiary services ought to be directly provided at regional level – again, with as much operational self-management by tertiary providers as possible, in whatever location. Some tertiary services are of course provided in standard 'district general hospitals' (as used to be).

In the context of the debate about whether and which type of planning is necessary in the National Health Service, a practical example arises in the case of specialized services. Recently, the media highlighted the case of a boy with a rare genetic disorder who could not receive NHS treatment (until a political row ensued) as a result of the specialized centre (previously regionally funded) being closed because of 'rationalization' of hospital care in London.

Many other examples exist (Clinical Standards Advising Group, 1993). On one interpretation, such situations could be the result of formal rationing or decision-making procedures which declared such treatment not to be a priority. Alternatively, leaving the provision of scarce and specialized regional or national services to the decisions of individual purchasers (rather than regional or national planning) could simply result in unforeseen consequences. Long-term investment in such services might not be forthcoming as a result of purchasers' decisions – yet purchasers collectively and individually might desire to maintain the existence of such services. In other words, 'short-termism' might be the source of such denial of care.

COMMUNITY CARE

Concerning community care, a number of significant problems are emerging, which have been well discussed elsewhere. In the context of this discussion, the main need is to create a genuinely unified purchasing framework here also. The Community Care Act (part of the NHS and Community Care Act), implemented late, merges local authority and social security budgets (albeit at the major cost of replacing certain social rights with cash-limited rationing).

This 'new unity', however, only applies to purchasing on behalf of clients requiring certain forms of community care. The initial, wider choice of 'care package', based on client assessment, might involve a choice between institutional or community care – ranging from hospitalization (long- or short-term), through nursing or residential home care, through community services, through to various alternatives generally grouped as 'community care'.

The development of GP fundholders' responsibility for community services – and an impetus towards the fundholder as purchaser generally – means an alternative purchaser is also emerging with responsibility for the community.

There is a need to unify the budget for community services and community care. It would make sense for the new health-care authority to hold such a budget. Ideally, these authorities should have responsibility for all services which have a direct effect on health outcome. If yet more 'reorganization' (to the detriment of local authority social services departments, in particular, which have just accepted new responsibilities!) is not palatable, then joint purchasing by coterminous PHCAs and local authority social services departments is desirable.

As with health care generally, some of the services would be directly employed and provided – for example, community services. The state of flux currently whereby some community services are becoming self-governing providers and some are being 'swallowed up' by GP fundholders would thereby be clarified.

Other services would be provided through contracts of the purchasing authority – for example, long-stay home care and hospital care. The bias to privatization created by the present legislation should be ended, as should the bias against NHS and local authority nursing and residential homes respectively.

COTERMINOUS AUTHORITIES

In order to unify the planning or purchasing of services which affect health status, it is argued that (ideally) one global purchaser ought to take responsibility for health-related purchasing and planning. One view argues that local authorities ought to take over all the relevant purchasing, as many local authority

responsibilities (for example concerning housing, the environment and social services) affect health arguably as much as, if not more than, 'the health service'. My view, however, argues that the health authority ought to take over as many of these responsibilities as possible, including community and social care. At the level of pure theory – ignoring politics – it may not matter which institution plays this role. What is clear is that it will be some time – if ever – before such a wholly unified purchasing or planning authority emerges. It is therefore important in the meanwhile that health authorities and local authorities be coterminous. New health authorities ought therefore be designed on the basis of being coterminous with local government. Ideally, a system of regional government could be coterminous with regional health authorities; local (primary-care-oriented) health authorities could be coterminous with local government units. Centrally, however, health authorities ought to unify planning and purchasing within the current health field.

HEALTH LOCALITIES

Within such health authorities, 'health localities' based on GP practices (or groups of practices) ought to be granted as much devolved management as is compatible with the overall purchasing and planning decisions of the authority. Thus, the advantages of GP fundholding may be retained without the disadvantages, in terms of fragmentation and social inequity, of actually continuing with fundholding.

'Locality purchasing' is actually in conflict with consortia of GP fundholders, an increasing trend. Only the federalism of the global health authority, incorporating devolution to locally-sensitive 'providers and referrers', can provide a coherent model for accountable strategic planning. (Likewise, on such a model, hospital trusts would become responsible to the new health authorities, while retaining Boards to ensure operational autonomy.) Thus localities would feed into plans by authorities, and the consequent funding of providers would flow from regions. This would be a democratic planning process.

A NEW 'HEALTH MAINTENANCE ORGANIZATION' (HMO)

In essence, the new health-care authorities would become what in the United States are known as 'staff HMOs'. The purchaser/provider split would not exist where it was actually harmful to the effective control of providers in the public interest. On the other hand, where there was a case for relatively more autonomous providers and contracting relationships with the health authority, such arrangements could be instituted – by local choice rather than political dogma.

In the United States, health maintenance organizations were specifically created to end the purchaser/provider split and the problems of the third-party payer. In other words, direct ownership (or tight control) of providers by financiers (i.e. by the HMO, a special kind of insurance company which unites the provider and financier) is a move in the opposite direction to the institutionalization of the purchaser/provider split as we have known it in the UK since 1992. The recommendations of this chapter argue for a health authority which replicates the best type of HMO.

GENERALIZING FROM GP FUNDHOLDING

As a result GPs could manage funds while being responsible to the health authority, without the disadvantages of GP fundholding (a two-tier service; fragmentation in purchasing). In essence, the incentives provided to the GP fundholder would be replicated at the level of the health authority, while responsibility for feeding into health authority plans would be devolved more than in the pre-reform NHS.

It might be asked, why not simply give budgets to GPs and allow them to be the purchasers? The answer has already been provided: in order to ensure adequate purchasing and planning power *vis-à-vis* secondary providers, such GP fundholders would form themselves into consortia which would become health authorities by any other name – but with only GPs as the decision-makers on the authority. This is a narrow model of accountability.

A RADICAL BREAK FROM CURRENT COMPLACENCY

It is always open to those who seek to belittle the significance of new ideas or new approaches to adopt a strategy (which might appeal to Sir Humphrey Appleby) along the lines of 'don't worry, it's happening anyway!' It can, for example, be pointed out that, already, Government ministers are asking for the purchaser/provider relationship to be 'cosy' rather than based on a rigid split. (It should of course be recognized that this is in order to force cost cutting in providers, by direct fiat rather than the market, which is always an unreliable and unpredictable ally!) Nevertheless, moves to increase competition (see NHSME, 1994) contradict such cosiness. Secondly, there are moves to 'strengthen purchasing', to seek to jam a lid on to the boiling pot of provider self-interest, which ironically has been increased rather than diminished by the reforms. Thirdly, it can be pointed out that there are moves afoot – in different ways, in different places – to increase links between FHSAs and DHAs, and even to merge them. Fourthly, just as purchasers and providers are supposed to live in a cosy relationship, it is argued that GP fundholders and DHAs ought to coordinate and get their act together.

Nevertheless, evolving policy is unclear as to its priorities. Firstly, whatever the language which is politically convenient at any one time, markets and even private markets are being encouraged. The problem is that nobody really knows 'what trusts are' in a theoretical sense, and therefore no-one knows how they will behave. If they are profit maximizers in some theoretical sense, only perfect competition and purchasing with perfect knowledge could ensure their compliance to the overall objectives of the service ('public good from private vice'). If they are not maximizers, however, they become rather messy 'non-profit but autonomous institutions' operating in a similar grey area to that in which US non-profit hospitals operated. This grey area has been criticized from both left and right in the United States as failing to provide rationalization or the capacity to deliver according to purchasers' or clients' needs in a coordinated and economical manner.

Secondly, the adoption by the Secretary of State for Health in 1993 and 1994 of a significant portfolio of policies to encourage private provision and private management of services meant that the amalgam of public and private provision operating in the context of a quasi-market will further diminish the capacity for effective relationships between purchasers and providers.

Thirdly, the fundamental attraction of GP fundholding in its current form is its separateness from district health authority (or regionally-driven) purchasing. Ironically, a significant regional role is emerging, to seek to set up incentives and mechanisms whereby GP fundholders can coordinate their aims with overall regional objectives. The Director of Primary Health Care in Wessex region, for example, wrote in the *Health Service Journal* concerning how this might happen (Meads, 1993). The fact remains that such policies reflect an attempt, inevitably bureaucratic, to police vaguely-constituted pluralism and fragmentation – not least in the conflicts between formulae for district purchasers' allocations and those for GP fundholders. Chapter 7 outlined, especially in the further reading, some regional and district strategies to coordinate purchasing.

Fourthly, overall purchasing objectives under current conditions are inadequately concerned with equity, let alone equality, in seeking outcomes defined in terms of health status. The pressure upon public finance and the re-restructuring of the welfare state (almost with overtones of yet another 'Prime minister's review' on the future of the National Health Service) means that the overall context in which the Secretary of State for Health operates is severely constrained.

Fifthly, constraints on finance mean that – on the one hand – purchasers are using contracting to regulate providers' processes rigorously (where possible – and sometimes more directly than under the pre-reform direct management of providers!) yet – on the other hand – are susceptible to provider definition of business – (often under pressure from political or elite public preferences).

Sixthly, the 1993 Functions and Manpower Review of all of health care's strategic bodies (above the level of districts and trusts) and the 1994 'follow-up' reviews were a rather shadowy operation – rather than an exercise in Government leadership. As a result, debates about whether a market (managed or not) was possible at all, given regional and governmental control of investment in line with purchasers' priorities, were stifled. The purchaser/provider split was becoming a somewhat artificial tool for 'macho' contracting rather than a real recognition of 'free' provider competition. In essence, allowing the NHS to operate with enough 'excess' capacity to allow competition would be too expensive, in a public system. Even if the NHS is 'over-bedded' in some areas, this is not the case by international comparison. Hence the need to 'create' excess capacity. But the question arises: is competition a means to an end (rationalization) or an ideological end – in itself – sought through creation of systems capacity. And in any case, competition is a temporary phase: as in most markets. Eventually, stable monopolies emerge, especially where fixed costs and start-up costs are high.

Seventhly, the NHS reforms have spawned a significant 'interest group culture' within the National Health Service. The Association of GP Fundholders on the one hand and the Federation of Trusts on the other are but two examples of this. Even where (for various reasons) economic markets are not allowed to work, a US-style political and bureaucratic pluralism and fragmentation renders strategic planning more difficult. It is all very well to realize, a little late, that 'real freedom' for GP fundholders may lead to the loss of the local provider (forever, given the barriers to entry and re-entry in health service markets). But it is one thing deliberately to foster what Maynard Keynes called 'animal spirits' in health service professionals; it is quite another to seek to tame these spirits just as they are developing.

ACCOUNTABILITY

In (re)recognizing the need for accountability in the National Health Service, the Conservative administration was signally failing to define coherently what such accountability should mean. Two particular needs are: accountability to the public and accountability of providers to purchasers. If there is a significant purchaser/provider split and it is believed that market discipline makes providers accountable to purchasers, the first type of accountability (to the public) is an accountability by purchasers.

With a purchaser/provider split but lack of clarity about the market, the scope for provider self-interest may actually be greater than in the pre-reform NHS. For that reason, it is better to see a linked accountability of providers to purchasers and purchasers to the public. In essence, in the pre-reform NHS, the purchaser was the national government operating through regions (and in part districts) and the providers were managed by districts responsible for catchment populations (based on flows to providers) rather than residential or self-contained geographical populations.

Planning of services, service mix and changes to service (such as development and contraction) was of course undertaken jointly by districts and regions. Thus it is perhaps a matter of some theology as to where the conceptual purchaser/provider split lay.

In the pre-reform NHS, often needs-based service planning (what would now be called purchasing translated into contracts), was inadequately carried out. On the other hand, examples of good practice also existed. Where health authorities (districts and/or regions) saw themselves as responsible for changing service mix in relation to need, direct control of providers offered a mechanism to do so in the sense of enforceable accountability. It was for reasons of professional power and often bureaucratic inertia and 'culture' that 'better planning' did not occur.

In the post-reform NHS, we have a rhetoric (and more than that – a culture) of needs assessment and needs-based contracting, but ironically have created some economic and behavioural incentives which render that more difficult. The challenge therefore is to re-establish accountability of providers to purchasers yet maintain and indeed extend operational self-management for providers.

ACCOUNTABLE BOARDS

Accountability of providers to purchasers may best mean operational rather than wholly independent boards for providers. If there are to be non-executive members such non-executives ought, however, to include some community and 'purchasing' representatives. This is only inadmissible if the fiction of perfectly competitive providers is used to argue that economic incentives replace the need for political and bureaucratic accountability.

Although concerned with operational matters rather than (say) strategies for marketing, such boards would be constituted formally, with prescribed powers. Their role would be to take responsibility for devolved management, rather than for provider autonomy. They would also be responsible to the health-care authority in whose territory they lay.

ACCOUNTABILITY TO CITIZENS

Accountability of purchasers (health authorities overall) to the public is a central concern. One might ask, should representation on health authorities be on a geographical basis or on a functional basis? At one extreme, health authorities could mirror a model (if not necessarily the current reality) of representative local government. On another approach, appointed health authorities could include representatives of the most significant agencies whose activities have a bearing on the health of populations – social services, housing, voluntary agencies and others. Currently, a narrow business model means that it is fair to characterize appointments to health authorities (especially Chairs) as being top-heavy with Conservative-sympathizing businessmen (in the main, men!).

If an elected tier of regional government were to emerge in the future, it would make sense for regional health authorities – re-established from the centralist regional offices created in 1993/94 – to be strategic bodies coterminous with such tiers and for regional health authorities to comprise a mixture of elected, appointed and executive members.

Meanwhile, at the level of the health-care authority, a major decision would be whether to have a single-tier or two-tier board. That is, should the current system of unitary boards (comprising executive and non-executive members) be retained, or should we move to a further developed model (of a previous system) in which the health authority was in effect a non-executive tier to which a second tier – the management board – was responsible.

Any particular structural solution for the long term would depend on significant

reforms, if any, to subnational government throughout the UK. Meanwhile, in the shorter term, minimizing change could argue for the retention of unitary boards comprising executives and non-executives, yet a mixture of functional and geographical rights to representation as non-executive members of primary health-care authorities. This would diminish the stark 'democratic deficit' which currently exists, whereby centralist patronage (increasingly on a single party basis) prevents (certainly) democracy and (arguably) accountability to the public. This chapter does not engage in the details of the argument as to whether elected, indirectly elected or appointed health authorities are best. Restoring meaningful representation is, however, an important challenge.

It would be problematic to retain a national system of resource allocation and promote directly elected health authorities at the level of the health-care authority. The present author, therefore, would eschew the option of direct election while reforming significantly the discredited politically motivated centralism of the current arrangements. Why argue for 'local voices' yet remove them structurally (or marginalize them, as with community health councils)? This is arguably a very 'British' hypocrisy.

ROLES AND INCENTIVES

Although the new primary health-care authority would resemble what in the United States might be called a 'staff health maintenance organization (HMO)' (see above), the authority would be responsible for the health of its population, on a geographical basis rather than on a subscription basis as in US HMOs. The incentives to doctors and other providers in primary health care could be developed in line with the incentives facing the authority. The authority would seek to maximize health care and tackle health gain – on an equitable basis – within its budget, and would offer programmes and responsibilities with money attached to non-hospital providers as a 'first conceptual option'.

There would not be a bias to primary health care so much as a system that was genuinely neutral as between primary health care and secondary care, in which decisions were made on the basis of appropriateness and cost-effectiveness.

It would be a 'staff health maintenance organization' in that the organization would directly employ – including GPs – providers for core services at the primary level. Long-term service agreements with accountable secondary providers would complement this picture. There would be a significant role for regional planning of tertiary services; and regions would ultimately finance all services, in a plan based on districts' plans, in turn based (where relevant, e.g. for primary care) on localities' plans.

PROVIDING CARE LOCALLY – IF POSSIBLE

An important issue – which on first glance seems to be a rather arcane operational matter – is the question of the reimbursement of what used to be termed 'cross-boundary flows'. In other words, if health authorities and providers are to have stable relationships, and the market is to be a marginal contribution rather than a key mode of delivery in health care, how are plans for episodes of care outside the host health authority of the patient to be determined, and – for example – at what price and at what quality?

It is proposed here that providers be reimbursed on the basis of long-term service agreements for stable patterns of 'flows'. It is as well to call this a planning process to be free of the jibe of 'a rose by any other name'. It is well known that the concept of planning does not smell sweet to the current administration. Nevertheless it is a major challenge for any left-of-centre government to reconcile a democratically informed system of health planning with appropriate incentives to providers.

Then the model proposed in this chapter is that care should be provided as locally as is possible, consistent with health authority choices regarding equity and access on the one hand and both effectiveness and affordability on the other hand. The model proposed is for overall health-care authorities large enough such that so called 'cross-boundary flows' – in other words patients who are resident in one health authority yet treated in another – are minimized. (Within the health authority, of course, locality-based input into purchasing decisions will inform the pattern of flows.) Nevertheless 'cross-boundary flows' will still exist: firstly, in some cases, it will be a short distance for patients to travel to care outside the boundaries of the residential health authority. Secondly, for specialized services and where the quality of the provider dictates preferences, certain cross-boundary flows will be both desirable and inevitable.

LONG-TERMISM

It is suggested here that long-term service agreements at agreed regional prices be employed to cope with such situations. Otherwise, providers cannot invest for the future and rely on stable income such that they can provide services in line with purchasers' wishes. In other words, if there were a genuine element of democracy as well as 'managerial planning' in determining such patterns, then the price of such democracy is stability to allow expressed choices to be catered for in the medium term and long term. 'Short-termism' in switching contracts may aid short-term consumerism, but it does not aid longer-term social choice on the basis of democratic citizenship.

The development of 'patients' voices' consistent with health authority decisions and management constraints (in a system where public finance dominates and where purchasing is not on the basis of individual market choices or vouchers) will require that health authorities reimburse providers at regionally agreed costs – arguably the specialty cost or even diagnosis-based cost of that provider. If a provider has high costs, yet for other reasons that provider is 'the correct one', then performance review between purchaser and provider is the best means of 'sorting out' such problems. It will inevitably be the role of regions to monitor such agreements, through a performance review of health authorities.

This is considerably less bureaucratic than policing the market in an incremental manner – in line with regional objectives, nonetheless – as occurs in the current environment. It would still be up to regions to authorize such flows through service agreements. That is, one would be moving towards a regional planning model but without current levels of bureaucracy and ensuring that funds flow in line with GP and local (district) health authority preferences. Regulating such a system openly, with a regional role, is preferable to backdoor interference on an undemocratic basis, which is a perhaps inevitable temptation in the present system.

It would – using strict logic – be possible to abolish health authorities and use regions to allocate funds to providers. But it is probably sensible, on grounds of their size and capacity to represent the public, to retain subregional health authorities as (1) planners, (2) coordinators of local providers and (3) funders of providers, under regional tutelage.

MANAGEMENT RESPONSIBILITY, NOT MARKET SCAPEGOATS

Thus health authorities would receive funds on the basis of residential capitation, but would make service agreements which would be reviewed by regions. The pre-reform, allegedly 'bureaucratic' means of calculating catchment populations would not be required. Under such a system, it is the local health authority's job to set standards for its providers (including efficiency and costs as well as effectiveness and quality). These standards – and costs – then apply to 'incoming' patients also. It remains the provider's job, therefore, to 'come in on line'. The challenge, however, is to ensure that the performance which is rewarded under such a system is for a balanced range of objectives, not the finance-driven or politically driven performance reward we are currently seeing. 'Voice' by the authority, rather than 'exit', is the best means of preserving morale and 'loyalty' on the part of providers.

Thus the region mandates funds for providers based on (district) health-care authority plans, and channels these funds through the health authority.

In such a system, the money follows the patient, with patients, GPs and other primary actors and managers at health authority level all having some say. It would be a façade to pretend this is an easy task. Constructing a system which enables this is a necessary and not sufficient task for achieving the wider objectives. It should, however, be pointed out that, currently, the reconciliation of economy and 'market-based purchasing' is an intensively bureaucratic task. In many respects, the evolving orthodoxy in the NHS is a kind of regional planning.

A VALID REGIONAL ROLE

Again, one may hear in some quarters that 'this is going to happen anyway'. But to assume it will happen 'for the best, in the best of all possible worlds' is a Panglossian pipe dream. The trends to regionally mandated 'planning' (purchasing) in the present system have to live alongside fragmentation and therefore 'back-door' means of achieving objectives.

Under the system proposed in this chapter, regions would have the significant, clarified and legitimate role of funding and monitoring health authority/provider links lower down the system.

THE NEW PLANNING

A defence of planning is anything but a defence of a 'bureaucratic paradigm' in which central planning consists in rules and regulations administered throughout a system. For example, in the NHS, 'bureaucratic planning' might at its worst involve centrally prescribed norms for provision of services, with staff agencies (such as personnel, supplies, information and so forth) accountable to central sources. This would tend to produce inflexibility and a lack of responsibility and accountability by 'line' employees who did not have enough decentralized control over resources to be responsible for their 'product'.

In their new book, already showing signs of creating a cult, Barzelay and Armajani (1992) argued that it is important to replace such a bureaucratic paradigm with a 'post-bureaucratic paradigm' which is user-oriented and which 'empowers' employees, in that they are allowed to see the importance of their work as having consequences for other people, being subject to improvement through information and contributory to improved outcomes through employees' own efforts and initiatives.

In a nutshell, decentralized management on 'non-bureaucratic' principles is an important adjunct to 'the right type of planning'. In the health service context, a defence of planning means a defence of coherent strategy to meet need; coherent and stable links between what have recently been termed, in the UK, purchasers and providers; and a minimum of necessary bureaucracy or unnecessary centralization in management, and particularly within service provision (the public sector analogue of production). Far from being reliant on 'private sector insight' to improve such service provision, the public sector has a unique opportunity to take the lead in 'non-bureaucratic' planning and management. In the private sector, much production is of 'goods' – inevitably a separate process from the distribution and consumption of such goods. Often the 'production' of a service such as health care is inseparable from its distribution and exchange. For an example, one need only think of community services, the essence of which is their 'distribution' by (for example) district nurses and health visitors who collaborate directly with the 'consumer' in order to produce the service.

A critique of bureaucratic planning is not a critique of the need to plan services and ensure the accountability of providers who are responsible for meeting such plans. Misapplying market mechanisms (often through uninformed use of the market metaphor, in the first instance) may simply lead to inadequate control of providers, who in turn may not be accountable as the theory of perfect competition – in all its sparsity and inadequacy – would have it.

In short, one may often meet the paradox that the most altruistic believers in 'central planning' are deeply 'unbureaucratic' people who would wish neither to advocate centralized 'command and control' systems nor to work within them! If central planning means strategy setting and integrated purchaser/provider links, then it need not involve 'command and control' management of service provision. Nor, of course, need it involve markets as opposed to service agreements.

Motivating employees through genuinely participative management and the 'creation of value' rather than simply the minimization of costs in a rigid production process may – in a context such as health care – necessitate, rather than militate against, stable links with customers. Local populations are the natural 'customers' or rather users, in a health service. If a misapplied market model leads, for example, to patients being sent in a mechanistic manner around the country or around the county in pursuit of a 'more efficient producer' (perhaps a shorter waiting list) rather than performance management to improve local conditions, then a valuable lesson from the new 'customer-oriented' business has been lost.

Diminishing operational bureaucracy is a prerequisite for successful strategic planning of services and their satisfactory delivery to the customer. In that sense one may truly proclaim 'planning is dead; long live planning!' – if one is pointing to the death of centralized command and control systems allied to rigid central planning according to primitive norms and to the birth of customer-oriented delivery systems involving genuine employee participation in service delivery, allied to flexible plans to meet changing needs.

Different perspectives on 'the management of human resources' stress different factors for either controlling or motivating employees. 'Scientific management' stresses the control of employees – or where it merges with the perspective of 'economic man' it stresses the provision of direct economic incentives for production. 'Human resource management' stresses the motivation of employees in a more humanistic manner by offering meaning to their work and preferably as much autonomy as possible to the employee in making decisions which enhance the product, itself linked to a desired outcome for the customer.

If such 'altruism' is to be more than a sham, however, and phenomena such as 'total quality management' more than mere propaganda or manipulation, there must be a genuine desire to please the 'customer' beyond simply the resultant effect upon one's firm's income and therefore one's job or profit share. Public services such as health services are ideally suited to create this type of altruistic commitment.

The organization with shared values – for example, in providing health services, may be more than a myth: the unitarist enterprise in which shared values are more important than conflict between say managers and employees, may be based on more than coercion, economic incentive or simply the use of power in propaganda and manipulation. To be so, however, egalitarian principles have to inform the relations between the various categories of producer; and relations with the 'customers' have to be based on identification of need rather than identification of income-producing markets.

DISCUSSION

The challenge now remains – as before the reforms – to ensure that planning services on the basis of need leads to hospitals and other providers being funded in relation to service agreements (including possible incentives for efficiency through flexibly allocated 'top up' resources). This could involve the following arrangements:

- general practitioners and others based in localities feeding into the commissioning authority's plan (both abolishing fund-holding and allowing GPs' desired referral patterns to be built into the planning process more effectively than in the pre-reform NHS);
- commissioning authorities' plans being reviewed by regions to assess the implications for 'cross-boundary flows' (i.e. people referred outside the boundaries of their local health authority);
- a regional capital programme compatible with service plans made in the above way (which requires regional planning, but is based on a 'bottom-up' planning process – from localities through districts to region);
- the funding of hospitals and other providers in relation to the workload implied by these plans, translated into service agreements;
- thus compatible capital and revenue (running cost) policies, channelled through health authorities to providers, in service agreements (for 3 or 5 years at a time);
- thus no distinction between the reimbursable costs of caring for people locally in their own districts, on the one hand,

and the costs of cross-boundary flows (the biggest problem of the pre-reform NHS and one of the arguments used in favour of provider markets); such a system would enable regional regulation of costs; the use of such costs in calculating providers' 3- or 5-year service level agreements; and the use of the same costs irrespective of whether the patients were local or 'cross-boundary flows' into their health authority (actual costs for services would of course be subject to detailed work to combine appropriate reimbursement and performance management, equity and protection of specialized and teaching services where relevant);

- thus providers' funding would not be dependent on either where the patient lived (a problem in the pre-reform NHS, as cross-boundary flows were funded at average specialty cost whereas the RAWP formula for local residents did not necessarily allow similar costs for local patients) or who the purchaser was (obviously a major problem in the 'reformed' NHS, as, for example, between district purchasers and GP fundholders).

Another problem with the pre-reform NHS arose when districts were allocated money in their 'targets' for their catchment populations, but did not pass that money on to the providers who were doing the extra work to increase targets. A further complication arose in that targets were often purely academic.

Although the RAWP formula was successful in allowing regions to reach their targets over approximately a 10 year period from 1976 to 1986, districts which were over-target or under-target often remained so as the political difficulty of 'robbing Peter to pay Paul' in times of financial stringency led to targets never being achieved.

A major challenge, therefore – and a very worthwhile one – is to abolish the purchaser/provider split yet to retain the capacity for hospitals and other providers to

be funded according to their workload. This requires a distinction between the health authority and the provider – a distinction which is achievable in terms of the provider being funded according to workload; managing itself on an operational basis; yet being responsible to the health authority in which it is situated.

This (to use a discredited cliche!) is actually an opportunity rather than a problem! For in such a system, providers are rewarded according to workload; health authorities have a geographical/residential basis as planners; yet are a clear locus for provider accountability. That is, even if providers 'do work' for non-local health authorities, the local health authority is the overseer of the health services in the locality, i.e. is responsible for the health services for a catchment population, in terms of its accountability function; while being planner for the health need for its local residential population.

This has a major advantage: the health authority is responsible for hospitals, community units and all primary care providers (GPs and others) in that it is a unified health authority in coopting the current FHSA. As a result, it can coordinate appropriate care and appropriate relations between hospitals, community units and other providers while allowing these to be managerially distinct in an operational and financial/budgetary sense. Thus the pre-reform NHS disadvantage of inadequate differentiation between hospital and community is avoided; yet the even greater disadvantage of the 'reform' NHS is also avoided – namely, the disadvantage that hospitals and community units compete and jostle with each other, and often dump patients on each other for financial reasons, in a competitive environment.

Thus there is a clear role for the health authority as the coordinator of local planning, in turn feeding into regional strategic planning (i.e. coordinating health authority plans). There is a purchaser/provider **distinction** – if one wishes to keep the language of purchasers and providers at all – but not a purchaser/provider **split** in order to run a market. There is also accountability of providers to their local health authority, acting as coordinator of health care for a catchment population. And such a policy changes and improves the current approach, improves on the pre-reform NHS but minimizes yet more reorganization.

An important challenge is to ensure that innovative behaviour by providers is not stymied. The problem with encouraging such behaviour through a market is that providers are encouraged to market themselves (either to fundholding general practitioners or to non-fundholding general practitioners, in the hope of 'bouncing' health authorities' contracts) in a disaggregated manner. This can have two bad effects. Firstly, different providers will spend a lot of effort simply trying to steal each other's business in a zero-sum game. Secondly, GPs and other decision-makers who ought to be contributing to the purchasing plan are instead encouraged to come to agreements with providers without reconciliation of such agreements into a rational purchasing plan. As a result, prioritization and indeed choosing the correct providers in the correct location in order to 'meet the whole picture' is less likely.

Instead therefore it makes sense for GPs and other decision-makers to be a formal part of the planning process, which should also involve provider representatives – but in a coordinated and single forum, not through disaggregated 'special pleading' and marketing.

This may in practice occur in a number of stages. For example, hospital and community providers may have forums with GPs as a preliminary process to the overall planning process. As long as the procedure is coordinated, this can reflect local wishes and local energies (or lack of them!)

It is also important that the health authority plays the role of coordinating the different providers within the district. This is not the same as direct management, but does involve responsibility for the providers. Otherwise, the dangers of turf-protection, aggressive behaviour and non-cooperation between providers (whether between hospitals or between hospital and community) are increased. Furthermore, treating providers as autonomous, with separate and (for example) annual financial targets, decreases the possibility of flexibility in the light of unforeseen workload. One should not encourage providers to think they can simply steal each other's budgets in times of difficulty. But moving from too great laxity to inflexibility through contracts is not the answer either. There will be times when cross-subsidization is necessary (due to client group mix or to unforeseen problems) and the health authority is the logical actor to mandate this. To do so through a process of rigid contracting, and making and breaking contracts, is unnecessarily cumbersome.

The system proposed here would overcome the disadvantage of over-decentralized contracting, which is destructive not only of providers' ability to plan (and in some cases survive) but also of providers' willingness to admit patients irrespective of where they come from. The different incentives set up by different contracts and different purchasers obviate against this. Admittedly, decentralized purchasing can help to target resources on those identified as in need. But this assumes 'correct' resource allocation in the first place. It may be better to monitor use of services, once they have been funded: no contracting system can ensure the social change necessary to change usage patterns, in any case.

The paradox created by the NHS reforms, whereby trusts become more 'autonomous' yet purchasers become more domineering, would also be replaced by a more balanced system of cooperation. Operational autonomy for trusts currently means 'autonomy' for managers to force clinicians to change their behaviour in order to win or maintain contracts from purchasers, or to force pay cuts under the guise of 'local bargaining' in order to ensure financial survival.

Devolution must be more than this travesty if the altruistic culture of the NHS is to be re-born after the depredations of the market.

REFERENCES

Barzelay, M. and Armajani, B. J. (1992) *Breaking Through Bureaucracy: A New Vision for Managing in Government*, University of California Press, Berkeley, CA.

Black, D., Townsend, P., Morris, J. *et al.* (1980) *Inequalities in Health*, HMSO, London.

Clinical Standards Advisory Group (1993) *Access to and Availability of Specialist Services*, HMSO, London.

Galbraith, J. K. (1992) *The Culture of Contentment*, Sinclair Stevenson, London.

Meads, G. (1993) The five commandments. *Health Service Journal*, 6 May.

NHSME (1994) *Local Freedoms, National Responsibilities*, Department of Health, London.

Paton, C. R. (1992) *Competition and Planning in the NHS: The Danger of Unplanned Markets*, Chapman & Hall, London.

Whitehead, M. (1987) *The Growing Health Divide*, Health Education Council, London.

Willetts, D. (1993) *The Opportunities for Private Funding in the NHS*, Social Market Foundation, London.

INTRODUCTION

It is instructive to compare the UK's health-care choices with those of another 'advanced capitalist' nation often seen as at the other end of the public/private spectrum, yet with an alleged convergence taking place around the principle of 'managed competition'. This chapter therefore considers current US health policy and the political factors conditioning it. Yet again, in the 1990s, a proposal for major health-care reform was presented as 'the answer' to the major health and health-care problems of the US. The Clinton Plan proposed universal coverage of the population for health care, with 'managed competition' allegedly to hold down costs and promote what economists would call technical efficiency. It seems sensible to hang a discussion of US health policy generally upon such a major proposal, as there has in the 20th century been a cycle in American politics from periods of proposed reform (whether successful or not) through periods of disillusionment to periods of quietism and acceptance of the status quo, whether reluctantly or not. Cycles in US politics may be reflected in health policy. Whether one accepts the 'liberal/conservative' cycle of Arthur J. Schlesinger, Jr or the more complicated cycle of Samuel P. Huntington (1982), or neither, US political institutions may accentuate or even cause such cycles. That is, institutional barriers to social reform may bring about disillusionment with reform even if it is incomplete or unsuccessful – and channel reformers' zeal elsewhere.

US health policy still stands at a crossroads.

On the one hand, there was, until 1994 at least, the Clinton Plan which holds out a partial convergence with European health-care systems. This convergence would be accentuated, were the Clinton Plan to have long-term success in changing US health care significantly, in that European health-care systems are also looking – in many cases – to 'managed competition' to control costs and manage the clinical process involved in care to that end. (One reason for this is that the same advisers who have been influential in providing the intellectual background to the Clinton Plan, such as Alain Enthoven, have also been influential in advising European governments – not least the 'English-speaking' governments in Sweden, Denmark and the Netherlands, as well as in the UK.)

On the other hand, the United States could continue on the path of frustrating, if occasionally innovative, pluralism in health-care financing and delivery (especially at the state level) – failing to fill the gap left by the absence of a national health system based on the principle of equity and equal access to health care. One cannot be too sanguine about the possibility of radical reform in US domestic politics generally, let alone in health care with its additional complexities (Paton, 1990). The early 1990s, after the election of the Clinton administration in November 1992, were not the first time that radical reform in health care had been promised.

There have been moves since early in the 20th century to establish national health insurance to provide widespread access to health care in the US. A presidential campaign of 1912 saw the independent candidate (and former Republican president) Theodore Roosevelt adopting plans for extended access to health care as part of a 'progressive' ticket. In the 1920s, the American Medical Association – the main interest group representing doctors, although by no means the only one – had not yet acquired the ultraconservative reputation it came to have in the 1950s and 1960s, and in those days it took a much more liberal stance on the question of comprehensive health insurance. There was a move to include national health insurance as part of the Social Security Act in 1935, but this was defeated in Congress. The social legislation of the 1930s promoted under the New Deal had provided a stimulus to the idea of health reform as well as general economic and social reform.

After this episode in the 1930s, it was only in the early 1960s that the question of national health insurance received significant political attention once again. Unlike in the UK, the immediate post-Second-World-War period did not see activist liberal or social democratic legislation, and the first liberal era in politics after the New Deal was in fact that of the Great Society under President Lyndon Johnson, especially during the Eighty-Ninth Congress of 1965/66. Yet in 1965, although Medicare and Medicaid were passed, this legislation represented a political compromise. Various moves to salvage national health insurance were promoted in Congress between 1968 and 1974 (and later, although with less chance of success). Nonetheless by 1990, after a growing conservative climate in domestic policy from the later 1970s throughout the 1980s, no solution was yet found to the problem of inequity in the financing and provision of health care for those in greatest need of it in the US.

By now, the problems of US health care at the macro level are well known, and consist primarily in inequitable access to health care (which seems to produce, along with other social factors, inequity in health status throughout the US nation) and rising costs which continue to spiral out of control. The US's traditional 'exceptionalism' in social policy (although a contested concept in political science) seems to be alive and kicking in the realm of health care. There are, however, recent arguments that attempt to mitigate this assertion. Changing trends in European health care – primarily involving the increasing use of markets and lesser attention to social equity than in the 1970s – may suggest that, to some extent, 'Europe is copying the US' rather than (as perceived especially by US liberals up to the 1980s) there being a need for the US to copy Europe.

To put it somewhat whimsically, the US has hitherto never been seen as a market leader in health policy. There are, however, some arguments which might suggest – descriptively rather than prescriptively – that things are changing. That is, like it or not, the inequitable pluralism of US health care (reflecting the US's inequitable pluralism in the general polity) and its reliance on both private provision and private financing may represent the future as well as the past.

THE LEGACY

Prior to the 1960s, US health care was largely in private hands, although not dominated to any significant extent by the laws of the marketplace. Non-profit hospitals and autonomous 'office physicians' predominated on what economists would call the 'supply side' of health care; and most health care was privately financed. In the 1970s, weak and decentralized 'indirect' planning structures were introduced in an attempt to rationalize provision and control costs prior to further expansion of equity (as those on the liberal side of the spectrum such as Senator Kennedy sought). The landmark 'planning' act was the National Health Planning and Resources Development Act of 1974. Federal legislation at this time also sought to encourage health maintenance organizations (HMOs), which were seen in the 1970s as part of a regulatory initiative rather than as part of a market initiative. HMOs act as a special type of insurance company which directly own or manage providers (hospitals, etc.) and therefore avoid the tendency of providers to pass high costs on to insurers.

The 'Reagan revolution' in the 1980s tapped into a political and public mood at the time which suggested that planning did not work. Mainstream liberals (in the American sense of the term) were disappointed at the lack of results from attempted social planning. Both conservative and radical critiques argued that planning did not work. The conservative critique is familiar; the radical critique tended to argue that planning was subverted by dominant interests and was too weak to challenge those interests (Paton, 1990).

In the 1980s, health policy was policy by default. While there were one or two significant initiatives (at the technical rather than political or ideological level) such as the introduction of 'diagnosis-related groups (DRGs)', the philosophy of the Reagan administration was to let market forces rationalize the system if they could. To some extent this was wishful thinking. American health care has traditionally not been characterized by market discipline in provision, but by inefficient subsidy of fee-for-service medicine, operating through local monopolies (whether for profit or non-profit), by the mechanism of third-party insurance. A *laissez-faire* approach was not likely to lead to the rationalization of the system. Market-oriented health reformers saw the need for competition in provision, and furthermore also an end to traditional fee-for-service medicine in the private sector. Such market competition was – in the eyes of many reformers – to come through health maintenance organizations (HMOs), which would enrol patients and guarantee their health care for the year. (That is, HMOs were a special type of insurance company, which would own their providers and end the tension between the provider and financier which led to spiralling costs when allied to rapacious consumer demand for everything available in health care, whatever the cost.)

By the end of the 1980s, it was clear that costs had not been rationalized at all – and that markets had only worked patchily and to a limited extent in controlling costs. Indeed much of the research-based literature implies that for-profit corporations delivering health care were in fact more costly rather than less costly by comparison with traditional providers.

THE RE-EMERGENCE OF REGULATION

The decline and fracturing of the right-wing coalition that produced Reaganism led in health care to a re-emergence of interest in regulation. It was never likely, however, that a recourse to the approaches of the 1970s would occur. The election of President Clinton in 1992 put squarely on the agenda the concept of 'managed competition'. The person credited with originating this phrase is Professor Alain Enthoven, Professor of Public and Private Management at Stanford University and a health economist who had previously been a young Assistant Secretary of Defense under Robert McNamara in the early 1960s. Disillusioned by what he saw as the inefficiency of Government, yet with a commitment to some version of social equity, Enthoven argued that managed competition was the best means of rationalizing the health-care system while permitting (both fiscally and politically) greater equity than had hitherto been either affordable or seemingly politically possible. He has subsequently sought – less appropriately – to export this blueprint to many European countries, aided by right-wing 'think tanks' and journals (after an earlier period of less political advocacy).

RECONCILING EQUITY WITH COST CONTROL

What is meant by equity in health care? In the UK the Resource Allocation Working Party in

1976 defined equity in terms of 'equality of opportunity of access to health care for those at equal risk' (Department of Health and Social Security, 1976). The concept of equity in health care – a necessary concept, although difficult to define – has implications for allocating resources and planning services. Equity can be defined in geographical terms, in terms of social class, or – most usefully – in a comprehensive manner that also provides practical guidelines as to how to allocate resources (Paton, 1985).

In the United States, there is no central authority that allocates available finance for health care on the basis of need. Naturally, this does not distinguish the United States from most countries in the world, as countries which both rely on public finance for most health-care spending and allocate resources 'scientifically' are rare: the UK is exceptional, although not unique. In the US, it is more useful to think in terms of demand rather than need. Health care is demanded by those who have the available finance and who wish to use it to buy health care or health insurance. Health care is delivered in a regulated marketplace, with supply and demand determining output and price.

The major difference between the buying of health care and the 'textbook' marketplace is that the consumer is not the key decision-maker as to the employment of resources in providing care. That role has traditionally fallen to the doctor. In the US, one major reason for cost explosions in health care (to the point that it now absorbs almost 14% of the US gross domestic product, approximately 1.5 times higher than the UK's), is that the 'consumer' or patient does not play a significant role in the reimbursement for services. The doctor makes decisions on behalf of the patient, in the context of a culture which is very demanding of expensive services, and the costs are passed on in most cases to a third-party payer – the insurer. Recently there have been moves to prevent this 'problem of the third-party

payer', as economists put it, by uniting the provider of health care and the insurer. The argument is that, if the insurance company that collects the premiums has to provide health care out of the resulting fixed pool of available money through a legal contract to the consumer/patient, then incentives promoting economy will exist. This is the essence of what has become known as the health maintenance organization, an early example of which was the Kaiser Permanente organization in California. The HMO is characterized by the insurer and the provider being part of the same organization.

In the UK, of course, attempts to replace the doctor as a significant allocator of resources at hospital level have been made via the NHS 'reforms', and their boost to governmental and managerial rationing.

If one wishes to begin from abstract principles and design a health-care system for the United States that acknowledges the need both to control costs and to provide equity in the sense of access for those who need care but cannot afford it, then creating a system in which care is provided through health maintenance organizations and similar forms of institution and financed by Government for those who do not have adequate access otherwise, is an obvious route to take. The most constructive and also practical proposal for reform of American health care have indeed followed this route, although often with a strong 'market' bias.

A FORERUNNER TO THE CLINTON PLAN: ENTHOVEN AND THE JACKSON HOLE GROUP

THE MAIN PROPOSAL

Enthoven's most recent proposal for US health-care reform has been devised in coordination with the so called 'Jackson Hole Group', the name deriving from the fact that the group meets at the home of Paul Ellwood, a long-time health policy analyst and Government adviser. The essence of the approach is to seek to combine greater efficiency in provision of health care with some degree of equity in purchasing on behalf of various stipulated populations (such as the poor).

To this extent Enthoven is a free market economist who nevertheless sees a need for Government regulation to ensure that specific 'problems with the market' (market failure) are addressed in devising a meaningful reform. One such problem is 'risk selection'. Insurance companies will seek to exclude those in higher risk brackets such as the poorer and sicker (unless they are fully recompensed for the higher costs of care which such groups are likely to incur when properly covered). Managed competition seeks to minimize the incentive for health plans to select risk by establishing:

- a single point of entry for all subscribers/citizens;
- a standardized benefit package;
- risk-adjusted premiums;
- agreed standards for access to care, including tertiary care.

These stipulations are made in the context of rules to ensure coverage of all in a sponsored group. It is argued that small employer groups seeking health care for their workers need to be pooled into large purchasing cooperatives, in order to:

- spread risk;
- achieve economies of scale in purchasing;
- acquire expertise;
- manage competition by allowing enough purchasing power *vis-à-vis* the power of providers;
- offer choice to individuals to change plans.

The Jackson Hole Group has proposed a health insurance purchasing cooperative (HIPC) which would play the just-described role of pooling small groups of employers and also coordinating the purchase by Government of health coverage for the disad-vantaged in society. These HIPCs would contract what Enthoven calls 'accountable health partnerships' (AHPs), which would in effect either be health maintenance organizations or other organizations offering what is increasingly known generically in the health policy literature as 'managed care'. This last concepts refers to the alleged need for care plans for specific diseases and conditions, to allow both cost control and standardized 'health planning' at the micro-level within the hospital or community setting.

Accountable health partnerships can allegedly produce better care at lower cost, on the following principles. Firstly, they will allegedly produce loyalty, commitment and the responsible participation of their physicians. Secondly, they will render compatible the incentives confronting doctors, the interests of patients and the interests of society in high quality yet economical care. They will do this primarily by ensuring that the incentives of their enrolled physicians are directed to making them work within the budget of the organization that pays them.

That is, in the terminology increasingly current in the UK, there will not be a split between the purchaser and the provider, in that the health maintenance organization will be the purchaser which also owns or directly controls the provider. (If, however, by the purchaser we mean the HIPC operating on behalf of citizens, employers and Government, rather than the HMO with the HIPC contracts, then, of course, there is a purchaser/provider split.)

Thirdly, the AHPs will allegedly have an incentive to produce information systems adequate for the purpose of monitoring the effect of health care – what is known in the literature as health outcomes. They will study variations in clinical practice and increasingly move towards adopting cost-effective patterns of care. Fourthly, these organizations will in effect do a kind of decentralized health planning, in that they will match provision (for example numbers and types of doctors) to the needs of their enrolled populations. One particular need in the United States is to increase primary care at the expense of both secondary and complex tertiary care. Resources generally should be matched to needs of population served, of course – not just numbers and types of doctors.

Finally, and most prescriptively and aspirationally, such organizations will allegedly indulge in what has become the buzz phrase of 'total quality management' (TQM) which, shorn of the jargon, means 'do it right first time rather than rectify mistakes'. This approach allegedly cuts costs and renders compatible both quality improvement and cost reduction.

In pointing to some current problems in US health care not addressed by traditional private-sector-based fee-for-service provision reimbursed by third-party insurance, Enthoven and the Jackson Hole Group can, of course, make common cause with more general critics of US health care. Firstly, inability to control costs, or even the rapid rise in costs, sits fair and square with gross inequity in terms of access to care by those who need it. Very selectively, some more specific characteristics of the latter are: a lack of primary care and an excess of specialists; an excess of facilities even after 'competition' has supposedly rationalized the system; wide variations in clinical practice, medical uncertainty and a lack of data on outcomes; and a lack of preventive, promotive and 'social' care: in particular, a record on childhood immunization which, as Enthoven points out, in a debating point no doubt intended to sting his fellow analysts, produces a record worse than that of Cuba. (The prescriptive implication – if it's worse than Cuba, it must be bad indeed – is, of course, very unfair, given Cuba's impressive record in health care for a previously underdeveloped country – at least until the collapse of Cuba's trading partners in the former Soviet block.)

The Jackson Hole reform proposal thus seeks to set right the problems of the traditional fee-for-service system, consisting in solo practice and remote third-party insurance. The incentives of the traditional system are (rightly) considered to be wrong. It creates a costly adversary relationship between provider and payer; there is no planning forceful enough to match resources to population needs; and the financial separation of the various components of the traditional system prevents rational resource allocation.

The key question is, can a 'pro-competitive regulatory framework', to produce managed competition, put right such wrongs? It is significant that universal coverage for care is very much the final element of the Jackson Hole prescription.

Admittedly the prescription offers comprehensive care to enrolled populations, on the basis of per-capita prepayment either by individuals or their employers – or by Government on behalf of the poor. The proposal also puts providers at risk for costs and poor quality and makes them publicly accountable to some extent in these realms. It is nevertheless very much an open question as to whether 'managed competition' would in fact rationalize the US health-care system.

It is certainly true that one of the major problems in US health care, from the viewpoint of the economist, is that demand is 'price-inelastic'. Where all expenses – however excessive – are tax-deductible and where a lot of insurance policies involve 'the employer paying all', then there is certainly little incentive to control costs.

When one adds to this the fact that existing benefit packages are not standardized, competition is even more difficult: the market is segmented and even HMOs may not compete in that, for example, some will be renowned for good care in one specialty and bad care in another. The perfectly rational fear by consumers of exclusions 'in the small print', whether in traditional medical insurance or in health maintenance organizations, means that – in the absence of regulation –

genuine competition by providers on an equal basis in the 'same market' may be difficult to achieve.

To put it another way, neither consumers nor Government may have adequate information on providers, in a seg n. market, to allow effective competition. Thus the Jackson Hole proposals may contribute something to improving the prospects for a market in provision.

Furthermore, the proposal at least acknowledges that 'risk selection' is a problem in health insurance. If insurers can discriminate among the population, they will seek to exclude 'bad risks' (i.e. the poor and sick) wherever possible. If insurers and the providers that they own (or contract with) are not regulated to 'take all comers' on the basis of annual open enrolment and full reimbursement of the actuarially calculated costs of those they cover, then either the poor and sick will simply not get coverage or the insurers who cover them will increasingly run into financial difficulties. Consequences of the latter will be that either they will go bust or will provide inadequate care for those they cover. In other words, there will be 'poor HMOs for the poor' – at best.

THE POLITICAL ENVIRONMENT

But, overall, the political environment within which any meaningful health policy proposal must find a niche makes it difficult to envisage an effective and equitable version of managed competition being implemented. The Clinton Plan, for example, challenged too many vested interests yet is a bureaucratic and labyrinthine structure of policy ('rationally' devised, without concern for the interest-group politics of the US). If part of it is removed, owing to political compromise, it tends to fall apart. For example, if HIPCs (alliances) are removed, or if equity is not adequately protected, it becomes simply a conservative and partial – yet bureaucratic – policy. Ironically, the insurance industry has opposed the Clinton Plan by posing as the guarantor of the people's freedom!

Even if private insurance is able to adapt to play a significant role in the new financial/purchasing arrangements without subverting them in the direction of the traditional system (a very dubious proposition in any case), the fact that the Jackson Hole proposals do not call for a redistributive payroll tax will make it difficult to ensure that the needs of those hitherto excluded from the system are adequately financed and covered through any reform, even if fully implemented. It is of some significance that the name of Enthoven has been identified with tentative health-care reform proposals throughout the duration of the Reagan and Bush administrations as well as in the early days of the Clinton administration. Healthcare is not seen as an exceptional need which transcends income so much as simply another good to be purchased in a more cost-effective manner, in the eyes of mainstream 'market' reformers. To expect the inequity of health care to be addressed without fiscal redistribution is to expect a lot.

Furthermore, there is no specific advocacy of the effective and comprehensive 'group health maintenance organization' as opposed to what are known as 'individual HMOs', which are more loosely organized and controlled, and which have, as suggested by research in the 1980s, a poorer record in cost control let alone in promoting social equity. The aim is to keep coverage in the private sector and to ensure that there are 'no free riders' that is, to ensure that those who can pay (whether individuals or firms) do pay. The role for Government is therefore a peripheral or tidying role.

The importance of the insurance industry in sponsoring Democrats as well as Republicans (such as Lloyd Bentsen, Clinton's first Treasury Secretary, when he was a Democratic Texan Senator) means that replacing pluralistic private insurance with a quasi-public national health insurance, as in Canada, is effectively off the agenda. The insurance industry is now more powerful than the 'doctor lobby'. The American Medical Association is now more of a toothless tiger than it used to be when physicians were scarcer.

TOWARDS THE CLINTON PLAN

It is arguably because Enthoven's earlier reform proposals have been mediated in a right-wing direction to produce the current Jackson Hole reform proposal that a schism opened up between 'conservatives' and the 'liberals' advising what was – in 1993 – the President's Healthcare Commission, headed by Hillary Clinton. Furthermore, liberal Senators such as Howard Metzenbaum (Ohio) were opposed to 'managed competition'. Health reformers such as Jay Rockefeller (West Virginia) are concerned about equity.

The conservatives seek a pro-competitive regulatory framework in the context of weak proposals to increase social equity, and the liberals seek a greater role for Government in pursuit of greater social equity as well as cost control.

While pro-competitive regulators admittedly argue for a Health Standards Board to define 'the uniform and effective health benefits' which would be eligible for tax favoured coverage in the private sector and also an 'Outcomes Management Standards Board' to ensure that information is available to help purchasers and HIPCs, these are in effect technical (albeit important) regulatory functions to ensure that money is not wasted in the marketplace.

In mainstream US politics, the choice has recently been not really between the traditional system, managed competition and socialized health care but between various fairly weak versions of managed competition as opposed to a traditional system. The question is, can the 'Clinton Plan' (White House, 1993) go beyond traditional incrementalism in reconciling equity (a national health insur-ance) and cost control?

Some prominent 'market-oriented' health-care analysts (such as Professor Mark Pauly of the Wharton School in Pennsylvania) have even argued for significantly less regulation than that inherent in the Enthoven proposals, let alone the Clinton proposals. Pauly argues that 'risk selection' by insurance companies is an over-rated problem; that the alleged crisis caused for companies' costs by health-care coverage for their workers is also an over-rated problem (on the grounds that it is simply an economic choice between higher wages and less health care on the one hand and lower wages and more health care on the other); and that traditional regulation is not likely to succeed. As with many who embrace the right-wing version of public choice economics, it is argued by Pauly that the incentives for regulators to do the right thing are not evident. In other words, according to this perspective, in analysing health-care reform, we should be considering a narrow version of economic man. At the end of the day, however, any debate, implicit or explicit, between Enthoven and Pauly is in effect a debate between a strong version of managed competition and a lesser version of regulated competition.

THE CLINTON PLAN

The Clinton Plan consisted of:

- guaranteed comprehensive health-care benefits for all Americans;
- a series of geographically-based, states-administered Health Alliances (descendants of the health insurance purchasing cooperatives), which would enrol all citizens, whether paid by employers themselves, or the state;
- a choice of health plans for all Americans, to be purchased by the health alliances (ranging from traditional fee-for-service medicine to health maintenance organizations);
- cost incentives to choose economical plans, but allowance for extra payments by

individuals (and firms) to pay for 'freer' plans;

- fixed payments to health plans, to control costs;
- coverage at the same rate for all participants ('community rating'), with 'purchasing' alliances adjusting payments to health plans (from their general revenues) to ensure that the more expensive (poorer and sicker) are properly covered;
- a National Health Board, to regulate and mandate standards for coverage, quality and service;
- allowance for large firms to set up their own health alliances;
- incorporation of existing schemes (such as Medicare and Medicaid) in the new structure;
- an enforceable 'price control' policy (the 'enforceable cap') which controls costs by regulation if market forces do not work; and therefore
- the replacement of the existing weak system with incentives for cost control by genuine provider competition, as well as equity.

THE CLINTON PLAN IN CONTEXT: VARIETIES OF REFORM

The last time it was even conceivable that national health insurance would be passed in Congress was in 1974. At that time, the various approaches to extending access to care ranged from the full national health insurance proposal of Senator Kennedy and his collaborators; through weaker NHI proposals embodying less regulation; through plans which merely subsidized access to medical care through tax relief or the like (such as the American Medical Association's proposals); through to piecemeal or incremental plans which attempted to 'count in' particular groups currently excluded from full access to the system (Paton, 1990).

By the early and mid 1990s there was a similar spectrum of plans – with the major proviso that the national health insurance approach of

Kennedy had been replaced by the universal coverage yet 'managed competition' approach of Clinton and others. The main difference between 'Kennedy' and 'Clinton' is that the former (in its 1970s guise – not its pragmatic 1990s guise) mandated universal access to a system which still retained private provision and in many cases fee-for-service provision, but which sought to control costs through regulation. To that extent the Kennedy Plan mirrored some of Europe's national health insurance enactments, whereby regulation rather than competition was used to reconcile equity with cost control.

The Clinton Plan seeks to embrace the ideas of competition, in that health plans compete to be included in the list of plans which local health alliances license in effect for approval. These health alliances receive their money from companies, (employers), individuals, and the Government (for those individuals unable to pay for themselves), and in effect act as a kind of purchaser, which channels the money (weighted for health risk to some extent) to lower level purchasers or health plans, which then either own or contract with providers such as hospitals.

Already we can see that the managed competition approach might be even more regulatory and bureaucratic, involving more administrative costs (what economists might call transactions costs) than a policy of regulation on a national basis. The need to provide an entry (for political reasons) to private insurance and indeed top-up payments from individuals and companies for more generous health plans, prevents the Clinton Plan from realizing the cost-efficient policy of a 'total cap' (both national and local) on health-care spending.

As a result, it is less likely to combine equity and cost control than a fully socialized model such as the British National Health Service (pre-reform) or indeed a fairly socialized model such as a European-style national health insurance of, for example, the Dutch variety.

The weaker proposals in the 1990s reflect the weaker proposals of the 1970s in a generic sense. For example, in response to the political imperative to produce an alternative to the Clinton Plan, Senator Bob Dole (in collaboration with John Chafee) and also Senator Phil Gramm proposed weaker models that did less to achieve equity and relied more upon either voluntarism in subscription or competition or both. The Dole proposal at least mandated universal coverage on paper; the Gramm proposal simply ignored this requirement. A more conservative or moderate version of the Clinton Plan was proposed by Cooper and Grandy; and only the McDermott–Wellstone Plan sought a European-style socialized system which relied on regulation (for example, fee schedules for doctors and hospitals) yet which in practice might well have been less bureaucratic than a plan relying on managed competition. The latter involves the bureaucracy of both planning and the market (sceptics of both left and right would describe this as the worst of both worlds).

ACTION OR INACTION?

The 1980s was a decade of inaction at the federal level concerning health-care reform, although significant state initiatives to develop innovative patterns of delivery and in some cases to increase equity were beginning to occur during that time. (In 1993, for example, Oregon and Washington states were seeking to combine cost control and greater equity.) Whatever version of health-care reform is adopted at the federal level – and this includes the Clinton administration – it is likely that the effects of both congressional behaviour and any subsequent implementation throughout the federal system would render reform incremental rather than comprehensive.

The most significant change is likely to occur in terms of what is publicly covered for those populations depending upon Government for their access to health care. Formal 'rationing' devices such as the so called Oregon formula are likely to increase in salience.

The state of Oregon has been developing various versions of its proposals which in effect 'cover more of the poor for less procedures or medical problems' (Strosberg *et al.*, 1992). That is, allegedly on the basis of both expert definitions of which procedures produce 'health gain' (better health status) and which do not, on the one hand, and popular participation in making hard choices, on the other hand, a schedule of allowable and non-allowable procedures as regards publicly financed health care is drawn up. The state's Medicaid programme is then extended to include all those hitherto excluded rather than simply the traditional Medicaid population. This is rendered affordable, however, on the basis that previously reimbursable procedures will in some cases no longer be available through public finance.

On the one hand this can be presented as a progressive proposal (supported by Clinton during the campaign in 1992), yet can also be presented as contributory to a two-tier system in that it is only the poor who are 'rationed'. (Vice President Al Gore, during the campaign, opposed the Oregon approach.)

It is therefore less a radical change in the financing of health care or even the provision of health care (that is, structural change) than in the changing role of the consumer and the expert that one might see significant changes in the 1990s in US health care. It is perhaps in this realm, to return to the introduction of this essay, that the US is a 'market leader' rather than market follower. The role of the consumer is now much more part of the rhetoric, at the very least, in British and European health care than previously, partly as a result of US influence. Furthermore, debates about 'who should make the hard choices in a context of rationing health care' – the expert or the consumer (technocracy or democracy) – is a live debate in the more publicly financed systems of Europe, where such decisions are at least more fairly and squarely social decisions. In the United States, however, such decisions tend to affect only those segments of the poor dependent on the public purse, and are an anathema to the bulk of the population.

One of the significant impetuses for national health-care reform (which has been a non-starter in effect since the 1960s) has been the increasing discontentment, at a time of economic recession, of what Galbraith would call the 'contented majority' (Galbraith, 1992). That is, middle-class people as well as working-class people have been losing their jobs and finding out what it is to suffer from insecurely held health insurance. The most likely political source of health-care reform is to ensure that 'the richer pay' – on the basis that, if they cease to be rich, they will still get coverage.

At bottom therefore, it is by giving the better-off a stake is what might broadly be called the social welfare system of the country that significant welfare reform in the United States may be achievable. To that extent, the US health-care system may therefore be belatedly catching up with Europe.

There is a problem here, however: if the aim is increasingly to ration expensive care, then one can ration on the basis of income or on the basis of access to services irrespective of income. If one chooses the later, the poor may suffer for those excluded services for which they cannot afford to pay in the private sector. If, however, one rations on the basis of income (assuming heroically even that the US political system is able to handle such a significant process in a coherent way), then one is in effect creating Government finance or Government programmes on the basis of either a formal means test or on the basis of a sliding scale of income.

This removes the 'stake in welfare' for the better-off, which is necessary to sustain 'healthy' welfare programmes in a society such as the US, where the atypical social manners of the faddish politically correct sit uncomfortably alongside a highly inegalitarian and conservative political economy.

AN INTERNATIONAL COMPARISON

All health systems fall into one of three categories – whether they are public or private. Category One is what might be termed third party reimbursement, whereby either public or private money is used to reimburse care sought by the individual or directed by a primary care doctor such as the general practitioner in the UK (especially before the NHS reforms). Whether or not it has regulation of the fee schedules of hospitals and doctors, such a system can be characterized as third-party reimbursement because there is free referral of the patient to care. Either the private individual or the insurance company (in the private sector), or the Government acting through health authorities or other financiers (in the public sector), reimburses the cost of the care to the provider.

If such a system is a public system, there is no overt 'purchasing' function, whereby a health authority or insurance company or whatever decides what form of care is to be provided for its population and makes a contract with providers. Such a public system may, of course, have planning of services, in response to GP referrals, to patient wishes, or indeed to other political or managerial imperatives (for example, through a capital allocation policy conducted on a national basis). In the latter scenario, the general practitioner would then refer patients to care as made available through such a policy. At best, such systems involve a creative and flexibly planned interplay between referral and regional planning.

Category Two involves contracts between purchasers and providers. For example, in the Clinton Plan, health alliances in line with individuals' and companies' preferences – purchase care from health plans, which in turn purchase care from providers if they do not directly own them. In the fully private sector, there is no overt purchasing function – only reimbursement as in Category One. In the fully public sector – as in the UK's public health authorities post-reform – purchasers (health authorities) contract with self-governing trusts.

Category Three is a situation whereby individuals are enrolled in organizations (whether geographical health authorities, insurance companies or health maintenance organizations) which directly own their providers. In this sense, there is overt purchasing or overt allocation of money either through individual purchase or through Government allocation, but the providers are not a separate organization from the purchaser. Comprehensive HMOs (of the public sort) in the US fit this category.

ASSESSMENT

There are political as well as analytical differences, of course, between such alternatives. Free referral in a private system has been the essence of the pre-reform United States health-care system. But it is generally the right wing (Republicans who resent the 'managed care' and bureaucracy of the Clinton proposal) who seek to preserve free referral. It is thus paradoxically the right wing who are less directly interested in cost control through managed care. Where health-care costs are out of control, it is up to businesses to pass costs on to their workers, or for copayments at least by workers to share costs. Some free market theorists (such as Mark Pauly of the Wharton School) deny that there is as much of a crisis in American health care as is alleged. It is alleged to be a legitimate free market decision that as much is spent on health care as actually is currently spent, and it is up to individuals and insurance companies – if they so wish – to mandate downward pressure on costs in the marketplace. (Enthoven, on the other hand, is less a fiscal and political conservative in this 'hard' sense than a constructive neoconservative.)

Such hard conservatives are less concerned with extending equity than with preserving the choice of those who already have it, and they are less worried therefore about the hypothetical cost implications of extending equity.

There is a somewhat ironical parallel between such believers in 'free referral' or unregulated care and defenders of the pre-reform NHS in the UK – by and large the public as a whole; certainly those on the left of the political spectrum; and those in the professions who see management decisions usurping clinical freedom. They believe that a public National Health Service is both most equitable and most efficient by allowing free referral and public reimbursement. There is a politically decided national cap on resources, but then resources are subsequently allocated in line with the preferences of patients and their doctors in both primary and secondary care settings. It is at least arguable that this form of 'purchasing' is less bureaucratic, more efficient and fairer than the very bureaucratic system of 'purchasing' and using 'managed competition' in provider markets in the UK. What is more, the British system always had natural cost control by using the GP as a gatekeeper, as well as national budgetary control (Paton, 1992).

The irony lies in the fact that unrestricted access is favoured by both these schools of thought – by the right wing defending the already privileged in the United States and by the left wing or public voice defending the whole community in the UK. Nevertheless, an important issue of principle arises: should care be managed by 'bureaucrats' and 'purchasers' (with, at worst, clinical decisions being usurped by managers – often with a degree of ignorance as well as a desire to control costs) or should individuals have greater freedom? The latter might be in the context of either an equitable public system (as in the UK, prior to the reform of the National Health Service in 1991) or as would be envisaged in the United States by defenders of a British-style or European-style 'central regulatory approach' which nevertheless maintained free referral. There is conflict also between general fiscal conservatives in the United States, who tend to believe in managed care in order to reduce health-care budgets, and more general ideological conservatives who wish to preserve what the French would call *la médécine liberale*.

There was an interesting source of political prediction available from this characterization. If it is true that the Clinton Plan is unappealing to the right and to the left for the reason that it restricts either private-oriented or public-oriented liberal access to health care, then it will be attacked from both the left and right. Thus, in the long term, such a proposal may run alien to significant strands in the US political culture. Can the 'hard centre' of politics rescue it? This may be Clinton's constituency. Congressional Democrats are mostly liberal or conservative: there is not much ideological or practical coherence to 'neoliberalism'. Set against this, of course, is the perceived greater need to control costs than ever before, and a growing belief that equity and cost control require a mechanism other than European-style national regulation. Thus the Clinton Plan in the early 1990s threw its ideological and practical opponents on to the defensive more than earlier attempts at national health insurance in the 1970s. Senator Kennedy attempted in early 1994 to aid its passage by – ironically – relaxing its regulatory characteristics.

But the Republican capture of Congress in November 1994 ended the prospect of passage.

Even before that, the decline of the Clinton Plan in 1994 was partly due to the opposition painting it as (variously) 'socialistic' and also expensive. A simpler advocacy of Canadian-style health care might have been more successful – no more enemies, yet a clearer and less bureaucratic agenda. On this argument, 'managed competition' was always a sell-out to the conservatives, which ironically made a liberal plan more bureaucratic.

One can surmise that – were there no need to be pragmatic – the wife of the President, Hillary Clinton, might well have favoured the abolition of the private insurance 'middleman' and a more effective and indeed cost-efficient national health insurance programme of a more directly European sort. Nevertheless, the need to please a variety of political constituencies has meant that the main proposal for 'universal coverage and a national health policy' will include the idea whose time seems to have come – managed competition. It may well be that managed competition would represent an improvement on the status quo in US health care. What is considerably less clear is whether it is an improvement also for those European systems which have done fairly well in terms of both equity and cost control (such as the UK, Sweden and to a lesser extent the Netherlands and other west European countries).

Some commentators have depicted a convergence between the United States and the socialized health-care systems of Europe – based on the principle of managed competition, a greater role for the consumer and so forth. A lot of this is, however, rhetoric, as plans relying on managed competition tend to diminish the direct role of the patient/user/consumer. In this sense, the Clinton Plan is better than some of the 'internal market' and 'managed competition'-type proposals in Europe: at least individuals are allowed to select their health plan and access to it is achieved (on paper) fairly equitably. Systems which rely on management agencies to buy care indirectly on behalf of patients often reduce consumer or patient sovereignty in any meaningful sense.

In countries such as the UK and Sweden, the internal market may well be a solution in search of a problem. In the United States, the system of managed competition as in the Clinton Plan may admittedly be that more conventional phenomenon – a solution to a problem! The barriers to the enactment of a national health programme, which attempts to fit in with American values and which also attempts to reconcile the market and cost control, are, however, huge. (By enactment is meant implementation to achieve a socially effective result, and not merely passage in Congress in some compromised form.)

CONCLUSION

At the level of international comparison, one finds at least superficial agreement on the objectives of a modern health-care system – effectiveness in terms of better health for the people, whether or not subdivided into social classes and particular groups in need; equity in terms of humane access at times of need to health care; and manageable costs or cost control. In practice, a variety of factors render the differences in different countries' health-care systems which we recognize. In the UK, the combination of socialist aspirations for the NHS and the paternalistic welfare tradition in the middle of this century led to the National Health Service. In the United States, greater individualism (an absence of both feudalism and socialism), and also a part pragmatic, part ideological belief in the free market where possible, has led ironically to the present impasse where a superficially 'free' health-care system is both expensive and bureaucratic. To add significantly greater social equity into an already expensive bureaucratic mixture is a tall order – in the absence of a socialization that goes beyond the idea of 'managed competition' as in the Clinton Plan. This would involve a move towards public budgeting (involving overall control on total budgets), public planning and regulation and yet – or therefore – an ability to allow both clinical practice in hospitals and referral by primary care doctors to hospitals to be less regulated than in a system which has to control costs obsessively at the level of the individual clinical decision and referral (i.e. at the 'micro'-level). The latter obsession is also the orthodoxy of the day in health reform.

But its costs may well outweigh its benefits.

Systems that create incentives for cost escalation – such as market systems, whether free market systems, systems involving managed competition as in the Clinton proposals or systems such as the 'internal market' in the British NHS after the NHS reforms – require regulation to limit the incentives for providers to oversupply or supply unduly expensive care. Systems that work more informally, albeit within overall planning guidelines, relying on altruism as well as merely contractualism and market incentives, have in fact a better record of reconciling cost control and equity, if one looks at both the UK and Sweden as prime examples of such countries. Such systems are public. It is often claimed the taxpayer will not countenance extra public spending. But if such systems are more efficient, the rational taxpayer would wish more public care then more private care, if the latter is more expensive (unless, of course, the degree of tax redistribution, i.e. progressivity, is too great).

Whither then US health policy and more particularly US health-care reform? Progressive reformers in the US, in the 1960s and 1970s, often looked to the UK to provide an example of progress, if not (for political reasons) a model to be copied exactly. More recently, progressive reformers have often looked to Canada as an example of a system combining public control and regulation with equity and some degree of success in cost control. More recently, however, health-care restructuring in Canada has rendered that system a less clear model, certainly at the political level, in terms of 'lessons across the border'. It has sometimes been observed that, whether before or after its recent reform, the British NHS is more of a 'socialist, left-wing' health care system than the most radical variants of Senator Kennedy's plans in the 1970s would have produced for the US. This is both true and false. It is true in that the British NHS pre-reform relied almost exclusively on public provision of care and did not distinguish between purchasers and providers, i.e. health authorities on the one hand and hospitals or community providers of care on the other hand. It is also true in that the British NHS controlled costs by central public allocation rather than through regulatory means within a system of private provision. On the other hand, were an adequately financed version of national health insurance according to Senator Kennedy's original principles to be passed in the United States, then comparing such a plan with the UK after the NHS reforms produces a different perspective: the American system under such a scenario would be both more generously financed and allow equity along the lines of European national insurance schemes. There would be greater choice of doctor for the patient/consumer; less 'managed care' as decided by managers rather than doctors or patients; and reliance on macro- rather than micro-regulation of care to limit costs. To that extent, US-style national health insurance could be more generous than a post-reform 'welfare wedge' in the NHS UK.

Comparing the Clinton proposal with the post 1991 'reform' NHS, one finds that both are concerned with cost control; that both offer a variety of purchaser/provider relationships; that neither offers free referral for the patient to care of whatever sort desired (although, in fact, there would be more of this in the US than in the UK); and that the US system would be more generously funded in a real sense than the British system.

And therein lies the rub. Given the expectation for health care in the US, a national system would require a greater level of generosity – i.e. bringing the poor up to the level of the better-off rather than reducing everyone's expectations – than in the UK. Hitherto, the UK has 'rationed' by waiting times and in some cases availability of services in the public system, whereas the US has rationed by social class and ability to pay. There is often a debate as to whether, in the

context of scarce resources, it is better to focus on the poor and end the pretension of a universal service for all comers. It has, however, been memorably observed that 'a service for the poor is a poor service'. And, if private services are more expensive rather than cheaper, leaving the better-off to fend for themselves in the private sector may leave less residual tax money for the poor, who may be worth worse off both relatively and absolutely. The alternative in a country such as the UK therefore is a universal service (for all comers) but with a rationing of those services available. In the US, this would not be politically acceptable to the middle classes. (Aaron and Schwarz, 1984).

And that is why a universal national health-care system in the US would be a generous and radical reform – yet that is why it is also proving so difficult, especially given the US political structure. (Paton, 1990). The abandonment of the Clinton Plan, temporary or otherwise, in September 1994 represented yet again the complex interplay of ideology and US political structure in preventing either efficient 'socialized' reform or less efficient 'regulatory market' reform in health care.

ACKNOWLEDGEMENTS

I would like to thank the publishers of two articles on which I have (loosely) drawn for part of this chapter, one in Peele, Bailey *et al.* (eds) (1994) *Developments in American Politics*, Macmillan, London, and the other in Davies *et al.* (eds) (1995) *Political Issues in America: The 1990s Revisited*, Manchester University Press, Manchester.

REFERENCES

Aaron, H. and Schwarz, W. (1984) *The Painful Prescription*, Brooking Institution, Washington, DC.

Department of Health and Social Security (1976) *Sharing Resources (the RAWP Report)*, HMSO, London.

Galbraith, J K (1992) *The Culture of Contentment,* Sinclair-Stevenson, London.

Huntington, S. P. (1982) *American Politics: The Promise of Disharmony,* Harvard University Press, Cambridge, MA.

Paton, C. R. (1985) *The Policy of Resource Allocation,* Nuffield Trust, London.

Paton, C. R. (1990) *US Health Politics : Public Policy and Political Theory,* Avebury, Aldershot.

Paton, C. R. (1992) *Competition and Planning in the NHS: The Danger of Unplanned Markets,* Chapman & Hall, London.

Strosberg, M. *et al.* (eds) (1992) *Rationing America's Medical Care: The Oregon Plan and Beyond,* Brookings Institution, Washington, DC.

White House (1993) *The Health Security Act 1993,* US Government Printing Office, Washington, DC.

INTRODUCTION

At the conceptual level, different types of health policy regime exist which are useful for classifying health-care systems in European and other countries. One of the most useful approaches is to distinguish between the **reimbursement** model and the **purchasing** model. In some ways this distinction builds upon a typology presented by Altenstetter (1992). This distinction is particularly useful to remember in the UK today, where the concepts of purchasing and in particular the purchaser/provider split have become both modish and faddish. There is an assumption both that overt purchasing is the best way forward for any health-care system, and that the purchaser/provider split is both an inevitability and a desirability. This final chapter suggests that neither analytical considerations nor a review of the political reasons for health sector reform lead necessarily to this conclusion.

TYPES OF HEALTH-CARE SYSTEM

Consider the following typology.

Firstly, a health-care system may allow the patient/user direct access to any services, and the bill is paid by a third party – whether private or the Government. Simplistically, the traditional US health-care system has consisted in private third-party payment, of the costs incurred by those lucky enough to

have generous insurance. There has not even been a 'primary care gatekeeper', in most instances, until recently in certain types of health maintenance organization. That is, the patient has access to specialized services and a third party picks up the bill.

In the UK, one means of characterizing the pre-reform NHS was as an 'open access' system whereby a public third-party payer reimbursed whatever care the patient/user sought. Major qualifications to this simplistic but useful characterization are of course necessary: there was a primary physician gatekeeper known as the general practitioner, who in most cases had to sanction referral of the patient to secondary and other services; there was a planning process based on health regions, in the main, whereby new services were developed within limited resources; and of course in practice – given the GP gatekeeper – referral was made to those services which had conventionally existed or which had recently been developed by regions and other planning bodies. That is, given an absence of generous financing, it was not simply a case of the patient or user stimulating a response to his desires for care from providers (whether competing in a market place or not) – more likely, services developed as a result of an interplay between GPs' desires for patient referrals and a Government (regional) planning process. Then local districts 'directly managed' their services, and presumably had the responsibility of giving them resources appropriate to their workload. This was of course the problem: there was not enough money to do this!

Secondly, there are health systems which rely on overt purchasing. In such a model, purchasers of health care – who are in effect a special kind of reimburser, taking a more active role in determining the services to be purchased – may contract with providers which are (probably) institutionally and (certainly) functionally distinct from the purchaser. Again such a purchaser may be public or private (mostly not for profit). Here a significant difference between health-care systems depends on whether or not the individual citizen chooses which purchaser to belong to or not. In the post-reform British National Health Service, for example, leaving aside the question of fundholding by general practitioners for now, purchasers are geographical entities – and are in effect agents of the Government.

If one makes what is another useful distinction, between the financier of health care and the purchaser, the Government is the financier (drawing on mostly general revenues) and the purchaser is the district health authority or health commission.

In the Netherlands, on the other hand, a central idea associated with recent health-care reforms there (partially implemented) is that of competing purchasers (sick funds and insurance companies, increasingly merged): the citizen decides which to join. There is still, however, a role for the Government, or quasi-Government agencies, as financier: public money (raised through social insurance) is channelled to purchasers (insurance companies and sick funds) in proportion to the estimated social need, as measured by the age and mobility structure of different purchasers' enrolees.

In a similar way, the proposed Clinton reform in the United States allows the citizen to choose a health plan, but there is a role for a financier (called a health alliance, a deriva-

tive of the health insurance purchasing cooperative (HIPC) proposed by the Jackson Hole Group). This spreads risk and adjusts for need in allocating to chosen health plans or insurances – in a manner analogous to the Netherlands although (as one would expect) with a less overt role for the Government in so doing for political and ideological reasons. (Hence 'health alliances' – are they quangos or are they independent institutions?)

Another model, which is less common in welfare capitalist countries and which has been proposed in (for example) Turkey as part of World-Bank-inspired health reform, seeks to unify the purchasing function without abolishing separate non-profit insurance schemes. That is, individuals join these schemes, but the purchasing is carried out, in the proposed model, by regional health authorities which purchase on behalf of the various insurance schemes. That is, unlike the above Netherlands/Clinton model, where the state intervenes to adjust subscriptions to individual purchasing insurance companies which then transact their own business, the autonomy of the individual insurer is superseded altogether in the proposed model.

Thirdly, there is the integrated model (with vertical integration between third parties and providers). In the United States, the health maintenance organization is an example of this model: it enrols subscribers and carries out a purchasing function in the sense of deciding which services to procure but (in the comprehensive HMO model) directly owns the providers. Some would characterize the British NHS pre-reform as a public integrated model in that the health authorities that 'reimbursed' the provider owned or were directly integrated with that provider. It is a matter of debate, however, as to whether there was an overt purchasing function at all (as with the comprehensive kind of health maintenance organization). If one characterizes the British NHS pre-reform as dominated by 'free referral' by general practitioners, then the public reimbursement by the Government/health authority to its directly owned providers was not overt purchasing but simply the money attempting to follow the patient (albeit often bureaucratically). In particular, non-local referrals were reimbursed under the formula (RAWP), which sought to make money follow the patients. Interestingly, between 1974 and 1982, there was a functional, but not institutional, purchaser/provider distinction between areas – which planned services – and districts, which provided them.

If on the other hand – as was certainly the case in many situations and in many regions – there was an overt regional role in planning services in conjunction with assessed need for the future (within limited resources), then there was a purchasing function, which shaped (as well as was shaped by) GP referrals. To call it an overt purchasing function would probably not be useful, however, as it would blur a distinction between the pre-reform NHS and the post-reform NHS. This distinction is based not on a black and white distinction between 'non-purchasing' and purchasing, but on a rather grey distinction between implicit purchasing (pre-reform) and explicit, decentralized purchasing (post-reform) carried out by districts and GP fundholders (albeit within a morass of direct political interference from ministers and both national and regional priorities which severely constrains local purchasing).

Abstracting from the typology just provided, one finds the following determinants of 'who gets care how'.

- The patient/citizen decides (albeit as conditioned by existing facilities and existing culture) and the provider is reimbursed.
- The GP decides and the provider is reimbursed.
- Services are planned and financed publicly, and either free referral by GP or self-referral by patient occurs (in practice, the pre-reform NHS was an amalgam of this and the previous method).

- Overt purchasing is carried out by the citizen/patient (using a voucher).
- Overt purchasing is carried out by doctors (as in GP fundholding).
- Overt purchasing is carried out by managers (as in the district purchasing model of the post reform British National Health Service) (Paton, 1992a).

Where the individual has choice of purchaser, it is likely that this purchaser will develop strong relations with providers over time – as in all stable 'markets' where the transactions costs of constantly renegotiating links are bound to be high, and where indeed the conditions for perfect competition or anything remotely resembling it (absence of entry costs to the market, and so forth) are not satisfied. Thus in choosing between different purchasers, the citizen is choosing between different providers.

This accounts for the confusion when discussing – for example, in the context of the Clinton reforms in the US – what is the purchaser and what is the provider. In essence, there is the finance for health care, provided from society (individuals, companies, general taxation and so forth), organized by Government and quasi Government agencies in a public or quasi-public system, and passed on to...to what: purchasers or providers?

If, for example, the health alliances in the context of the Clinton Plan allocate their money to health maintenance organizations, one can describe this as allocating to competing purchasers who have enrolled individuals, or allocating in some cases directly to providers. Where the purchaser and provider exist in a vertically integrated organization, the allocation is to both purchaser and provider.

In a pre-reform NHS allocations from central government and region to districts were allocations arguably to both purchaser and provider, in that the district both received monies on behalf of its population to meet the needs of that population and also to run the services of the providers for which it was directly responsible. That is, there was an implicit or tacit purchasing role carried out by the region, but also by the district. The complication lay in the fact that the district was also a provider – and allocations to the district took account of geographical need (as in the RAWP formula) but also took account of the district as catchment area provider.

Ironically, an attempt to develop a health maintenance organization-style model in the UK would not lead to a situation as created by the NHS reforms, but would lead instead to either an acceptance of the pre-reform NHS or a creation of competing purchasers vertically integrated with their providers!

In other words, there is finance for health care; there is a reimbursement role which may translate into overt purchasing or may not; and there are providers of health care, which may or may not have stable relationships with purchasers; which may be directly integrated with purchasers; or which may not have anything to do with the purchasing function but may simply be reimbursed from either public or private money.

POLITICS AND IDEOLOGY: ASSESSING THE BRITISH REFORMS

In comparing the pre-reform NHS with the post-reform NHS, there has hitherto been little perspective. Obviously, at the level of rhetoric from the UK's Conservative Government, the reforms represent efficiency in targeting rather than 'vagueness' and 'provider capture' in the pre-reform NHS. Some academics go along with the view that the reforms are all about effective 'needs assessment' for populations (a reinvention of epidemiologically based social medicine), whereas services in the old system were hijacked by 'professional interests'. Whether at the level of ideology or analysis, however, this approach, in my view, conceals more than it reveals.

One of the difficulties is that there was no single 'old system' in the UK. In some cases, regions either had or were developing (in the mid-to-late 1980s) effective means for allocating resources and providing services in relation to need as gauged by relatively sophisticated methodologies. That is, regions were undertaking needs assessment, in those parts of the country where regional health authorities took an activist role in planning and then seeking to allocate resources to fund these plans – what was known as planning-led resource allocation. In some parts of the country, where less imagination was employed at health authority level, of course, services were no doubt simply 'funded because they always had been', and internal monitoring of the usage of resources (for example, within hospitals or within hospital departments/specialties) was inadequate to achieve 'the meeting of social need'.

Many comparisons of the old and the new NHS compare a dismal stereotype of the old with a naively optimistic stereotype of the new, implying that a vaguely funded, poorly planned, 'provider-captured' NHS has been replaced by a more efficient, better targeted service. This is what one hears respectively (in different ways) from the Government; from senior health service managers (arguably not particularly distinct from the Government, given the tight political control of senior management); and a variety of health policy commentators. It is presumably an alleged 'irreversibility' of the reforms which allowed Professor Julian Le Grand to claim in 1994 that 'most health policy academics were in favour of the reforms.

The paradox is that, contrary to this view, the view held by huge swathes of the public, most of the professionals and certainly the lower-paid employees of the NHS is that the reforms are a disaster and that the NHS is seriously undermined as a result of them. In other words, there has been a huge polarization in British society concerning the NHS. Arguably the polarization now – although organized on very different fault lines – is as great as at the time of the NHS's creation between 1945 and 1948.

The alternative caricature of the change from old to new (reformed) NHS would run as follows: we have moved from a relatively unbureaucratic system that indulged in flexible planning and free GP referral to services as provided, to a system where not only is there a GP gatekeeper affecting access by the patient to services, but a managerial gatekeeper acting through contracts with providers, in a service that is more tightly budgeted than ever before. That is, one has moved from a needs-oriented but unbureaucratic service to a finance-dominated and 'philistine' service where professions are Aunt Sallys to be attacked and where the politics of euphemism (concerning primary care; needs assessment and the rest) hides a dismal reality.

It is unlikely that either stereotype is wholly true. It is as well therefore to do two things: to situate the NHS reforms in a comparative context and to look at current political trends affecting the content and progress of the NHS reforms.

INTERNATIONAL COMPARISON AND INTERNATIONAL TRENDS

One can distinguish between the following international variants of health-care system in order to measure current trends in a variety of North American and European countries (as well as wider):

- expensive systems that have difficulty in reconciling cost control with equity, such as in the USA;
- European social insurance models with cost-control problems;
- European social insurance models with a relatively satisfactory combination of equity and cost control;
- European health-service models.

The United States fits the first category. It is therefore conceivable that a system combining greater equity in financing (based on at least a partly redistributive financing system, involving Government funding if not redistribution from rich to poor) and managed competition in the provision of health care, can both increase equity and increase cost control in the USA.

European health-care systems which have had difficulty in reconciling equity and cost control have frequently resorted to greater central regulation of doctors' fees and hospital charges (if not incentives for new modes of care) in order to keep their health-care systems within the bounds of what is both politically and fiscally possible within a capitalist welfare state of the 1990s. Examples are Germany, Switzerland and – arguably – also the Netherlands, which has recently witnessed a political compromise between managed competition on the one hand and greater central regulation on the other hand. France is also an example of a country which has sought greater regulation in order to control costs without fundamental restructuring of the system.

European systems which have been relatively successful in reconciling equity and cost control tend to have a health services rather than health insurance model: primary examples are, of course, Sweden and the UK. This latter category of countries are those which have unequivocally the least need to resort to a model of managed competition in the provision of health care (and arguably also in the financing of health care, i.e. competing purchasers).

The intermediary category of countries – national health insurance models with some difficulty in cost control – are interestingly enough those which could on theoretical grounds be considered to require 'market discipline' from the viewpoint of those who believe that neoclassical economics are applicable to the health-care sector. Yet such countries, because of their political and cultural traditions – not least in their particular health-care institutions – are those which have least inclination to do so. And who can blame them: managed competition contains an unverified, and indeed untested, hypothesis (to the extent that is a theory at all) as to the possibility for equitable cost control in health care.

It is the final category – Sweden, the UK and the like – which *prima facie* is most likely to view managed competition as 'a solution to a problem which does not exist'. Cost control and equity are already being achieved without the bureaucracy of managed competition. Sweden admittedly spends considerably more (as a percentage of GNP) on health care than the UK. But this is, to the extent that such things can be gauged, a political choice rather than an unintended consequence of the particular incentives operating within the health-care system. Not least, Sweden has at least hitherto chosen to integrate its social policy with the goal of full-employment (including the public sector's contribution to that).

The question therefore arises wherein lies the trend in the UK and possibility in Sweden encouraging the adoption of 'internal markets' and other examples of managed competition rather than public regulation.

BRITISH POLITICS

Particular politics behind the British NHS reforms ought to be set alongside the so-called underlying factors encouraging health sector reform.

The review of the National Health Service which led to the British reforms was a political accident, announced by the then Prime Minister Mrs Margaret Thatcher as a defensive response to criticism of underfunding of the National Health Service. The British reforms were an attempt to divert attention from alleged underfunding of the Health Service to so-called 'efficiency factors' on the supply side of health care. Some particular factors concerning the adoption of the NHS reforms ought to be noted.

Firstly, the Government did not have a mandate to introduce the reforms. There was no prospectus for health-care reform in the 1987 Conservative election manifesto. It is at the very least arguable, therefore, that the Government which announced a review of the NHS in 1988 (in the form of the Prime Minister rather than the cabinet or whole executive) had a mandate neither for a radical new health policy nor for a restructuring of a health service which had hitherto operated (warts and all) on the principle of bipartisan political consent.

Secondly, the Government had even less of a mandate, on this argument, to create an ideologically motivated health policy, involving an ideologically motivated restructuring of the health service, along the lines of market competition in the provision of health care. There was also an end to consent in relations between Government, the professions and indeed health service managers – who, after the reforms, have become 'line agents' of the Government rather than quasi-autonomous public administrators.

Thirdly, it is in this context – or indeed in any other context – illegitimate for the Government to use the more neutral and accepted structures of public administration for tactical political interventions in pursuit of the new policy. In this context, it can be noted that the structures of general management introduced as a result of the Griffiths Enquiry of 1982/1983 were also introduced, like the NHS reforms after 1987, after the general election of 1983 without having been heralded in the manifesto of that year by the Conservative Party. To be generous towards the Conservative administration, however, the Griffiths Enquiry had been instituted towards the end of 1982 and any avid constitution watchers could have spotted the likelihood of the adoption of any principles emerging from the Enquiry after the election of 1983. (This is generosity indeed!)

What is perhaps more important is that the institution of general management – whether politically legitimate or not in terms of the way it was introduced – is not an ideologically motivated reform so much as a move from public administration to public management of the sort which genuinely is part of an international trend, and not unique to the UK.

What is certainly illegitimate is the means by which the structure of general management – originally devised a means for devolution of management autonomy – has been used by recent Conservative administrations as simply a conduit for political directives. And this brings us to the final act of illegitimacy: under the guise and rhetoric of devolved management, and therefore in an attempt to disguise the political content of top-down directives, recent Conservative governments have subjected the Health Service to direct political control of a tacit and therefore of an arbitrary and tactical sort. What in the rhetoric is 'scientific management' in the sense of neutral management is in reality political intervention, carried out through the willing or unwilling subservience of health service managers.

To talk of illegitimacy in such a manner may seem strong – although less so, I suspect, to an audience of political scientists than to an audience of health service managers in the UK, who live in a world of the NHS reforms and have already forgotten both the previous situation and the possibility of alternatives. But the terminology is justified: a Government has the choice, in a democratic political culture, of operating through the doctrine of mandate or through the subsequent creation of political consensus.

A political party may reorganize itself through internal majority rule (mandate) or through the creation of unanimity or at least consensus. And when a political party promotes policy or an attitude towards the restructuring of public institutions beyond its own control (such as the Conservative or Labour Party proposing constitutional reform) it should seek the consent of wider social institutions and interests (political parties and

other institutions) through either mandate (majority rule) or again consensus-building.

Likewise, a political party controlling the Government – especially in a strong, centralized state such as the UK, where the capacity for 'one-party rule' is strong – may introduce new policy or may restructure social institutions beyond itself as a result of mandate (such as proposals in an election manifesto, with all the imperfections that this doctrine has notwithstanding) or through the building of consensus. Where the restructuring concerns the institutions of the state (as, in a public health-care system such as the NHS, health-care institutions such as purchasing and providing authorities undoubtedly are), in the absence of a mandate, then consensus-building within that state ought to be achieved. This was conspicuously absent in the case of the NHS reforms.

Arguably the Prime Minister imposed the policy on the cabinet. Arguably the cabinet imposed the policy on the executive. Arguably the executive imposed the policy on Parliament. And arguably the policy was imposed on the Health Service (indeed before being passed by Parliament, which was the subject of a lawsuit by the NHS Support Federation).

Unfortunately the consequence of this has been a politicized reform operating under the guise of depoliticization and 'neutral management'. The political result of this is exemplified by the exchange between the former minister of State for Health, Dr Brian Mawhinney and the former Shadow Secretary of State for Health, Mr David Blunkett – **Mawhinney**, 'We have taken politics out of the health service'; **Blunkett**, 'You have certainly taken our party out of the health service!'

THE INTERNATIONAL COMPARISON REVISITED

There may well be an international trend towards 'managed competition' in health care. However the countries adopting such policies may have greater need of such policies than countries such as the UK and Sweden. Moreover, it is important to consider the level of financing of health care – and therefore the benefits available to the people – as well as the structure of financing and provision. Differences in spending *per capita* (and percentages of GNP and so forth) on health care may reflect differences in efficiency. They may, however, reflect real differences in spending on health services, whether or not these health services lead to what is now called 'health gain' for the people. Additionally, cheaper health services may reflect greater exploitation of (possibly) the professions and (certainly) the poorer Health Service ancillary workers. The UK finds itself in the latter position.

The question then arises: are competitive mechanisms, which may be suitable for generously funded health-care systems that do not 'exploit' their health workers, also suitable for a tightly funded national health service such as the UK's? The danger is that corners will be cut both in the provision of services and in the conditions of employment of workers, in order to run a market, in the particular context of the UK's internal market.

Whether one is talking about the funding of specialized services, secondary services or primary care; whether one is talking about management techniques to reduce labour costs (so-called 'reprofiling of the workforce'); whether one is talking about management techniques within hospitals, such as 'business process re-engineering' (a philistine euphemism if ever there was one): the prospect for the NHS is for a standardization of services and an increased rationing that will provide the greatest disbenefit to those unable to exit to the private sector.

Whether or not the NHS remains a univer-sal service in the sense of access by those of all incomes, the poor will still suffer disproportionately. If the NHS becomes 'a service for the poor', in an attempt to target resources upon those least able to pay for themselves, the poor will suffer as the rich and middle classes leave, find private health care less economical and therefore have less money available to redistribute to the poor, even if they were willing to do so to a similar extent as in the old NHS.

But if the NHS remains open to all, but on the basis of heavily rationed services, again the middle classes will leave it, find private care and private insurance more expensive; and therefore reduce the amount available *per capita* to the poor in the absence of a suddenly discovered greater middle-class generosity to redistribute tax income to the poor.

In other words, a bloated and generous health-care system which requires to increase equity, such as the United States, may be able to get away with efficiency measures which a system such as the UK's cannot. It is as if one expects to transplant American shopping malls to the crowded British conurbations and precious British countryside and achieve the same effect: it simply is not possible, as any view from a train window in 1990s UK informs one. One needs space to begin with if one is going to encroach upon it. Alain Enthoven saw the market as a means for rewarding high-quality providers (especially London teaching hospitals!) more effectively. This did not foresee the use of the internal market as a mechanism for ever-increasing squeeze.

PARTICULAR CONSEQUENCES OF THE NHS REFORMS

The essence of the NHS reforms is the concept of the purchaser/provider split, created in order to run an internal (and external) market. In the traditional NHS, the general practitioner was the 'gatekeeper' and also the referrer to available services. This contrasted with the traditional US system of direct access to specialists (for those insured and so forth) and what might be termed the traditional European system of publicly funded direct access. The essence of the change in the UK is to replace the non-fund-holding GP gatekeeper with (primarily) the manager gatekeeper based in the purchasing health authority and (secondarily) the GP fundholder for a limited number of procedures – likely to be operating increasingly under regional guidelines. (Considering 'ideal types' of health reform, rival options in the US might be to move to a system of managed competition based on health alliances as in the Clinton Plan or the primary care gatekeeper system and greater socialization as in the pre-reform NHS.)

The choice for the UK, however, was whether to remain with a GP gatekeeper system, improved where necessary to ensure that the planning of services (by regions and districts) reflected GPs' and patients' wishes within available resources, or to move to a system of managed competition British-style, whereby an ideological justification was provided for a market mechanism and a technical justification was (*ex post* rather than *ex ante*) provided for a formalized purchasing function.

The irony is that, in many cases, this formalized purchasing function is simply bureaucratizing what could have been done more naturally under the old system. In other words, 'consulting GPs as to preferred location of services' and 'making choices on the basis of quality and cost-effectiveness' was the essence of the better variants of regional planning which were evolving in the UK throughout the 1980s, prior to the NHS reforms.

The fundamental criticism of the old system (again made *ex post* rather than *ex ante* in most cases) was that it was a theme park for lazy doctors: 'provider capture' allowed public and (what would now be called) purchaser (i.e. health authority) desires to go unrequited.

The alleged advantage of an overt purchasing function is to allow a combination of public wants, cost-effectiveness criteria in purchasing services and a transfer of power from the consultant to the general practitioner. A lot of this is, however, Panglossian rhetoric and an attempt by those working within the system – including academics – to make the best of things.

Traditional typologies of health-care systems may be falling short in their ability to explain reality. For example, it is a common observation that, despite the recent changes in the UK, it still has a fully public system by comparison with what even the more radical versions of the 1970s Kennedy Plans would have proposed for the United States (Paton, 1990). This is, however, misleading. For while there is more direct public provision in the UK, even after the creation of quasi-private self-governing trusts, and also much greater proportionate public financing, there is less meeting of public demand than there would be in a more generously funded and more equitable US health-care system.

Table 13.1 ranks a variety of health-care systems, for illustrative purposes, according to five dimensions: equity on the 'core' definition of universal access at least to a defined range of services; free referral as opposed to restricted referral or managed care; institutionalized cost control; public provision or close purchaser/provider relationship rather than contracting with private or quasi-private providers; and, financial stability in the light of growing need or demand.

Table 13.1   Characteristics of various health-care systems

Characteristic	US now	US à la Clinton Plan	US à la Kennedy Plan,1974	UK pre-'reform'	UK post-'reform'	Sweden	Netherlands now
Core equity	✗	✓	✓	✓	✓/?	✓	✓
Free referral (no rationed purchasing)	For well-off	✗	✓	✓	✗	✓	✓
Cost control intrinsic	✗	✓/?	?	✓	✓	✓	?
Public provision or close purchaser/provider relationship	✗	?	✗	✓	✓/?	✓	?
Ability of system to meet growing need/demand	✗/?	✓	✓/?	✓/?	?	✓	✓

The table allows a rough and ready comparison of the UK pre-reform and the UK post-reform on these criteria, albeit somewhat arbitrarily; also by comparison with other systems. In terms of Altenstetter's typology, the old British system was an interesting amalgam of third-party reimbursement of the public variety, regional planning ('purchasing' in the new language), especially of large capital projects and a role for integrated purchasing and provision (in the new language) by district health authorities. In other words, GPs referred to the services that were planned and provided; and services were in return planned and provided in line with appropriate consultation with GPs and others, in the more imaginative systems of regional and district planning.

The new British system, on the other hand, moves to an overt as opposed to covert purchaser/provider split, and in effect decentralizes the purchasing function from regions to districts and to GP fundholders, at least on paper. In the old system, regions were not purchasers officially, but there is insight provided by a characterization of the old British system as regional purchasing and district provision.

The element of the old British system which allowed a surrogate 'consumer choice' was the assumption of free referral by the GP, albeit in the context of inadequate funding (and arguably inadequate efficiency) to meet all legitimate demands within the system. Nevertheless if it works as the theoretical model intends, the new British system prevents patient choice in the light of the more direct cash nexus introduced – by contrast with (for example) the Netherlands, where choice of insurer/sick fund in a better funded system is an important aspect of the reform.

This produces a paradox, whereby 'left-wing' critics of British reforms might therefore be tempted to seek competing financiers of health care. This would, however, be a chimera to pursue as – given the restricted British financing – nominal choice of purchaser/insurer by consumer/patient would in practice be more a choice of consumer/patient by purchaser, i.e. institutionalized cream-skimming.

MARKETS AND QUASI-MARKETS

The origin of the NHS reforms lay in a desire by the then Prime Minister to move from the defensive to the offensive about health policy and to change the terms of debate from one about levels of funding to one about levels of technical efficiency. This was the context in which the market evolved as 'the answer'.

It was apparent, however, to even the most right-wing advisers to the Prime Minister with any sense of political pragmatism, that a fully marketized health service would be unfair, inefficient and ineffective. Health-care markets do not obey the necessary and sufficient conditions for the achievement of a whole range of *desiderata*, such as access on the basis of clinical need rather than ability to pay; efficiency in line with the ideal type of perfect competition; and coordinated purchasing on a large enough scale to guarantee (for example) the effective provision of specialized services. Health-care markets are difficult to enter (barriers to entry), especially in the hospital sector, have a tendency to produce monopoly (as do many markets in varying degrees) and generally create severe difficulties due to market failure.

Defenders of public sector markets (sometimes called quasi-markets or mimic markets) point to a range of conditions for the successful functioning of markets, i.e. the achievement by markets of the familiar *desiderata* such as equity, quality and efficiency. These necessary conditions include the correct market structure (i.e. competing providers and possibly competing purchasers); adequate motivation (i.e. institutionalized selfishness whereby the public good is produced from private vice); perfect or at least adequate information so that 'gaming' by other purchasers and providers does not subvert the intentions of policy-makers; manageable costs (transactions costs under control); and attention to equity in the context of a right to health care of various sorts (Bartlett and le Grand, 1994). These are necessary rather than fully sufficient conditions, as other conditions for the effective functioning of markets apply.

The main paradox for a market such as that created by the NHS reforms is that using Government regulation and management *Diktat* to seek to achieve these necessary conditions – which are not achieved by the natural functioning of markets – leads to an almost inevitable breaking of some of those very conditions in order to fulfil others.

Most obviously, administrative costs (including the transactions costs of contract-ing rather than dealing through direct management) are almost inevitably high. Some commentators put the eventual cost of the NHS reforms at £1.5 billion start-up costs and £0.5 billion annual costs. These costs are incurred through seeking to regulate providers to be both decentralized, 'selfish' businesses yet also accountable public hospitals and providers generally; creating an appropriate distribution and quantity of hospitals, hospital beds and other services (for example, eliminating surplus capacity) yet maintaining or developing spare capacity (a different thing!) in order to allow a market to function.

For, even where there are many providers within a given locality, specialty by specialty, a market may not naturally exist – if the seeming potential for competition between specialties is belied in practice by the fact that the different specialties have different subspecialisms within them. More importantly, simply observing the conditions for a spatial market (Robinson and le Grand, 1994) does not mean a market can function, unless there is adequate spare capacity and adequate speed of reaction on the part of providers – as well as familiar factors such as ease of entry and the political possibility of exit by providers.

In other words, creating the necessary conditions for a successful market – as opposed to merely a market – is a very bureaucratic exercise indeed. It can produce absurdity in the context of a public health service. The example of the British government aspiring to close 40% of acute beds, yet maintain spare capacity in order to run a market, is one prime contemporary example.

When one adds to this the politics of the NHS and of the NHS reforms, one ends up with not so much an expensive 'quasi-market' as simply a *mélange*. Some political characteristics of the environment in which the NHS reforms are implemented are:

- severely limited finance, unlike in the kind of market eulogized by Professor

Alain Enthoven (the father or godfather of the reforms);

- the fact that the patient (or consumer, or unit as the 'efficiency index' of the Department of Health has it) is not the purchaser;
- the real political agenda on the part of many Conservative policy-makers – cost cutting and at least partial privatization (Willetts, 1993, 1994);
- the obsessive regulation of providers in line with political and public disquiet as to the local implications of the market;
- the perfectly legitimate use of public policy, rather than private markets, to define not only desired outcomes but behaviour within the Health Service in order to produce these outcomes.

It is such characteristics that lead the self-appointed ideological high priests of the reforms (such as various self-governing trust chairmen and the former NHS Personnel Director Eric Caines) to claim that more markets rather than fewer markets are the answer. A recent quote from Caines suggests that 'only where a green field operation is offered to tender can competition start to provide benefits' (*The Times*, June 1994). This might be paraphrased as, 'only then can staff conditions be worsened to such an extent that a market seems on paper to be efficient'! It may, however, be more sensible to interpret the current semi-marketization of the NHS as a half-dug hole rather than a half-plotted green field site, and one is reminded of the aphorism that, when one is in a hole, one should stop digging.

A variety of commentators have suggested that the Conservative government in the UK in fact has a Marxist approach to business: whether public or private, enterprises can only prosper by extracting surplus value from exploited workers. Even doctors are allegedly to be put on performance-related pay. The problem with such a scenario within a public

service such as the NHS is as follows: what performance is to be rewarded? Is it for doing more, (for example when waiting list monies arrive like manna from Heaven to allow extra procedures to be carried out on a political agenda); or is it for doing less, when block contracts run out of cash and consultants are encouraged not to be 'overactive'?

More likely, performance-related pay is for doing what the Government and their line managers tell doctors to do – marginalist economic theory and euphemistic prescriptions from the field of the 'management of human resources' are of little help in either predicting or prescribing within such a political context. PRP in the British Public Sector is a charter for toadyism rather than a scientifically tested scheme.

THE REAL AGENDA

The internal market in the UK is better interpreted as a management tool to bring direct pressure on providers, using a variety of techniques and 'learning' from a variety of dubious case studies drawing on the Japanese steel industry as well as the British private sector. Thus as well as local markets, we have regional directors within the British NHS plotting the ideal configuration of future hospital services; as well as alleged competition between providers, we have the euphemism of 'cosiness' between purchasers and providers. Rather than a return to the rather more friendly pre-reform NHS, this instead is a harbinger of the introduction of private-sector management techniques such as 'just in time management' and 'business process re-engineering' to bring direct pressure to bear on providers' processes as well as stipulation of their outcomes. The euphemism through which such politically inspired management is presented has been quite nicely described as 'the new English babble' (*The Independent on Sunday*, 12 June, 1994).

PERVERSE INCENTIVES – BOTH ECONOMIC AND POLITICAL

'GAMING' BY PROVIDERS AND PURCHASERS.

Firstly, there is an incentive for purchasers to 'pass the buck' to providers, where block contracts exist whereby a fixed sum of money is given by purchasers to providers for unpredictable quantities of service. Purchasers now have power without responsibility: they are responsible for stipulating the services to be provided (commissioning, in the rather newer sense of the term which points to outputs rather than processes) yet not for the direct operation of services.

As a result they can place unrealistic expectations (on behalf of the public) on providers and seek to imply that shortfalls are the provider's fault. On the other hand increasingly precise contracts (moving through cost per volume to cost per case, with increasing prespecification and increasing monitoring) are both expensive and subject to manipulation by the provider: in the absence of extremely sophisticated information, which is also expensive, providers can 'game the system' and either seek extra reimbursement on a per case basis or simply fail to provide the required service yet go undetected. Trying to prevent gaming means – for example – that purchasers have to keep providers in the dark as to whether, or for what, they will be reimbursed. For example, only certain conditions, or severities, or particular protocols for treatment, are reimbursed, in certain US 'managed care' organizations. If such schemes are mirrored in the UK (and they are already), then seeking to avoid the downside leads to bureaucracy, lack of trust between purchasers and providers and uncertainty for patients, doctors and managers. Providers seek to 'game the system' – as do purchasers – especially during disputes over 'extracontractual referrals' (i.e. care provided without a contract through free referral by GPs, permitted previously). Even with contracts, both purchasers and providers seek to avoid expense. To the extent that they collude, it is likely to be at the expense of the needy but unintentional patient.

Government is responsible itself for a 'buck-passing' culture, with its Citizen's Charter for the Health Service, known as the Patient's Charter. Instead of relying on purchasers to make local contracts with providers, central intervention has recently created a series of league tables for hospitals, on a number of incomplete, partial and often misleading criteria as to hospital performance. In turn, purchasers are then constrained to obey the national agenda rather than any local agenda they might have in making contracts with hospitals.

Without resorting to the wilder shores of conspiracy theory, it is not difficult to see that the indicators used by the Government have been designed to fulfil the Government's desires as regards which hospitals to close and which to remain open. Putting the percentage of operations carried out through day case surgery is an indication of good performance as a case in point. Leaving aside the obvious point that day surgery may not in itself be good and that there can be inappropriate as well as appropriate day case surgery (not least for the poor and those with difficult home conditions), if the Government has a political agenda to save money through closing large percentages of hospital beds, then rewarding hospitals that have high rates of day case surgery will obviously provide a boost to 'merging or closing' the less successful hospitals.

Some argue that the challenge is to produce better information rather than to criticize what information exists. While in certain cases this may be true, it assumes a benign Government rather than diagnosing the political agenda underlying the British government's health policy in the early 1990s. The social costs of a 'sausage factory' healthcare system are ignored: there is an assumption that unpaid voluntary care by families and communities will pick up the pieces within such a scenario. Despite the assertion that the 'priority services' include the non-acute and in particular the chronically sick, it is worth noting that now only 10% of long-stay elderly beds are in the National Health Service as opposed to other sectors, whereas even 10 years ago the figure was 30%.

Such a squeeze on hospitals also increases inequity through creating an incentive to avoid expensive cases and – unless there is specific earmarking of funds – expensive services.

CONTRIVED COMPETITION

Providers have service knowledge but purchasers have money. Ideally they would therefore work together. Otherwise the purchaser has to commission knowledge from non-local providers, which is expensive as well as often fatuous in a public service. Treating the provider as the local market enemy is necessary if a market is to work properly, but also runs foul of the Government's other policy objectives. Government intervention in this area as elsewhere is not so much to create the conditions for a successful market be regulation, as to create the 'worst of both worlds' whereby there is politically inspired and tacit planning yet 'market uncertainty' at the same time.

THE DESTRUCTION OF PROVIDERS' VIABILITY AND ABILITY TO PLAN

GP fundholding and other sources of unstable purchasing prevent long-term planning, as well as creating the problem of inequity and a 'two-tier service' which has been pointed out frequently in the media. It has also proved in some locations a boost to unfair competition, as hospitals market themselves to GP fundholders on a loss-leading basis in order to undermine competitors, creating non-competitive situations in the longer term.

COST-SHIFTING AND PATIENT-SHIFTING.

Part of the rhetoric underlying the NHS reforms (although not related to the market) concerns 'effective purchasing' and 'seamless care' for patients – another piece of jargon which is intended, to the extent that it points to anything, to point to the need for integrated care for patients whose episodes of care require (for example) both hospital and community services.

The creation of autonomous hospital and community trusts, however, gives these trusts an incentive to shift costs (i.e. people) to each other. Hospitals that are financially squeezed seek to get people into the community. Community providers that are financially squeezed seek to get people into hospital.

Purchasers have in some cases sought to get round this problem by designating either the hospital or the community as 'lead provider', subcontracting to their partner (or competitor) community or hospital. This, however, can produce an incentive to under-fund services from the subcontractor.

It can also undermine hospitals if community trusts are hired as lead provider. Some community trusts in the UK are contracting with doctors (indeed sometimes on a private basis) by the session, at marginal cost. This is part of a 'short-termist' strategy whereby the 'fixed costs' of the medical profession and services generally are not paid for, and hospitals are put into financial difficulty. In the longer run, the infrastructure which enables such a tactic is then destroyed.

These perverse incentives can, of course, be dealt with through regulation. However, opening up a Pandora's box of perverse incentives and then creating even more administrative costs and bureaucratic complexities to regulate the situation does not seem a particularly efficient way to run a public service.

MARKETING BY PROVIDERS TO THE PUBLIC

This phenomenon is one whereby hospitals

and providers generally seek to impress local publics with their services, and to create a political 'head of steam' through local media to ensure that purchasers contract with favoured services. This may be desirable, given the dynamic of the system, as a means of protecting legitimate interests. On the other hand, it subverts the notion of the NHS reforms as about coordinated and strong purchasing, with providers 'red in tooth and claw' when it comes to competing financially for contracts yet passive when it comes to promoting their service interests. Only a naive or optimistic reading of markets would provide such a notion.

Senior policy-makers often admit in private that the post-reform NHS is therefore not about 'local purchasing'. It is about both national priorities and dealing efficiently with acute demand, leaving little scope for autonomous local priorities, which are squeezed between these two constraints. Policy-makers of this orientation see national targets for health prevention and so called 'primary care' as but one thrust of national policy, not involving large sums of new money. Long-term significant savings can be made in acute care – on this view – as a result of shorter length of stay and more day-case surgery, more intensive use of capital and labour and significant changes in skill mix. Initial research on the opportunities available to local purchasers to 'follow their own line' – even by those sympathetic to such a notion – suggests that this is fairly minimal if defined in budgetary terms. (Heginbotham and Ham, 1992).

On this interpretation, providers can market their value for money as well as their service mix to meet both public and Government targets.

DESTRUCTION OF CENTRES OF EXCELLENCE

Both the market and planning processes (as in London) are being used in the UK to reconfigure services generally. This often involves the closure or merger of centres of excellence in tertiary services. Closure of famous hospitals in London is but the best known example of this phenomenon. Sometimes these closures reflect new priorities for the health service, however contentious.

Specialist centres are, however, more often closing by default. The essence of the NHS reforms is to devolve planning (now called purchasing) from regions working with districts to districts, and GP fundholders. (This is planning in the sense of procuring care, not making priorities in the broader sense.) As a result there is a problem of collective action, whereby coordinating the purchasing of specialized services in rendered more difficult and services are resultingly lost by default. A report from the Clinical Standards Advisory Group (1993) entitled *Access to Availability of Specialist Services* pointed to some of the problems.

THE MARKET AS MANIPULATION

A fundamental question is whether the market is seen as a short-term means to an end (the end being a new configuration of services) or whether it is the end in itself – rather the reverse, with planning mechanisms often being used to bring about the 'correct' configuration of services in order to enable a market to work in the longer term. Confusion around such basic questions helps to produce the 'worst of both worlds', and a practical example is the paradox whereby regions (now operated as regional offices of the NHS executive) often have their vision of the future, yet on the ground people feel with some justification that they are running a market.

The existence of two different agendas probably explains the reality: on the one hand there is what is now called the 'right-sizing' of the hospital sector (a euphemism to replace the earlier discredited euphemism 'downsizing', itself a euphemism for cuts);

and on the other hand, there is an agenda of using local purchasing (especially GP fund-holding) to reconfigure services in a more short-term and opportunistic manner.

Examples of the latter include the already cliched 'hub and spoke principle' whereby hospital trusts are intended to 'take over' other hospitals – or indeed to subcontract consultants to units in the community (at the behest of fundholding general practitioners, in the main). As with so much development in the NHS, this is, however, an act of faith rather than a policy developed as the result of attention to desired outcomes and cost-effectiveness.

Overall, regions are increasingly 'coordinating purchasing' through the euphemistically named 'market meetings', to ensure concentration of services and economies of scale. (Otherwise 'local purchasing' could prevent cost-effectiveness.) Overall, the patient has to follow the money, even where GP fundholders are nominally increasing. In this context, 'the market' is a centrally controlled competitive tender to survive. There are planned winners and losers – only an intermediate tier of 'possibles' is really operating in a market of uncertainty. Otherwise, it is a game designed centrally to cut costs.

PURCHASERS AND PROVIDERS – WHEAT AND CHAFF

The 'wheat' of the purchasing function is the creation of appropriate services in a cost-effective manner, ideally with public consultation (although this is difficult, in that public preferences are very often intransigent). This requires flexible planning and stability for both providers and general practitioners. The 'chaff' is the institutional purchaser/provider split as opposed to the more useful functional distinction between 'needs assessment' epidemiologically based (planning) and the operational management of services. It is interesting to note that the health mainte-nance organization, one of the better ideas to come from the United States, closes the purchaser/provider split in its most effective form and certainly does not make a fetish of it in general. In the United States, where there is choice of HMO or insurance company, such purchasing organizations have direct ownership of, or close long-term relationships with, providers. Indeed the closing of the split between the insurer/financier and the provider, in the interests of cost control, was the imperative behind the amendment of traditional, third-party reimbursement.

WHAT FOLLOWS WHOM?

The rhetoric introducing the NHS reforms was that the money would follow the patient. The reality is, of course, that the patient follows the money, in line with contracts placed. As a result patient choice is the embarrassment of the reforms, and various direct interventions by the Government reflect a need to present patient choice at least at the level of rhetoric: witness the recent 'star system' for hospitals accompanied by the myth that patients can now choose the hospitals they prefer.

In the context of pre-purchased, contracted care, establishing patient choice is often a bureaucratic nightmare rather than simply a means of flexible joint planning of services by health authorities and GPs, as in the pre-reform NHS. The 'Alice Through the Looking Glass' nature of some ideas presented to establish such patient choice illustrates the point. One example (Ward, 1994) recently suggested that a lesson from the private sector was the creation of 'secondary markets' whereby health authorities entering into block contracts with providers might buy or sell part of the contracted workload on a secondary market just as options are traded on shares or commodities. 'If markets can readily be established in pig belly futures, why not in hernias?' Less market-oriented 'patient choice' schemes, it was suggested in the same article, could mandate purchasers to set aside a number of cases within the block contracts for trading with other purchasers, in a 'patient mobility scheme'. It was suggested that the 'clearing house service' would probably be operated 'by a lead authority on an agency basis'. Oh what a tangled web we weave....

THE PUBLIC SECTOR CULTURE OF THE 1990s

The NHS reforms are the product of a government that believed – or wanted to believe – that the British public sector was wasteful and bureaucratic and that market-based motivation, whether or not through overt privatization, was necessary to improve performance. Such a political project of 'marketization' involved strong central political control to 'attack the traditional institutions' of the old system. (Observers of the British political scene will see some irony in the greatest enthusiasts for the market, such as Mr Michael Portillo, senior cabinet minister, lamenting attacks from the liberal left on great British institutions. Presumably he means those policing and deference-inducing institutions necessary to maintain order in an atomized market society in which traditional professional and public intermediary institutions have been undermined.)

As with the rest of the centralizing–decentralizing public sector reforms in the UK, a rhetoric of devolution has been preached by the Government and its own *nomenklatura* within the new 'patronage state', which has replaced either elected local officials or, in the case of the health service, the less rigidly controlled public administrators and indirectly elected health authorities of old. Some signposts along the route concern the partisan political appointment of health authorities and self-governing trust boards; the centralization of regions into regional offices of the national health service executive; the use of general management structures for tactical political interventions and the

creation of a 'tight ship' in the NHS. There is a gulf between the Government and (in public at least) its senior managers, on the one hand who initially believed their own sunshine stories about the NHS, and the public and NHS staff on the other hand.

The *nomenklatura* British style operates by creating a climate of accountability upwards yet inadequate devolution downwards so that – as in the old eastern Europe – there is a paralysis of effective decision-making as decisions are referred upwards for approval and instructions are awaited from the centre (the opposite to the rhetoric surrounding the reforms). One difference, however, in the British public sector of today is that operational decisions have to be taken at the ground level – there is a genuine operational devolution – but this is accompanied by a rather demoralizing system whereby blame is devolved and credit is centralized. NHS managers are the necessary servants of the new cultural revolution, when it suits the Secretary of State for Health, but the traditional wasteful bureaucrats, when it suits the politicians' rhetoric.

Thus no sooner has the army of managers been hired or reclassified to run the new internal market, than the politicians are complaining about excessive numbers of managers and management costs. Managers are now being encouraged to speak out more to explain their policies to the public. The problem is that managers do not have an effective voice in formulating policy in an open manner, either at the national or local level, and are now afraid to speak out – unless ordered to do so! – since 'local management decision-making' is in fact the implementation of a centralist agenda.

All in all, we have less the invisible hand of the market than the visible fist of political administration. This produces some gains in technical efficiency, but ironically less because of the market than by planning (such as though earmarked funds from the Department of Health for reducing waiting times for patients; special allocations for the NHS prior to the 1992 general election; and so forth) (Appleby, 1994).

Evaluation of the reforms is likely to prove very difficult, as the reforms are now taken to mean virtually any major policy initiative conducted since 1989. In their latest incarnation, the NHS reforms are suddenly all about primary care and health promotion. There is, of course, a paradox that, if primary care is a successful strategy, the long-term need for secondary care is greater – as older people die of more complex morbidities and comorbidities! But, in any case, the Government does not have a coherent 'health of the nation strategy', as some of the major causes of ill health – social inequality and environmental factors – have worsened considerably in the last 15 years. In consequence, the pressure for a patch-you-up NHS will increase, not decrease.

THE MEDICAL PROFESSION

The disaffection of large sections of the medical profession has increased, after a temporary lull in attrition between the Government and the medical profession from approximately 1990–1993. A more militant leadership is again back in control of the British Medical Association, as in 1989, which is opposing the consequences of the reforms. Albeit as a bargaining chip, the British Medical Association has recently proposed resignation of doctors and the contracting-back to the NHS of their services (on the model of the barrister and his chambers) in line with the contract culture propagated by the reforms! Presumably this is based on the notion of the contract as representing a diminution of trust rather than simply an economic transaction. The problem for the British Medical Association is that this could presumably afford a ruthless government the opportunity to 'reprofile' the medical workforce, with the result that many doctors would find themselves not as much in demand as they expected.

Longer-term problems, however, concern demoralization of general practitioners and an apparent inadequacy of entry to general practice by young doctors; revived concern over junior doctors' hours and working practices; and the reliance upon non-career specialists, often on short-term contracts, to plug the gap filled by reducing junior doctors' hours to some extent yet not significantly increasing the number of consultants or doctors generally in training.

It seems a paradox that, as the medical profession is being called to greater accountability within the public sector in terms of exact workload, performance targets and sessional appearances, the private sector is also being encouraged by the Government. From the early 1980s, restrictions on private practice by NHS consultants were relaxed, and this remains the case. It may, however, not be such a paradox. While chief executives of hospitals may find the desire of consultants to emphasize their private practice tiresome or productive of difficulties in terms of management control of their workload, it is probably an informal 'political fix' whereby the Government relies on the lush pastures of private medicine for senior doctors to damp down some of the anger created by worsened working conditions in the NHS (based on squeezing more out of diminishing budgets for hospitals). In other words, James Morone's characterization of doctors in the US as 'the new proletariat' may have its British parallel – and the Government is probably wise enough to realize that private practice provides an exit from frustration. Without it, the future of a quality medical profession altogether would probably be threatened, under current conditions such as proposals to pay doctors according to performance (discussed above) or for senior consultants to be on call to relieve junior doctors of their excessive responsibilities.

It is also the case that the traditional private sector in the UK is responsible for a certain section of the medical profession earning significantly extra income – for example, doubling their salary as a result of 10% extra work due to generous reimbursement from BUPA and other private payers. This is again partly an informal political fix, doubtless, whereby 'the market rate' is thereby paid to senior doctors without expanding the NHS budget.

Again ironically, these practices are threatened somewhat by the phenomenon of self-governing trusts seeking to force doctors to bring their private practice into the hospital as 'trust business' rather than having autonomous private practices. This does not threaten the private insurance industry, but it threatens the traditional private hospital industry. There may be a logic to it, however, if it is genuinely the case that trust hospitals are capable of being more economical than private hospitals, yet private insurance is growing in the context of a limited NHS budget.

The question then arises, why not simply channel the finance as well as the provision through the public sector? If the tax system to finance public health care were not significantly redistributive, the middle classes might be willing to spend more on the NHS and to eradicate swathes of even the existing small private sector. Indeed a hypothecated health tax might be a route to achieve this, given the reduction in the progressivity of a British tax system since 1979.

POLITICS, LEADERSHIP AND MANAGEMENT

A relatively neglected area within international comparison of health reform is that of the relationships between political decision-making, structures of accountability within health services, management structures and behaviour and the nature of the representation of interests in health management.

The NHS reforms, for example, produced yet another structural reorganization of the health service, to some extent building on the Griffiths Enquiry of 1983; but in other respects going further and indeed arguably in different directions from that intended by the Griffiths Report.

International comparison of health-care systems tends to focus at the 'macro' level, on levels of financing, types of financing, type of reimbursement, populations covered, and so forth. Discussion of health management and institutional arrangements tends to be more parochial. While there are cultural and methodological arguments against simplistic 'lesson-learning' at the level of management, it is nevertheless worth considering management changes in an international context. After all, management structures are created or tolerated by political decisions or non-decisions.

It is within the context of particular cultures and their practices that incentives and 'laws of nature' (or norms underlying what seemed to be positive economic theories) actually function. It might therefore be interesting to trace the effect of similar institutions operating in different countries – to see if the interplay of similar institutions and incentives mobilize similar behaviour, or whether cultural and other factors produce differences.

One example might be purchaser/provider relationships and, more particularly, forms of contracting between purchasers and providers. A more specific example might be a comparison of decision-making by primary care physicians in US HMOs and within British GP fundholding. Contracts with community health providers in the US might be compared with models in the UK where a district health authority purchaser, for example, contracts with a 'lead provider' in the form of a community trust. As will all case studies, the problem of induction is a real one. Nevertheless insight may be shared.

The importance of institutions (including management structures, which reflect political and management cultures) is that they may both channel and alter behaviour. If, for example, management structures are changed as part of an ideologically-based policy initiative – such as the NHS reforms in the UK – then new modes of behaviour may emerge. This is another way of stating that the 'laws of human nature' apparently underlying 'sciences' such as neoclassical economics, may be created, strengthened, abolished or diminished by political and management structures if these are both conditioned by and condition norms of behaviour.

To put it simply: man may be rendered more aggressive and competitive (in the work environment at least) by operating within the NHS internal market, by comparison with the previous NHS culture in which public policy was based more upon a public administration ethos than upon a part-prescriptive, part-descriptive 'micro-economics'-based incentive culture.

That is where leadership comes in. It is no coincidence that the NHS Executive in the UK, under instruction from politicians, adopted 'leadership' as its latest fad concept in 1991. First we had had administration. Then came management, reflecting the need to make hard choices within resources, rather than simply run systems. However management is fundamentally about rationality, control and consistency. This turned out not to be enough to 'turn around' the culture of a national health service. Leadership, by contrast, is concerned with direction-setting, inspiration, vision, creativity, legitimacy and consent in public affairs (Altshuler, 1990). Perhaps this is the difference between management science and political management: 'total quality management', for example, requires an analytic and qualitative focus for its operation but a leadership focus for its instigation and legitimacy.

The main problem with leadership, of course, is that it is context-dependent. Fidel Castro has been in the past a great leader in a Cuban context; Adolf Hitler was temporarily a great leader in a German fascist context;

Margaret Thatcher is to some a lost leader for the UK; various industrial entrepreneurs have been accredited with leadership status in the business world. It is from the last category that public sector leaders are now sought in the UK.

The main problem with this is that the prescriptive and scientific elements are blurred; the ideological basis of change is blurred with the technical agenda. It might, for example, be easier to get agreement on appropriate goals for purchasing in a health service (difficult though this is in itself) than to get agreement on whether or not market mechanisms are either culturally or 'empirically' the best means for running health-care systems.

In other words, one man's leadership is another man's propaganda. Is the aim of leadership to impart values or to embody universal or majoritarian values? If leadership consists in imposing unpopular policies, it is unlikely to have legitimacy with the led. As a result, one or more of either material incentives, authoritarian measures or 'totalitarian' means of changing hearts and minds (rather than communicative means of changing hearts and minds) will be necessary.

It is unfortunate that the lack of consent around the health reforms in the UK has created a schism between Government and those associated with it, on the one hand, and swathes of the public and NHS staff on the other. In this context, techniques for 'the management of human resources', 'efficiency' and the like become infused with an ideological agenda and therefore a often involve a need to 'divide and rule'.

In other words, is leadership about changing people's values? And if it is, on what basis is this project a legitimate one?

This may seem a far remove from the management changes instituted by the NHS reforms. But consider the following. On paper, health authorities and self-governing trusts (hospitals and other providers) are respectively to be accountable to boards.

These boards comprise a chairman plus five non-executive members, plus five executive members (strategic managers). This does two things. It replaces the former unitary system whereby health authorities were directly responsible for providers. It also replaces a split between the authority and the management board, in the previous system. Now there are unitary boards combining executives and non-executives, and there is no mechanism for accountability to the local community.

It could be argued that, if a market is to operate, the accountability to the local community ought to be exercised by purchasers and not providers – and therefore this lack of accountability does not matter at the level of providers. This, however, is a rigid and naive interpretation of providers as 'market actors' rather than local hospitals. This is certainly a cultural change as far as the British public are concerned, and not one to which either they or most NHS staff have given their consent. It is in this context that recent exhortations to 'consult the community' raise a wry smile: all 'consultation' on whether or not hospitals should become trusts was ignored.

The logic behind the unitary board is to ensure greater decision-making by managers and allegedly greater accountability for decisions. It is argued that, in a system wherein top managers are responsible to a separate authority or board, they can pass decisions upwards rather than take them. This is not to be confused with consensus management, which is the absence of a 'chief executive' or overall general manager and which therefore is either group decision-making or informal deference to a natural leader or general manager. At its best consensus management does what it says – generates consent for decisions. At its worst it allows decision-making 'at the lowest common denominator', i.e. the fudging of important decisions by postponement or log-rolling. It is no coincidence that general management was therefore seen to be

necessary in a British context at a time when tough decisions about resources were arising, owing both to expansion of medical technology and a Conservative government hostile to the public sector.

Even with general management or a chief executive, nevertheless, it was argued that unitary boards would guarantee effective decision-making. In some cases this may be true. The problem is that the chairman and also the non-executives of such boards are appointed by the political bosses of the day. The Secretary of State appoints all chairmen, and all non-executives are appointed through a consultation process dominated by the rulers of the day, which makes health authorities and trust boards in part the creatures of ministers and in part quangos. In this context, executive managers do not always take greater responsibility for their decisions, without referring them to non-executive boards or board members, so much as clear their lines automatically with such non-executives (especially the chairman) on all matters of strategy. In other words it is self-policing rather than self-discipline that may frequently occur.

It is also no coincidence that, in such a system of patronage, the chairman of the health authority and of the trust has had a tendency in the last two or three years to become over-powerful. Chairmen are the creature of ministers and of the 'centre' and chief executives are dependent upon them. Although working relationships between chairmen and chief executives vary widely, as in the private sector, the overarching chairman is more of a problem in today's NHS that the inert chairman who does not even play the role of overseer and source of accountability.

There is in other words no source of local legitimacy for local decision-making about matters of (local) strategy. There ought, of course, to be a place for national policy-making in a national health service, and an expectation that national policy is implemented locally. Nevertheless recent demands by ministers that managers take more responsibility for communication with the public miss the point, or – worse – are based on a rather severe hypocrisy. Since managers are creatures of 'the centre', by a not very complicated chain of command, it is unrealistic to expect them to take the initiative in local debates when, in nearly all other circumstances, ministers seek to keep a lid on such debates. It was after all because of a hostility to such local pluralism that the new health authorities and trust boards were constituted in their current form in the first place. Ministerial pleas for management visibility ought to be seen therefore as a plea for central political decisions to be presented as local management decisions.

POWER AND HEALTH-CARE SYSTEMS

The debate over the NHS reforms in the UK provides some insight into attitudes to health-care systems, health professions and health reform in other countries as well. In the UK, the main supporters of the reforms are the Government (of course); those health managers who see the current agenda as the eternal agenda (whatever the agenda is!); and a variety of academics who see the reforms as one or more of the chance to evaluate health outcomes, the chance to make a transition to 'primary care' whatever that means in practice, the chance to be more efficient, the chance to avoid 'professional capture' in the sense of doctors doing what they want rather than what the public needs, the chance to move power from hospital consultants to general practitioners, the chance to study markets, etc.

Ranged against 'the reforms' are most of the public (to the extent that they understand the issues); the vast majority of the medical profession, especially the hospital-based medical profession; the majority of the nursing profession; and significant swathes of other professions – as well as almost all lower

paid health workers, who feel permanently under threat. Added to this are the voices of some students of politics and journalists, on the one hand, who see the NHS reforms as one of the many manifestations of an over-centralized state which is abolishing intermediary institutions in British society and, on the other hand, 'voices of conscience' such as the Bishop of Birmingham, who sees the reforms as damaging the altruistic culture of the national health service *per se*.

The apparent paradox is that – on the one hand – the reforms were a historical accident for the UK, based on Margaret Thatcher's immediate reaction to a political problem in the winter of 1987, and yet on the other hand the reforms are seemingly part of an international trend towards managed competition and managed care (although these concepts mean different things in different environments). The apparent paradox is, however, based on a perception that **all** health-care systems require pro-competitive moves in the name of efficiency to an equal extent and for the same reason. There is also a tendency to 'be wise after the event' about the inevitability of the reforms. The same managers and indeed academic commentators who say that there is no alternative to the reforms (and that they require, if anything, a redirection rather than a fundamental change of route) are those same people who had never heard of the internal market or who had never dreamed of the concept prior to Alain Enthoven's sortie into British health care in the mid-1980s.

In an international context, the reforms – in the sense of the internal market and managed competition, rather than the general panoply of changes all of which tend to be subsumed under 'the reforms' – are often grist to the mill of those who argue that, having been the laggard in health policy for most of the 20th century, the United States is now the leader. Instead of a welfare statist model based on equality and planning, health-care systems are now seen as developing – in varying degrees

– pluralistic access; a stress on consumerism; use of pluralism if not competition in provision; and so forth. That by default makes the United States the 'market leader'. It is an irony, of course, that the United States is now earnestly seeking to move away from its historical niche at this very time.

Nevertheless, as a descriptive statement rather than a prescriptive assertion, it may be true that the decline of the welfare statist model is upon us, by this is meant a decline in paternalism and implicit trust in professions rather than a mixture of competition and regulation allied to consumerism, in a culture of greater scepticism towards professions (Moran and Wood, 1993).

The most fundamental reason for the reforms being seen as 'inevitable' is that they are supported by the economic right as an attack on 'guilds' (i.e. professions and professional autonomy, even where that is necessary or laudable) allied to a cost-cutting agenda; and by the left as a continuation of the process whereby the professions are brought to heel. A significant section of the so-called progressive left has been 'anti-doctor' for a long time, and a misreading of what Sir Douglas Black might call the 'false antithesis' between clinical medicine and social health care has often led left-of-centre commentators to view anything which is 'anti-doctor' as likely to be useful! What such commentators often do not see is that recent Conservative governments in the UK have been extremely capable of using this phenomenon to 'divide and rule': to set one group of doctors against another; to set nurses against doctors, especially former nurses-turned-chief-executives who see a Conservative agenda as progressive because it is anti-doctor; and to set advocates of primary care against 'centres of excellence' such as the UK's famous teaching hospitals. It would be a bit strong to employ Stalin's phrase, 'useful fools', but perhaps the warning is worth considering.

Just as, prior to the NHS reforms, the 'battle for the patient' (in a clinical world where doctors' autonomy was being challenged by nurses and other professions) was heating up, the battle is even hotter post-reform. In the setting of 'purchasing' priorities as well as within clinical directorates, what might be considered to be an opportunity for rational evaluation of clinical priorities is often the locus for politically based and culturally based battles over priorities and procedures. Far from removing politics from resource allocation at the macro-level and from resource management at the micro level, the reforms have institutionalized political battles as a *modus operandi*. Life in a clinical directorate in a large hospital trust in the UK is currently a life of crisis management and conflict, not a life of incentive-based smooth operating procedures.

CONCLUSION

The Marxist view of health services, and particularly of the British NHS, was expressed in a fairly simplistic form in the 1970s by Navarro (1978). A 1990s interpretation of the British NHS on Marxist lines would argue that, if one looks at the three most important questions – who finances health care?; who is employed is to provide it, under what conditions?; and who benefits form the services which are provided? – then an interesting answer follows. Health care is increasingly financed more regressively than in the past (due to changes in the tax system and due to greater limitations on public finance than in the past). The hospital or community unit is less a cooperative organization than a source of squeezing the maximum surplus value out of 'reprofiled' workforces – in the hope of contributing to, as well as providing less of a drain on, the capitalist economy. And finally, health benefit is increasingly judged in terms of QALY-related methodologies which tend to stress benefit in a functionalist or often economy-directed manner. Just as Marxism had fallen into disrepute, the Conservative government saw fit to reinvent it!

What is happening in the British NHS is to some extent symptomatic of a greater social trend – towards the atomization of society (Paton, 1992b) as a result of the unfettered reliance on market forces, yet promoted through a centralized state which is intolerant of civic institutions of an intermediary nature. The extent to which this is now perceived widely has thrown the more intelligent Conservatives on to the intellectual defensive.

Witness former health adviser within the No.10 Policy Unit and member of Parliament David Willetts, who seeks to put a decentralist and communitarian gloss on what are hard-nosed market reforms. He has argued recently (National Association of Health Authorities and Trusts Conference, June 1994) that hospital trusts are an example of devolution to communities, and that in many ways the hospital pre-1974 (the year of a bureaucratic reorganization of a the NHS) is the model for the hospital trust. This is, however, political analysis by soundbite rather than something more.

Prior to 1974, professions within hospitals – such as Guy's, the 'flagship' of the Government's reforms now known as the *Belgrano* on account of its having been torpedoed – acted with relative autonomy, despite low budgets by international standards. Indeed this was the essence of the political settlement: Governments did not challenge doctors, as long as doctors did not challenge Governments' allocation of resources to the service. Quite apart from the fact that Guy's on present plans will not exist at all in a few years time, the rose-tinted spectacled view of hospital trusts as cosy communitarian institutions is sheer ideological gamesmanship. Hospital trusts are free to compete in a rigged market place and free to do little else. While the reforms are unpopular, the Government has been relatively successful in diverting attention from its overall intentions by making local disputes within providers such an inevitable part of the new system that, without much exaggeration, the

time – let alone the political daring – for a wider critique is absent.

Health reform in the UK may be atypical rather than typical of reform in other Western countries. In the United States, there is scope for managed competition to provide an answer to both continuing cost escalation and an absence of equity (although it is much more expensive, in all likelihood, than a socialized model, as well as being more bureaucratic (despite the prevailing rhetoric). That is because managed competition is harnessed to more, rather than less, egalitarian purchasing power. European countries seeking to replace the rather expensive system of third-party reimbursement of private providers with either managed competition or central regulation may also find a less politically gerrymandered managed competition than the UK's more useful than the UK does.

In the UK, however, more ideologically motivated reform than elsewhere in Europe (except for the former Eastern Europe) is often justified by virtue of the fact that it is part of an inevitable international trend. The question for the future is whether, just as the middle classes threatened with economic insecurity in the United States are looking towards more socialized health care (despite Republican attempts to use US political institutions to stymie reform), the middle classes in the UK start to rebel against attacks on their socialized health care and on legitimate professional autonomy, attacks made in the name of accountancy; a somewhat philistine rhetoric of 'quality'; and the lure of private profit from public health care.

DISCUSSION

* In the present author's view, there are paradoxes and perverse incentives associated with the NHS 'reforms'. The paradoxes concern reactions to current trends; the perverse incentives flow from many of the mechanisms and structures created in the post-1991 NHS. I will deal with the

latter first and then outline the nature of the paradoxes.

It is increasingly taken as axiomatic that 'the purchaser/provider split' is a good thing. Criticism of the NHS reforms by policy analysts is thus usually tactical rather than fundamental. It might stress, for example: inadequate coordination in 'purchasing' (Ham, 1994a); a tendency by the Government to muddle through rather than act strategically (Ham, 1994b); or the fact that inadequate attention is paid to appropriate outcomes and that inadequate or inappropriate · uses are made of information (Bloor and Maynard, 1994). But these relatively gentle critiques ignore problems which stem from the heart of the reforms. A number of these problems are increasingly in evidence.

Firstly, the purchaser/provider split is being used as a mechanism by which purchasers pass the buck. This is not to malign purchasing authorities. Increasingly under pressure from the Government's ever tighter agenda, based on squeezing more output from less money, purchasers can now say to their main providers: 'We have the money; but it's you that runs the services. So here's the cash; here's our long list of requirements. Don't complain to us if you can't manage within the money. We're safe in the knowledge that it's hospitals to which the public complains. (They don't understand the theology of the purchaser/ provider split.)'

Incidentally, moving away from block contracts is unlikely to sort this out. For the Department of Health is speaking with forked tongue on this issue: the more contracts quantify cost, volume and cases, the more rationing is overt and the more the limits of existing finance are seen to block the Government's desire to increase productivity beyond the reasonably possible.

- Secondly, separate hospital and community trusts are increasingly seeking to 'shift' costs (i.e. patients!) on to each other. The purchaser/provider split is encouraging gaming by providers against each other as well as against purchasers. Additionally, attempts by purchasers to regulate this state of affairs are falling victim to short-termism. For example, purchasers are contracting with community providers for acute care and tenders are being won by community providers paying doctors by the session. But this pulls the rug from under hospitals, which face the fixed costs (and the major service costs of the medical profession) yet less activity and income. All in all, the aspiration of 'seamless care', hospital to community, is undermined by such behaviour.

- Thirdly, GP fundholding is threatening both hospitals' ability to plan and regional offices' strategies for rationalizing services to increase 'value for money' and the total productivity of the system. Thus backdoor planning has to be undertaken by the region – to coordinate purchasing on an area basis (euphemistically called market management) and indeed to scale the Chinese walls between purchasers and providers. Yet the transactions costs (the costs of mediating this rather than planning it) are very high.

  Even more seriously, some GPs are seeking to use the market to lure NHS consultants to do work in private hospitals. This would mean them competing with themselves, as part of the NHS tender!

- Fourthly, a combination of frenetic marketing by trusts (to fundholding GPs and also to non-fundholding GPs, to try to steer district contracts their way) and disaggregated purchasing, is leading to radical uncertainty in the hospital sector. Protecting appropriate centres of excellence, specialized services and indeed the appropriate local services is rendered much more difficult – and, again, becomes a surreptitious exercise by the 'back-door men' of the region.

- Fifthly, given that the logical essence of the reforms is to replace reimbursement of referred patients using public money with contracts whereby the patient follows the money, except for emergencies, the incentive is to reclassify patients as emergencies (compounded by fundholders' attempts to 'cost-shift' by getting emergencies out of their budgets).

- Sixthly, the transactions costs of the reforms are high enough that such costs have to be recouped through greater 'productivity' – which often means exploitation rather than efficiency. The so-called 'productivity gains' of the reforms are at least in part due to the extraction of surplus value from both workers and managers, working longer hours more intensely without reward. Just as Karl Marx is pronounced dead throughout the world, Mrs Bottomley had him turning in his grave.

- Seventhly, the domination of national productivity over local choice (questions in Parliament are best answered by statistics about the former) means that a defence of 'purchasing' as greater sensitivity to local needs is mostly hype. Neither services themselves nor their locations are being chosen by patients or citizens on any significant scale. Many commentators naively add to this, 'yet' – without seeing that the motor at the heart of the changes makes it less likely in the future. Regional Offices have to 'plan the market' – to squeeze more acute care out of less money and produce a 'shift primary care' out of existing budgets. In this context, communication with the public means in practice PR on behalf of the inevitable.

- Eighthly, the shift to primary care is in fact a move to 'acute care in the community' – a different thing altogether. The pressure which this will put on GP practices and community services is currently unquantified, but has the potential to make the debacle of unfunded community care seem a gentle aperitif by comparison.

- Let me now set out my view of the paradoxes tacitly shaping the future. This returns us to the key policy issues raised in the discussion sections in Part One.

Firstly, 'the market' is in fact becoming a competitive tender by hospitals to survive, not a mechanism by which money follows the patient. A 'managed market' is an oxymoron – one or the other takes over. Inevitably, in our centralized culture, management by regional offices will supersede any market recognizable by Alain Enthoven. This may even be desirable, albeit hypocritical and deliberate by the present government. But desirable or not, winners and losers are being planned by regions, and mergers and closures likewise. How is it, then, that at the 'sharp end' a fierce market seems to be operating?

The paradox is explained when one understands that only a middle tier of hospitals and services is actually competing openly (as much for regional 'waiting-list' monies as for purchasers' business). The rest are 'marketing' themselves to achieve expected targets. When the planned shake-out of hospital beds has occurred, there will be even less scope for a market. Thus the market is a transitional device, not a long-term feature.

After all, the hospital market has a tendency to monopoly, arguably more than most markets; and paradoxically only expensive regulation can preserve the trappings of a market in the long run (by which time the appropriate scale and location of services exists, begging the question, why bother with a market anyway?)

Public finance for publicly planned services is both more efficient and more equitable. But since the Government is forced by its own ideological agenda to apologise for this rather than proclaim it, it is equally forced onto the defensive when confronted by ultra-right ideas advocating greater privatization and more cut-throat markets.

- Secondly, since gaming as the result of an uncoordinated purchaser/provider split is at the heart of the problems engendered by the reforms, why are long respected managers now advocating even more autonomy and commercialization for hospitals? The reason lies in the oxymoron. The limitations of the 'managed market' are now evident. The choice is either increasing privatization or more effective management of the system, with a lot of the unhelpful rhetoric about markets dropped. Yet if the reforms are to be seen to have a dynamic of their own, there is a tendency to be bounced into the former (as, for example, in the contributions of Mr Peter Griffiths and Professor Sir Duncan Nichol to the BBC 'Public Eye' programme *The Health Business*, 8 Oct 1994).

- Thirdly, in light of the need for greater coordination of services and secure financing for the NHS, it is ironical to see elements of the left-of-centre (Coote, 1994) advocating that local government takes over health care. In 1948, doctors preferred Bevan's national model, as control by local politicians was considered highly unappealing. It is argued now that local government purchasing is possible, without intense opposition from the medical profession, as a result of the purchaser/provider split: in other words, hospitals and services would be split off from the local government purchasers even more fundamentally than they are from health service purchasers. But ironically the purchaser/provider split would thus be deepened, when the sensible challenge instead is to preserve the distinction but not the institutional split which has

actually proved harmful in a number of significant ways as described above.

Furthermore, local councils would be conservative in protecting local hospitals even when regional centres of excellence were a better way forward. As a result, advocates of a local government-purchased NHS often advocate a separate acute service, funded centrally, with local government concentrating on public health (Coote, 1994). A huge irony, however, exists here. The advocates of a holistically purchased health and social care would be responsible for more fragmentation than at any time since 1974, and arguably since 1948.

Financing the NHS would become subject to the tortuous and politicized financial wrangles between central and local government, and inequity between rich and poor councils would grow as the scope for a national resource allocation formula was diminished. Currently, reasonably objective measures of need are used to allocate resources to health authorities. While some local choice would be increased by giving budgets to elected local governmental authorities, central government would have to give money to poorer areas (as with the former rate support grant, later revenue support). But such grants would either be dependent on central definitions of need or subject to a complex 'revenue equalization' formula which would be difficult both economically and politically. General reflection and actual experience in the US with 'revenue equalization' (between federal, state and local government) suggests it is difficult to 'tax' richer areas for spending in poorer areas in ring-fenced policy arenas: it means (for example) Area 1's decision to spend compels Area 2 to subsidize it – if Area 1 is poor, with less local tax base and/or greater (locally-defined!) 'need'. Admittedly, such subsidy is limited to the total 'pool of money' generated, which ceases when the poorer area is subsidized such that the richer area then has to tax at an equally high level. (This is the analytical principle which defines pure 'revenue equalization'. The only alternative is for central government to find the money – this is unlikely on an equitable basis, especially if central government disagrees with the local definition of 'need'.)

Certainly we need a clearer strategy for health promotion, involving housing, transport, education and – especially – antipoverty policy as well as social services. But we also need a 'cure and care' NHS. Creating one agency responsible for all would make it easier paradoxically to diminish the total budget for health services and health-relevant public spending. There is a need both to prevent ill health where possible (through broader social policy) and to 'cure and care' as well.

- Fourthly, when so much requires to be improved, it is a paradox that sceptics who scent trouble on the road ahead are confronted by the fatalism which says, 'whatever the current situation, no future government should change much'. At one level this is understandable. Managers and professionals are suffering from an iatrogenic disease known as 'initiative fatigue'; and the irony, not lost on the Conservatives, is that a lot of harmful change makes 'change back' or further change, less tolerable even if *per se* desirable.

But the challenge is to improve and recoordinate the NHS without either huge structural reorganization or simply a return to 1979. The reforms actually consisted in an ideological answer to a practical problem. And now the ideology is of little practical help. That is why commentators who argued in 1994 that the Government was drifting were right – but almost to the point of truism (Ham,

1994b). Such commentators were, however, inadequately perceptive in that from the 'cock-ups' there was emerging a conspiracy: to use the state of flux created by the 'reforms' to impose ever tighter productivity requirements upon the NHS, and to reorient the NHS away from comprehensive goals without public debate. In this context, one can contrast the recent British apology for a debate about distinguishing health and social care with Scandinavian attempts to create consensus through open debate.

- We should readdress the original practical problem of the 1980s, in a practical way: how can we reward providers for appropriate workload, planned on the basis of communities' needs, within available resources? That certainly necessitates more sensitive commissioning, but not necessarily a market. There is now scope to diminish the costs of the malfunctioning market and use the dividend to invest in better services.

This can be done by investing in both egalitarian and 'pro-health' economic and social policy and a more generous 'cure and care' NHS. Structural change is only part of the story in providing effective health care – and better health – but it is important nonetheless. Stability must be established on a stable basis! That means planning services, on the basis of need and local choice of location where possible; funding their capital and revenue requirements together; and rendering the providers accountable for long-term plans to health authorities. Otherwise long-term benefit is lost in short-termism and fragmentation.

ACKNOWLEDGEMENTS

Much of this chapter was first presented to the International Political Science Association, Sixteenth World Congress, Berlin, 21–25 August 1994. This conference presentation is also to be published, in changed form, in Altenstetter, C. and Björkman, J. (forthcoming) *Health Policy, National Schemes and Globalizing Markets in Western Societies*, Macmillan, London and St Martins, New York. The Discussion uses some material published in the *British Medical Journal* Education and Debate section, **310**, 1995 13 May; pp. 1245–8.

REFERENCES

Altshuler, A. (1990) Teaching leadership. Paper to the Annual Meeting of the Association for Public Policy and Management, October 1990.

Altenstetter, C. (1992) Health policy regimes and the single European market. *Journal of Health Politics, Policy and Law*, 17.

Appleby, J. (1994) Evaluating the reforms. *Health Service Journal*, 10 Mar, 32.

Bartlett, W. and le Grand, J. (1994) *Quasi-Markets and Social Policy*, SAUS, Bristol.

Bloor, K. and Maynard, A. (1994) An outsider's view of the NHS reforms. *British Medical Journal*, 309, 352–353.

Clinical Standards Advisory Group (1993), *Access to Availability of Specialist Services*, HMSO, London.

Coote, A. (1994) Accountability is good for you. *The Independent on Sunday*, **30 Oct**, 21.

Ham, C. (1994a) The future of purchasing. *British Medical Journal*, **309**, 1032–1033.

Ham, C. (1994b) Where now for the NHS reforms? *British Medical Journal*, **309**, 351–352.

Heginbotham, C. and Ham, C. (1992) *Purchasing Dilemma*, Kings Fund College and Southampton and South West Hampshire Health Authority, Southampton.

Moran, M. and Wood, B. (1993) *States, Regulation and the Medical Profession*, Open University Press, Buckingham.

Navarro, V. (1978) *Class Struggle, the State and Medicine*, Martin Robertson, London.

Paton, C. (1990) *US Health Politics: Public Policy and Political Theory*, Avebury, Aldershot.

Paton, C. (1992a) *Competition and Planning in the NHS: The Danger of Unplanned Markets*, Chapman & Hall, London.

Paton, C. (1992b) *Ethics and Politics*, Avebury, Aldershot.

Robinson, R. and le Grand, J. (1994) *Evaluating the NHS Reforms*, King's Fund, London.

Ward, S. (1994) Too many beds on the block. *Health Service Journal*, **19 May**, 21.

Willetts, D. (1993) Social Market Foundation (Paper).

Willetts, D. (1994) Speech to NAHAT Conference, June 1994.

INDEX